A COMPENDIUM OF ESSAYS ON ALTERNATIVE THERAPY

Edited by **Arup Bhattacharya**

A Compendium of Essays on Alternative Therapy
Edited by Arup Bhattacharya

Published by InTech
Janeza Trdine 9, 51000 Rijeka, Croatia

Publishing Process Manager Ivona Lovric

Technical Editor Teodora Smiljanic

Cover Designer InTech Design Team

Additional hard copies can be obtained from orders@intechopen.com

A Compendium of Essays on Alternative Therapy, Edited by Arup Bhattacharya
p. cm.
ISBN 978-953-307-863-2

For EU product safety concerns:
IN TECH d.o.o., Prolaz Marije Krucifikse Kozulić 3, 51000 Rijeka, Croatia,
info@intechopen.com or visit our website at intechopen.com.

Meet the editor

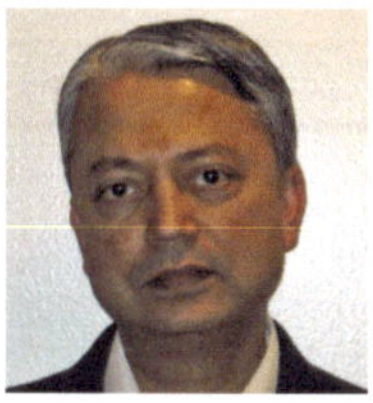

Dr Arup Bhattacharya is a practicing homeopath and a member of the research faculty at the Department of Cancer Chemoprevention, Roswell Park Cancer Institute in Buffalo, NY, USA. He has a Masters in Biophysics from the University of Mumbai, India, and in Psychology from Annamalai University, India. He completed his PhD in Molecular and Cellular Biophysics from SUNY at Buffalo with a full scholarship and fellowship in 2005. Thereafter, he completed his postdoctoral training in Translational Pharmacology and Physiology under the tutelage of Dr. Youcef M. Rustum, distinguished professor and Chair, Department of Cancer Biology, Roswell Park Cancer Institute, Buffalo, NY. He is a member of the American Association for Cancer Research (AACR), International Society for Magnetic Resonance in Medicine (ISMRM), American Association of Physicists in Medicine (AAPM), Homeopathic Medical Council of Canada (HMCC), National United Professional Association of Trained Homeopaths (NUPATH), Canada, and North American Society of Homeopaths (NASH), USA.

Contents

Preface

A Compendium of Essays on Alternative Therapy is a web based resource, encompassing some of the modalities of complementary and alternative medicine (CAM), such as homeopathy, herbalism, tai chi, cupping, and Feldenkrais method. While this e-resource deals with only a few of the popular CAM modalities, it is hoped that this will promote further insight, research, and exchange of ideas on the state of CAM modalities within the CAM community, CAM practitioners, conventional clinicians, and general scientists . The information presented will be of equal interest to researchers and practitioners of any modalities including that of conventional medicine. This e-resource is divided into different sections:

- Role of CAM
- Homeopathy
- Feldenkrais Method
- Qi jong and Tai Chi, and,
- Herbalism

The section on "Role of CAM" deals with the salient aspects of the influence of CAM in promoting well-being and health. Dr Robin Philipp, Consultant for Occupational and Public Health Physician, and Director of the Centre for Health in Employment and the Environment (CHEE), Bristol Royal Infirmary, England, discusses the critical elements for maintaining well-being in "Fostering the Art of Well-Being: An Alternative Medicine". These elements that utilize the innate healing power in an individual is what a successful CAM practitioner is often able to harness in order to bring about a rebalance back to health in the client. Patricia Fox et al from UCD School of Nursing describes the different perspectives of women with breast cancer, oncology professionals, and CAM practitioners regarding the role of various CAM modalities in a cancer setting in the chapter "The Role of CAM (Complementary and Alternative Medicine): the Different Perspectives of Patients, Oncology Professionals, and CAM Practitioners". Prof. Vaez Mahdavi Mohamad Reza et al. from Medical University of Shahed, Iran, provides insights into the effects of traditional cupping on the biochemical, hematological, and immunological factors of human venous blood in their review paper "Evaluation of the Effects of Traditional Cupping on the Biochemical, Hematological and Immunological Factors of Human Venous Blood". Drs S. Husain and F. Malik from National Institute of Health, Pakistan, discuss the use of alternative and traditional systems of medicines in Pakistan in "Alternative and

Traditional Medicines Systems in Pakistan: History, Regulation, Trends, Usefulness, Challenges, Prospects and Limitations".

Under the "Homeopathy" section, the second chapter outlines a new way of understanding disease and health in terms of basic units of life - "sensations". Dr. Banerji, a homeopathy clinician from Kolkata, India, discusses in detail some of the homeopathy protocol for treating cancer in the chapter "Homeopathy: Treatment of Cancer with the Banerji Protocols". The third and fourth generation homeopath father and son duo have been acknowledged by the National Cancer Institute in the U.S.A. under the Best Case Series Program for the efficacy of their treatment in treating certain cancer cases with complete remission. While their work strictly does not fall under the category of "classical" homeopathy, where medicines are individualized to the patient and not the disease, it has nonetheless generated a lot of interest in the scientific and medical community worldwide because these protocols allow reproducibility - a key element for clinical replication and scientific evaluation.

The use of Feldenkrais Method, as discussed by Prof. Patricia A. Buchana of Des Moines University in "The Feldenkrais Method® of Somatic Education", serves as an excellent introduction of this method for achieving a life time of creative fulfillment and satisfaction, leading to self-actualization. This is an integrative approach to learning and improving function among people of varying abilities across their lifespan to enhance an individual's function in various aspects of life, such as performance at work, in sports, or in the performing arts.

Under "Tai Chi", Dr Judy Yuen-man Siu from David C. Lam Institute for East-West Studies of Hong Kong Baptist University describes the use of qigong and tai chi among chronically ill patients in Hong Kong and the underlying factors that has made these CAM modalities popular with empowered individuals to take responsibility of their well-being in a proactive way.

The section on "Herbalism" consists of five chapters on different aspects of herbalism. In "Medical Herbalism and Frequency of Use", Prof. Behice Erci, of Malatya Health School, İnönü University, Malatya, Turkey, looks at the prevalence and use of herbal preparations worldwide. Dr. Arash Khaki, from Tabriz Branch Islamic Azad University, Iran, discusses the use of various herbal remedies in diabetes for prevention and treatment of diabetic nephropathy. Dr. Tülay Askin Celik of Adnan Menderes University, Turkey, highlights the genotoxic potential in vitro of widely used medicinal plant extracts, hence advocating safety and caution regarding their indiscriminate use by the population. Drs. José Roberto Macías-Pérez and Saúl Villa-Treviño, from the department of Cell Biology, Cinvestav-IPN, Mexico, writes on the use of caffeic acid phenethyl ester analogues found in various natural and dietary supplements as a chemopreventive agent in their research paper "Searching for Analogues of the Natural Compound, Caffeic Acid Phenethyl Ester, with Chemoprotective Activity". Finally, Dr Sakagami Hiroshi et al. from Japan summarize "Functional Analysis of Natural Polyphenols and Saponins as Alternative Medicines' the Use of Natural Polyphenols and Terpenoids in Alternative Medicine".

It is hoped that these collections from an eminent worldwide panel of authors on wide ranging topics within the field of CAM will be of use to readers and hopefully stimulate more research and dialogues for integration of CAM modalities into main stream heath care. Today, despite a burgeoning and out-of-bound increase in health costs worldwide, the main stream approach has not been successful or curative in many disease conditions where it is, at best, a palliative medicine. Integrating some CAM modalities and its principles in main stream health care is likely to improve universal health care and overall well-being.

Dr Arup Bhattacharya PhD
Department of Cancer Prevention and Control,
Roswell Park Cancer Institute, Buffalo, NY,
USA

Part 1

Role of CAM

1

Fostering the Art of Well-Being: An Alternative Medicine

Robin Philipp
Centre for Health in Employment and the Environment (CHEE), Bristol Royal Infirmary, Bristol, England

1. Introduction

This chapter addresses the physiological and emotional components of health and well-being. It aims to help people become more aware of their internalized frameworks and how they can be utilized so as to attain and enjoy a healthy outlook on life. In turn this can influence health-related behaviour and reduce consequently the likelihood of experiencing illnesses induced by aspects of modern living. These health problems arise from behaviours such as sedentary lifestyles, cigarette smoking and abuse of alcohol or drugs, exposure to excessive emotional pressures, or maladaptive coping mechanisms to life events. Fostering the art of well-being can therefore be seen as alternative medicine.

The medical model emphasises health care and remedial treatment. Greater importance needs now to be attached to primary prevention and health promotion and with which there is a heightened need for people to accept their personal responsibility and individual accountability. Traditional approaches to health have not encompassed sufficiently primary prevention. New models are needed for positive health. These models require a reassessment of value systems in society that enables improved understanding of the WHO slogan: *'health is our real wealth'*.

Unfortunately many people do not value their health until they lose it. It can be reasoned however that if people can understand and appreciate better the basis of human value systems they could be more likely to reappraise their values and thereby encouraged to address aspects of life and living which have more intrinsic and sustainable or 'real' value for them. If too they can become more aware of the ecological interplay of internal physiological and external environmental factors that influence their health and well-being and adopt healthier lifestyles, this will at the same time as ensuring their own health and happiness, contribute towards a sustainable future and the well-being of their society. This chapter is a contribution to that process.

2. The concept of health and well-being

The current World Health Organization (WHO) definition of health, formulated in 1948, describes it as: *'a state of complete physical, mental and social well-being and not merely the absence of disease or infirmity'* (WHO, 2006). It has however been suggested very recently that as this definition *"is absolute and therefore unachievable"*, it is *"no longer helpful and is even counterproductive"* (Editorial, 2011a). A new definition: *"the ability to adapt and self manage in the face of social, physical, and emotional challenges"* has been proposed (Huber et al, 2011). Nevertheless, both concepts imply *'a balanced relationship of the body and mind and complete adjustment to the external environment"* (Howe & Lorraine, 1973).

This balanced relationship is the basis of the underlying hypothesis of work undertaken by Arts Access International (www.artsaccessinternational.org). The hypothesis states that: *"the way, from within ourselves, we look outwards at the world around us influences our perception of factors in the external environment that impinge on us and how we respond to them. The relationship is dynamic and symbiotic"*. The hypothesis is developed to note that: *" greater understanding is needed of this interdependent relationship and of how the roles in it of creative endeavour and aesthetic appreciation benefit our morale, self-esteem, confidence, well-being, sense of belonging and personal development. This understanding helps to give pleasure, enjoyment, direction, purpose and meaning to our lives. There is an art to acquiring and utilising this understanding and its basis is in the arts. Appreciation of it and the culture associated with it are supportive of us and of society. They are worth fostering as they enable us in the art of living"*.

The English poet, John Keats, explored this relationship when he asked: "Do we retreat from the reality of the outer world into ourselves at times, or do we retreat from the pressures of the outside world into the reality of our inner selves?" (Philipp, 2001a). In taking this question further, the doctor-poet, Dannie Abse, musing on it in 1993, noted that: "imaginative daydreaming is an escape from the precipitous pessimism of living or dealing with problems and the sphere of sorrows, and it is used to restore balance" (op.cit.). Nevertheless, whichever way we look at it, as the English poet, T.S. Eliot noted: ..... "human kind cannot bear very much reality" (Laycock, 2003). It is therefore reasonable to explore in these present times of considerable global insecurity, uncertainty and rapid change, what we can each do, whoever we are and wherever we are, and how the arts can help us to:

- remain positive and feel more settled in life and living;
- understand and appreciate what we truly value and wish to give priority to;
- contribute constructively towards helping the world becoming a better place for all its citizens;
- allow everybody to be recognised for their own worth;
- help everyone enjoy and fulfil their own potential (Philipp, 2006).

These aspects of health and well-being and where the arts can contribute to them have evolved from early ideas in history of the worth of balance and harmony in life and living.

2.1 Early ideas of balance and harmony with respect to health

Early civilizations understood the importance to health of achieving a natural balance between people's body systems, their lifestyle and their environment. In Hippocratic medicine for example, illness was believed to be an imbalance between the four bodily humours: blood, phlegm, yellow bile and black bile. Although physicians would try to correct this by such means as bleeding, purging, cooling or heating, in order to restore the balance and thus the patient's health, people were considered to be responsible for maintaining their own balance, in order to remain in good health, by leading a temperate lifestyle with plenty of exercise and sleep, and no excesses of rich food, alcohol, sex or excitement (http://library.wellcome.ac.uk/). The four humours were believed to be linked to the seasons, and also to the four elements: earth, air, fire and water. Similar concepts of bodily harmony in tune with nature are central to other medical systems with ancient origins, including Ayurvedic medicine and Chinese medicine, both of which have evolved over 2000 years into complete medical approaches that involve diagnosis and treatment (http://www.familydoctor.co.uk/complement01).

Traditional Chinese medicine, which includes a range of practices including herbal medicine, acupuncture and Tai Chi, is based on the concept of Yin and Yang which for health must be perfectly balanced http://www.rchm.co.uk/ It remains a major part of healthcare in China and has gained popularity in the West over the last hundred years.

Ayurveda, which means 'the science of life' from the Sanskrit words ayur (life) and veda (science or knowledge), originated in India and is still widely practiced in Eastern countries. It uses a variety of products and techniques to cleanse the body of harmful substances and restore the balance and harmony of body, mind and spirit (http://nccam.nih.gov/he alth/ayurveda)

In Western medicine, the concept of health diverged from this model when in the 17th century Descartes described a dichotomy of matter and body on one hand and consciousness and spirit on the other (Rothschild, 1994). Although he considered the interplay between the two an essential aspect of human nature and was well aware of its implications for medicine (Capra, 1983; Gold, 1985), the idea that mind and body were separate entities became embedded in developing medical science.

With the rapid advancement of scientific knowledge and technology during the 19th and 20th centuries, the body came to be seen as a machine, and disease an external, alien entity which caused it to malfunction (http://library.wellcome.ac.uk/). Responsibility for health thus shifted to the medical profession who focused on disease, while the patient took his body for repair (Gold, 1985). Molecular biology drove the focus on treating and eradicating disease and for a period the biomedical model predominated, with medicine dealing almost exclusively with organic complaints (Engel, 1977). However, in the second half of the last century, it became increasingly apparent that this model could not account for a large part of the 'illness' seen by the psychiatric profession, i.e. the behavioural and psychological problems which had no somatic cause (Shah & Mountain, 2007). Also, in spite of a decline in the rates of many organic diseases, rates of disability and invalidity absence from work increased (Wade, 2009). Changes in the nature of work had led to new workplace risks (Fingret, 2000) and the concept of 'stress', itself a mechanical metaphor, was used to describe the result of perceived pressure on an individual which exceeded his or her ability to cope (French et al.,1982; Karasek, 1979). By 2005, in the United Kingdom (UK)'s annual national Labour Force Survey (LFS), stress was the second most commonly reported illness.

Clearly, the recognition of this type of functional illness, with no apparent organic basis, could not be explained by the linear and reductionist biomedical model which *'assumes disease to be fully accounted for by deviations from the norm of measurable biological (somatic) variables. It leaves no room within its framework for the social, psychological and behavioral dimensions of illness'* (Engel, 1977). A biopsychosocial model of health was proposed (Engel, 1977) in which biological, psychological and sociological factors are all considered to contribute to health or illness, and attention began to focus on what exactly is meant by the term 'well-being'.

2.2 What do we mean by 'well-being'?

In 2005, the Royal College of Physicians (RCP), UK, defined well-being as 'a *holistic notion of achieving a state of health, comfort and happiness*' (RCP, 2005). Other societies have however for a very long time throughout the history of Western society addressed the holistic aspects of health and the concept of '*feeling*' or of '*being well*'. For example, the Hellenistic Greeks such as Aristotle, in exploring questions of ecology and organic unity, referred to '*ataraxia*' (inner peace), and '*eudaimonia*' (a feeling that reflects a combination of well-being, happiness, contentment, pleasure and satisfaction and of living the best life possible) (Westra & Robinson, 1997).

In the Western world, the arrival in the 20th century of the Welfare State meant that the basic needs of citizens in terms of health, hygiene and socio-economic considerations were met to a greater extent than ever before. It soon however became apparent that, as Maslow's hierarchy of need predicts (Maslow, 1943), people continued to want more, they needed choices, and they sought opportunities to fulfil ambitions and goals. Affective well-being, or how we *feel* about our lives and situations, became the focus of empirical research and over the last 50 years a large body of work has explored the construct and its measurement.

Well-being is more than the absence of mental illness. One review of the literature (Ryan & Deci, 2001) describes it as '*optimal psychological functioning and experience*'. Precisely what constitutes optimal experience has been the subject of philosophical debate since the roots of the hedonic tradition in the 4th century BC when it was proposed that the goal of life was to experience the maximum amount of pleasure. Psychologists adopting the hedonic approach define well-being in terms of pleasure versus pain, and the maximisation of happiness, though it is conceded that this can be derived from the attainment of valued goals as well as from physical hedonism (Diener et al., 1998, as cited in Ryan & Deci, 2001). This paradigm assesses subjective well-being (SWB), with measures of affective state, which concern relatively short-term feelings, and a cognitive element of satisfaction with life, which extends to a longer-term assessment.

An alternative viewpoint, which has equally ancient antecedents, is that well-being consists of more than just happiness and requires the actualisation of human potential. This is based on eudaimonism, the belief that well-being consists of realising one's daimon or true nature (Ryan & Deci, 2001). Aristotle for example believed that true happiness came from the expression of virtue. According to eudaimonic theory, not all desires which are pleasure producing necessarily result in wellness, therefore subjective happiness does not equate with well-being (op.cit.). One model of eudaimonic well-being, which uses the term psychological well-being (PWB) to distinguish it from SWB, operationalises human actualisation on six dimensions: autonomy, personal growth, self-acceptance, life purpose, environmental mastery and positive relatedness (Ryff, 1989). It is claimed that these constructs also promote physical well-being through their influence on physiological systems. Although the hedonic and eudaimonic perspectives are distinct they also overlap to some extent and it is likely that well-being is a multidimensional construct which includes elements of both, with psychological well-being predicting subjective well-being (Kafka & Kozma, 2002).

In a definition from contemporary philosophy, well-being has three inter-related elements: **Welfare** - the provision of food, drink, shelter, medical care, and other requirements for 'bodily flourishing'; **Contentment** - an enduring and stable sense of satisfaction with one's life; and **Dignity** - the control of one's destiny and the ability to live a life of one's choice (Kenny & Kenny, 2006). It is pointed out that it is not necessary to have all three distinct components in order to be happy, so for example a well-fed, well-housed and well-treated slave may be contented, though he lacks the dignity of freedom. A devout and ascetic hermit may have contentment and dignity and consider himself blessed, even though he is undernourished and living in poverty (op.cit.).

The contemporary debate as to what constitutes well-being parallels the centuries old question of the nature of happiness. Studies have suggested that the pursuit of happiness, in the sense of pleasure seeking, does not increase life satisfaction, whereas eudaimonic pursuits such as personal growth, development of potential and contributing to the lives of others, do (Seligman, 2002). However, it has been observed that a law of diminishing returns appears to operate, in that as we realise one set of aspirations, we move onto another (Delamothe, 2005). As the Latin philosopher Seneca put it:

'the more we look for happiness, the less likely we are to find it. What we need is 'felicitatis intellectus', the awareness of well-being' (De Vita Beata).

2.3 Threats to well-being in modern living

Unfortunately, many valued activities in a modern lifestyle, which may bring 'happiness' in the short term, can result in threats to well-being (Philipp, 2006). Problems have arisen in society from a lack of understanding that apparently widespread, superficial, short-lasting values based on wishes for immediate gratification do not help longer term, to expand or otherwise exercise the mind, feed community spirit or nourish the imagination in sustainable, personally-satisfying and enduring ways (Philipp et al., 1999a; Santayana 1988). Examples include:

- alcohol and recreational drug use;
- cigarette smoking;
- sedentary lifestyles;
- poor nutrition and weight management;
- unprotected sex;
- standards of safety associated with behaviour in occupational and leisure time activities.

Other threats to well-being associated with values in modern living include:

- mental health and emotional well-being associated with working hours, work tasks, living conditions, isolation, peripatetic working, language barriers, sleep deprivation, and workplace stress;
- cultural alienation and lack of respect for the cultures and customs of others;
- uncertainty as to what lies ahead for society and for each of us personally in an at-present unsettled, insecure world.

The likelihood of experiencing these lifestyle health problems and of improved overall well-being can be influenced greatly by a heightened understanding of value systems in society and an increased sense of personal responsibility and individual accountability, greater awareness of the importance of balancing personal freedom and collective responsibility, and by wider appreciation of the personal enjoyment that can be attained from having a greater sense of citizenship.

In addressing the need for a reappraisal of value systems, it has been reasoned that the needs for improved understanding of individual accountability and personal responsibility can be addressed by greater attention to the interdependence and importance of:

- the quality of our surrounding natural and built environments;
- the aesthetic component of '*health*' which is included in the WHO European Charter on Environment and Health, developed and promulgated by the Ministers of Health and Ministers of the Environment in Europe (WHO, 1989);
- the need reported by a WHO Inter-regional Consultation on Environmental Health for the aesthetic aspects of recreational value and mental health within '*healthy tourism*' to be addressed (WHO, 1997);
- the roles of creative endeavour and aesthetic appreciation in mental health and emotional well-being;
- improved understanding of how our personal attitudes, outlook and behaviour are influenced by a combination of all our actual (externally derived), and perceived (internal) experiences;
- heightened awareness of the factors needed for sustainable, economic development of society and within this, the increasing importance for wider, on-going investment in social capital and emotional economics (Philipp, 2001b, 2003).

In 2004, this interdependence was addressed in the Brighton Declaration (Editorial, 2004). It identified five global health action areas:

- health as a global public health good;
- health as a key component of global security;
- health as a key factor of global governance of interdependence;
- health as a responsible business practice and social responsibility;
- health as global citizenship.

2.4 Well-being and government policy

Concern over the risks to the public health in modern living has led to well-being becoming a required outcome of government policy in countries as far apart geographically as New Zealand (NZ) and the UK. In NZ for example, with a framework which has been reported by the WHO, the Local Government Act 2002, requires Local Authorities to demonstrate on an annual basis what they are doing in support of four components of well-being, viz. economic, social, cultural and environmental (Philipp & Thorne, 2007). The WHO also initiated in 1991 a Quality of Life project aimed to develop an international, cross-culturally comparable, quality of life assessment instrument. It assesses the individual's perception in the context of their culture and value systems in which they live and in relation to their goals, expectations, standards and concerns. It has been translated into more than 20 languages and is widely used in many countries (WHO, 1995). Linked to it, in the UK, an instrument has been developed and validated for assessing mental well-being in a general population. The Warwick-Edinburgh Mental Well-being Scale (WEMWBS) is a 14 item scale designed to cover both hedonic and eudaimonic perspectives and it is also now widely used (Tennant et al., 2007).

As a further example of evolving government policy, in 2004 the Department of Health in the UK outlined a new approach to the health of the public, which reflected modern lifestyles, and responded to the needs and wishes of its citizens. The White Paper *Choosing Health*, outlined a new strategy to give people informed choices, and with services tailored to individual needs, with the aim of reducing inequalities in health and tackling the emerging problems of a consumer society. Areas prioritized for action included smoking, obesity and diet, alcohol, sexual health and mental health. The vision was that the National Health Service (NHS) would increasingly become a health improvement and prevention service, supporting individuals in the healthy informed choices that they make (DoH, 2004). In addition to the focus on individual choice and responsibility, the importance of organizations and communities working together was stressed. The report stated that:

'Organisations, including NHS organisations, will increasingly use their corporate power in ways that promote the health and wellbeing of their local communities, and people across all sectors of society will be encouraged to work together to improve health' (DoH, 2004).

Evidence is emerging of the worth of this policy. For example, there is growing evidence that regular exercise can help maintain cognitive function in later life and that therefore adults in midlife and beyond should be advised to keep moving for as long as possible (Editorial, 2011b).

Progress has been achieved. One useful model for measuring national well-being that has emerged from such government policy initiatives is the conceptual frameworks approach described by the Office for National Statistics, UK Government. It notes that:

- people who feel in control of their own destiny feel more fulfilled;
- having the purpose of a job is as important to the soul as it is to the bank balance; and that
- people have a real yearning to belong to something bigger than themselves (Office of National Statistics, 2011).

2.5 Well-being and work

The UK Government policy has evolved further. The report, *Choosing Health*, was followed by a further government strategy focusing on well-being at work. In response to the finding of the UK Labour Force Survey of 2004/05 that 13 million working days were lost due to work related stress in that year, *Health Work and Well being* (DoH, 2005) focused on the active promotion of health and well-being in the workforce. It was quickly followed by a review of the health of Britain's working age population, *Working for a healthier tomorrow* (Black, 2008) and a review of the health and well-being of the NHS workforce (Boorman, 2009). Reports from industry and the private sector suggested that appropriate interventions focusing on well-being could reduce sickness absence by as much as 30% - 40%, with consequent monetary benefit (Black, 2008; Boorman, 2009; Health & Safety Executive, 2005; Litchfield, 2007).

As one of the UK's largest employers, the NHS, it was suggested, could take an exemplary role in tackling health and well-being issues for its staff, at the same time making a significant contribution to the health of the population as a whole (Boorman, 2009). While some national programmes were rolled out to improve working conditions, it has been stressed that successful programmes need to be specifically designed to meet employee needs, since no one size fits all (PricewaterhouseCoopers, 2008). Each individual's response to stressors in the workplace is modified by personal and environmental variables, and accordingly, modification of workplace stressors can only go so far towards reducing risks to individual health (Keating, 2005). Again, the view is endorsed that individuals have a fundamental personal responsibility for maintaining their own health (Black, 2008; Boorman, 2009; Seligman, 2000). Many healthcare Trusts have consequently developed programmes which provide choice for the individual and help staff to have some control over their own health and well-being, for example raising awareness of self-help methods for reducing stress, and offering resources such as relaxation classes and other complementary therapies (Philipp & Thorne, 2008).

2.6 Science and the art of assessing well-being

Clearly, conventional medicine, in spite of its many advances in scientific knowledge and technology, has not met all our needs for complete physical, mental and social well-being. With this awareness, the focus of healthcare has broadened and begun to turn once more to promoting health rather than focus exclusively on curing illness. There is a renaissance of interest in many practices from ancient times and in support of well-being they are experiencing a growing popularity in the 'new' field of complementary and alternative medicine (CAM). But how best should their worth be assessed ?

CAMs, including different arts-based activities, are interventions used in areas such as:

- ways of reducing levels of perceived stress and of inducing relaxation;
- methods to help improve emotional well-being, productivity and effectiveness at work, so as to help reduce sickness absence, accidents, errors, low morale and poor performance (Philipp & Thorne, 2008);
- encouraging practical activities with creative endeavour and personal expression to help ease perceived distress, induce relaxation, and foster well-being (Philipp, 2003)

In association with the WHO 'Health for All' programme, it was noted in 2001 that the links between morals, personal ethics, art, aesthetics, well-being and environmental health deserved further interdisciplinary study (Philipp, 2001b). An *'Arts-Science Spectrum of Inquiry'* was developed and endorsed in publications of the Nuffield Trust (Philipp et al., 1999b; Philipp, 2002). It spans from:

a. the **subjective**, intuitive, individually inspirational, **artistically** expressive viewpoints to:
b. the **objective**, measurable, productive, logical and **scientific** perspective.

This model recognizes that both the artistic and scientific approaches are expressive and informative and that each has its own methodologies and ways of benefiting and extending the evidence base (Philipp, 2003).

Neuropsychology is a discipline that helps health professionals to link these two approaches. In neuropsychology it has for example, been noted that the neocortex of the human forebrain has been described as the thinking brain: " *the left hemisphere is Apollonian; verbal, mathematical, logical, deductive, and oriented towards the external environment ('outward bound'), whereas the right hemisphere is Dionysian; holistic, intuitive, spatial, pattern-recognizing, and concerned with inner spaces ('inward* bound' (Porteous, 1996).

The likelihood of personal and community well-being is associated with having both a personal, healthy outlook and ready access to healthy places. Enabling this requires recognition of the arts-science approach to evaluation, the utilisation of qualitative and quantitative research methods and recognition of the need to audit different interventions and activities (Philipp, 1997). To assist this process a '*Community Health Gains Model*' has been developed (Philipp,1997, 2001b, 2003). It reasons that:

1. A community is more than a collection of individuals in that it has 'synergy' and not just 'summation'.
2. Becoming actively and constructively involved in a community gives a sense of belonging and helps to increase personal well-being.
3. '*Self-esteem*' as a sense of personal value and worth, heightened morale and confidence, and '*well-being*' as a feeling of contentment, happiness and health, are interdependent.
4. Heightened self-esteem, morale and confidence are likely to lead to healthier lifestyles.
5. Creative expression through individual and group endeavour provides health-promoting opportunities that help individuals to improve their well-being, self-esteem, morale and confidence.
6. The art therapies and participation in '*arts for health*' workshops can produce beneficial changes in cognition, feelings and behaviour.
7. Improved well-being and self-esteem lead to:

a. reduced dependence and prescriptions for psychotropic medication;
b. less repeat attendances at primary care services for health care and support;
c. healthier lifestyles (less smoking, use of alcohol and addictive substances, improved diet and more physical exercise;
d. less delinquency and crime;
e. less sickness absence from school and work;
f. healthy leisure time pursuits;
g. greater participation in adult education and further learning courses.

In essence, the fostering of well-being needs a strengthened evidence base. Both arts and science approaches are being utilized. Wider awareness of the findings is in turn helping to justify different strategies, interventions and programmes that are, as complementary and alternative medicines, being introduced in society. The term, Complementary and Alternative Medicine (CAM) therefore deserves further study.

3. Complementary and alternative medicine (CAM)

The increasing incidence of non-organic illness, and subsequent focus in government strategy on health promotion and well-being, have led to a demand for new forms of treatment, which offer choice to the patient, and support well-being. There is increasing interest in what is termed in the West 'complementary and alternative medicine (CAM)', treatment practices which fall outside conventional medicine. In fact such treatments are not new but rather, in most cases, revivals of ancient healing practices.

The international Cochrane Collaboration, which systematically reviews primary research into healthcare to ensure that treatment decisions can be based on reliable and up to date evidence, has defined CAM as:

'a broad domain of healing resources that encompasses all health systems, modalities, and practices and their accompanying theories and beliefs, other than those intrinsic to the politically dominant health systems of a particular society or culture in a given historical period.' (CAM Research Methodology Conference, 1995).

The terms 'complementary' and 'alternative' refer not to the practices themselves, but to the different ways in which they may be used (Genders, 2006; http://nccam.nih.gov/hea lth/what iscam/).

3.1 Complementary therapy

Complementary therapies are non-invasive, non-pharmaceutical techniques which are used as an adjuvant to the primary, conventional treatment, to improve the general health and wellbeing of an individual in treatment for an illness or receiving palliative care. Such techniques are also commonly used to maintain health and improve well-being in the absence of diagnosed illness.

3.2 Alternative therapy

An alternative therapy is one which is used in place of conventional medicine (op.cit.), as for example those considered 'whole medicine systems'. A 'whole medical system' is defined by the National Centre for Complementary and Alternative Medicine in the USA (NCCAM) as: *'A complete system of theory and practice that has evolved over time in different cultures and apart from conventional medicine'.* Examples include traditional Chinese medicine, Ayurvedic medicine, homeopathy, and naturopathy (http://nccam.nih.gov/).

In some cases, where there is sufficient evidence of safety and effectiveness, a CAM treatment may be an integral part of mainstream treatment. An example of such 'integrative medicine' is the use of acupuncture by physiotherapists (http://www.familydoctor.co .uk/complement01).

The common denominator for CAM therapies is that each contributes to the concept of holistic healthcare, an approach which acknowledges the interaction of many interrelated components of health (Wade, 2009), affecting mind, body or spirit.

3.3 Holistic healthcare

The term 'holism' was coined in 1926 by Jan Smuts who defined it as: *'the tendency in nature to form wholes that are greater than the sum of the parts through creative evolution.'* This law of nature was implicitly understood in the healing traditions of the ancient world. Both Aruyvedic and Chinese medicine believed that life should be lived in harmony with nature and Socrates in the 4th century BC realized that it was no good to treat only one part of the body since *'the part can never be well unless the whole is well'* (Walter, 1999). In modern thinking, holism is related to General Systems Theory and to theories of complexity and chaos in which many relationships are not linear (Wade, 2009) since a whole is made up of interdependent parts (Walter, 1999). Applied to illness and health, this means that there may not be a simple relationship between cause and effect as the medical model implies. Holistic healthcare emphasizes the connection of mind, body and spirit and, as in the biopsychosocial model of illness (Wade, 2009), disease is understood to be the result of physical, emotional, spiritual and environmental imbalance (http://www.holisticmedicine.org). It recognizes four systems: organs, the whole person, behaviour, and social role function, and four contexts which influence these systems: personal factors, physical environment, social environment and time. The importance to health of free-will (or choice) and quality of life (or well-being) are also recognised (Wade, 2009) and, as in ancient times, in considering the whole person in interaction with his environment, the responsibility for making the right choices for health is recognized (Walter, 1999). Holistic Health has been described as an approach to living in which the absence of disease is merely the centre point of a continuum between premature death and maximum well-being, leaving plenty of scope for healthy people to improve their level of well-being (Walter, 1999). CAM therapies are therefore also used by 'healthy' people to enhance well-being and quality of life. Both conventional medicine and CAM aim to treat the whole person and in some cases an integrated approach is used which provides both. This is now quite commonly seen in cancer care.

3.4 CAM in integrated healthcare

An example of a holistic approach to treatment for cancer patients is that followed at the Penny Brohn Centre near Bristol, UK (http://www.pennybrohncancercare.org/). The centre was named after its co-founder, who saw the need to bring treatments for body, mind and spirit under one roof after her own cancer diagnosis in 1979. While exploring a range of different alternative therapies in various parts of the world, she realized that: '*it was really her soul and emotions that were in complete turmoil and desperately needed help*' (Cooke, 2003). Today the centre aims to help individuals with cancer to gain a sense of control and achieve the best possible health and quality of life by combining the support and complementary treatments available at the centre with their orthodox treatment (op.cit.). The ethos of the Penny Brohn approach is summed up in the foreword to its handbook '*The Bristol Approach to Living with Cancer*':

'*Medicine is an art as well as a science, and the healing art is holistic through and through. It must touch all aspects of the sick person – the mind as well as the body, the soul, spirit or feelings as well as the reason, and the unconscious as well as the conscious. And it must be interactive, a dialogue between the sick person and the healer. The word 'patient' comes from the Latin for passive, but it is vital that the patient should be an agent as well.*' Roy Porter, in (Cooke, 2003).

The recently formed College of Medicine in the UK holds a similar view, focusing on health improvement, wellbeing and self help as well as medical care (http://www.collegeofmedicine.org.uk). This new alliance believes that doctors, nurses, health professionals, patients and scientists should be on an equal footing in the healthcare team. A number of innovative projects which offer a patient-centred, integrative service are described on the website, including the NHS Bristol Homeopathy Hospital, The Complementary Therapy Service at the Christie Hospital NHS Foundation Trust in Manchester, the Culm Valley

Integrated Centre for Health, which is based in a general practice surgery in Cullompton, Devon, and the British College of Integrative Medicine, based in Bath, England.

CAM therapies are now quite widely offered as part of NHS cancer services, though it is not mandatory for such treatments to be made available to patients. However, the National Cancer Peer Review Programme has included Complementary Therapy (Safeguarding Practice) Measures in its Manual for Cancer Services (2008). These comprise clinical governance requirements to be applied where complementary practitioners work on NHS premises or are endorsed or cited in information for patients, and cover: clearance for working with vulnerable adults; qualifications; written information for patients; informed consent; and equipment and materials.

3.5 Evidence for the effectiveness of CAM therapies

Not all medical practitioners are in favour of CAM therapies being available on the NHS. In 2006 leading doctors in the UK aroused controversy when they expressed their reservations in a letter to The Times Online, suggesting that limited funds for healthcare should be spent on conventional treatment for which there was solid evidence of efficacy (Baum, 2006). The response from supporters of CAM was that since taxpayers funded the NHS there should be consumer choice in what treatments were available.

Choice is a key tenet of holistic medicine, and the eclectic range of complementary therapies now available, albeit not always on the NHS, does provide the choice of treatment which is essential to the idiosyncratic nature of non-organic illness. However, the UK healthcare system has to represent value for money and needs therefore to be evidence based. It has been suggested that multifaceted, individualized and holistic CAM therapies do not lend themselves to evaluation by the gold standard method used in conventional medicine for evaluating the efficacy of treatment interventions, the randomized controlled trial (RCT) (Hermann et al., 2006). The Cochrane Collaboration, which organizes the preparation, maintenance and dissemination of systematic reviews of the effects of healthcare interventions, has a Complementary and Alternative Medicine (CAM) field which in 2004 held 145 reviews (Manheimer et al., 2004). Therapies were not evenly represented, and barely one quarter of them showed a definite positive effect (op. cit.). Interestingly, some therapies which were widely used had few or no reviews in the database, whilst others for which there was strong evidence were not popular (op.cit.). In 2007 an attempt was made to improve the quality of the Cochrane CAM field (Wieland & Manheimer, 2009), and the number of systematic reviews has risen to 249 in 2011.

Sufficient evidence now exists for some CAM treatments to be accepted into mainstream medicine, but for many others there is still a lack of empirical evidence for their efficacy (Manheimer et al., 2004). Whether or not a treatment 'works' in quantitative terms is not the only useful evidence, since CAM treatments are concerned with more intangible and qualitative outcomes including empowerment and patient determined outcomes (Herman et al., 2006). It has been suggested that the 'whole systems' methods of health service research (HSR) might be more appropriate for exploring these outcomes, and such aspects as the interactions between patient, provider and system, or the impact of patient and provider expectations on outcomes (op cit). It is acknowledged at the Cochrane Library that evidence from qualitative studies can play an important role in adding value to systematic reviews for policy, practice and consumer decision-making (Noyes et al., 2008).

In the UK, the National Institute for Health and Clinical Excellence (NICE) provides independent guidance on promoting good health and preventing and treating ill health (http://www.nice.org.uk/). Its recommendations have rarely addressed CAM, although occasionally they have noted that a patient might find such a treatment useful (Ernst & Terry, 2009). However, recently, exercise, manual therapy or acupuncture were recommended as treatments for non-specific low back pain (op.cit.). NICE does however incorporate the resource database NHS Evidence, which includes a specialist collection on complementary and alternative medicine. This unique resource provides access to good quality, up-to-date information on CAM which includes research evidence and information on regulations, safety and best practice (http://www.uclh.nhs.uk/ourservices/ourhospitals/rlhim/pages/nhsevidence-complementaryandalternativemedicine.aspx). This can be accessed by the general public as well as professionals.

There appears to be no evidence that CAM treatments do any harm (Manheimer et al., 2004) but it has been pointed out that the potential danger of such treatments, particularly when used in the private sector, is that a patient may not receive appropriate conventional treatment because the non-medically qualified CAM practitioner is unable to make a proper medical diagnosis (http://www.familydoctor.co.uk/complement01).

3.6 How do CAM therapies work?

Until recently, little was known about **how** complementary treatments work, although it has been suggested that they mobilize '*the inherent capacity of people to heal themselves*' (Wright, 2005). It can be reasoned that there appears to be a dynamic relationship between our internal, physiological environment and the resonance that can be established with appropriate, extraneous stimuli in different supportive, soothing external environments, and that through the internal limbic system it supports our personal emotional resilience and coping skills. There are for example well-recognized benefits from engaging with the natural environment and the associations with physiological body rhythms that arise from rhythmic movement associated with activities such as walking, jogging, yoga and tai chi, or from engaging with natural sounds in the environment around us such as bird song, the sound of water in streams, rivers and waterfalls, and from wind in the trees. Such stimuli to the bodily senses are thought to help to foster an internal energy or chi flow which can result in a calming effect which brings peace of mind, and a feeling of being able to cope much more readily with what ever needs or pressures one may be experiencing.

Such thinking goes back to the Ancient Greeks. Plato for example, believed that in getting outdoors and walking along some pleasant pathway in the countryside and allowing the beauty of the natural surroundings to be absorbed into our consciousness, we should cultivate a gentle and even walking rhythm. He considered that the movements of the body would start to influence gradually the functioning of the mind (Puttock, 2000).

The associations of medicine and poetry, and of health with aesthetic appreciation of the natural environment, are well-expressed by the English poet, William Wordsworth, in his poem, 'An Evening Scene'

Come forth into the light of things,
Let nature be your teacher.
She has a world of ready worth,

Our minds and hearts to bless –
Spontaneous wisdom breathe by health.

Much more recently, developments in neuroscience have illuminated the bio-psychosocial medical model, demonstrating how psychosocial factors and interventions translate into biology, and thus how psychosocial interventions actually work (Shah & Mountain, 2007). The relatively new field of psychoneuroimmunology (PNI), defined as the study of the connection between the mind, the body and the immune system (Daruna, 2004) explains how the endocrine, immune and nervous systems react to stressors and how this can be mitigated by the physiological response to pleasurable stimuli, which is synthesized in the morphinergic processes of the limbic system. Endorphins and enkephalins are the body's natural opiates and it would seem that the CNS reward and pleasure mechanisms are implicated in the significant benefits which have been shown to be derived from therapies such as reflexology, massage, aromatherapy, Yoga, T'ai Chi and acupuncture. Similar benefits are experienced from exercise, or the experience of nature, and these encompass both physical and psychological symptoms and general well-being (Tait, 2008).

For many CAM treatments, the relationship between therapist and client, which involves trust, and belief and expectations about the treatment, suggests cortical involvement (Lundeberg et al., 2007). The same reward and motivation pathways have been shown to be common to different CAM approaches (Esch et al., 2004) and the release of oxytocin is known to reduce anxiety and stress levels and facilitate social interaction and trust in others (Carter, 2003; Esch & Stefano, 2005).

One common feature of CAM therapies is rhythmical movement, seen for example in the Eastern practices such as Tai Chi and Yoga. Occupational therapists who work with autistic children have found that rocking, swinging and balancing activities can help to initiate speech and this has been demonstrated in a study where slow swinging in a net swing stimulated the production of speech sounds (Ray, King, & Grandin, 1988). Horseback riding has many of the same motions and sometimes parents report that their child spoke his/her first words on a horse (Grandin, personal communication). Horseback riding has for a long time been used therapeutically with disabled children and has been shown to improve motor control of the head and neck (Engsberg & Shurtleff, 2007) and muscle symmetry and gross motor function (Snider et al., 2007; Sterba, 2007). More recently, riding or simply being with horses, termed Equine Assisted Activities (EAA) has become a popular therapy for improving social and cognitive functioning, particularly for autistic children. A pilot study in Florida found that children exposed to EAA exhibited greater sensory seeking, sensory sensitivity and social motivation, and less inattention and distractibility (Bass & Llabre, 2010). Other animal assisted therapy has been found to significantly benefit cognitive, psychological and social domains, influencing physiological factors such as lowered blood pressure, heart rate and decreased anxiety levels (Morrison, 2007).

In Germany, researchers at the University of Rostock are testing the hypothesis that the curative psychological effects which have been found to be associated with equine assisted activities - reduced anxiety, stress, aggression and depression, and the facilitation of social communication and trust in others - are based on the shared neurobiological mechanism of the hypothalamo-pituitary-adrenal axis (HPA) stress axis interacting with the oxytocin system (http://www.sopaed.uni-rostock.de/en/forschung/animal-assisted-interventio ns

/basic-neurobiological-and-psychological-mechanisms-underlying-therapeutic-efects-of-equine-assisted-activities-eaat/abstract/).

In ongoing controlled studies with insecurely attached children, the Rostock researchers are investigating whether contact with horses will help these children to engage in more secure and trusting relationships with their adult caregivers. A moving case study of the effects of riding on an autistic child's social functioning and attention can be found in Rupert Isaacson's book about his own son '*The Horseboy*' (Isaacson, 2009).

A very different modern therapy uses sensor technology to translate body movement into digitally generated sound and image (http://www.soundbeam.co.uk). Soundbeam provides a medium through which even profoundly physically or learning impaired individuals can become expressive and communicative using music and sound. A random, barely controlled movement from a severely disabled person, or the slightest wiggle of a digit from a sick child, produce aesthetically pleasing sounds. The sense of control and independence which this provides can be a powerful motivator, stimulating learning and interaction in other areas.

3.7 Arts for health and well-being

Similar benefits to those of CAM may be derived from engaging with the arts. The '*arts for health*' movement and the involvement of artists in health care became a public health strategy in the 1990s, targeted to mental health promotion and emotional well-being and for which the evidence base has being strengthened steadily by peer-reviewed published research (Philipp, 2006).

Art can though mean different things to different people. It can mean:

- expression of self;
- cultural expression and belonging;
- an escape from daily routines and as a way to relax and reduce stress;
- opportunities for socialization;
- access to new experiences and new skills;
- a source of enjoyment.

To ensure that an arts for health intervention is appropriately targeted and meets its specified aims, it is important for organizers to:

- acknowledge individual needs and abilities;
- recognize the characteristics (culture) of specific groups;
- understand the levels at which participants are able to appreciate and enjoy the arts;
- choose art forms relevant to the client group.

3.8 Poetry as CAM

One example of the way in which the arts can produce similar benefits to CAM, is the use of metaphor and imagery in poetry. It can result in internalised pictures with their associated emotional frameworks of thinking that promote relaxation and less rigid thought patterns. Such frameworks are nowadays used increasingly in clinical work to help people derive personal benefit from alterations to their personal perspective and personal outlook on what is going on in their lives, so that they can again move forward with living. In follow up to a small qualitative study exploring whether or not reading or writing poetry might benefit people's health (Philipp & Robertson, 1996), it was identified at 2001 costings that more widespread use of poetry as a health care intervention may result in annual direct health care prescribing cost savings for antidepressant medication in the UK which could amount to as much as UK£1.26 millions (Philipp, 2002). A subsequent study identified that poetry interventions may also improve emotional resilience and anxiety levels in cancer patients (Tegner et al., 2009).

More generally poetry, is considered useful as it has been likened to medicine in that it explores aspects of communication, and because "*the poet, using words as tools, demonstrates and communicates mankind's awareness of the complexity of the human situation. Like the physician, the poet tries first to grasp, then to control, the reality of the human predicament*" (Mathiasen & Alpert, 1980). Medicine and poetry were too, seen by the Ancient Greeks as having a common source of inspiration; to some extent because in antiquity healers and poets were widely assumed to possess some sort of magical power (Bax, 1989). They shared the same God, Apollo.

3.9 Music therapy

Music is another art form with a long tradition of therapeutic use. Music and poetry were closely related in ancient Greece and the word 'melos', from which our 'melody' is derived, indicated both lyric poetry and the music to which it was set (Storr,1997). Playing an instrument or singing in a choir have been described as life-enhancing activities which are irreplaceable but listening to music rather than making it also has a profound effect on the emotions (Storr,1997). It causes arousal which may be intense, but is not unpleasant (op cit).

3.10 Next steps with CAMS and the arts

Further studies and research on CAM with a focus on correlating specific treatments with specific symptom improvements are still needed (Tait, 2008). What these diverse treatments have in common is the personal benefit which is derived in terms of well-being. As with arts activities, participating in the use of CAM treatments restores a little control into people's lives and encourages better coping mechanisms, thus improving quality of life. By embracing these principles we are also accepting, as the ancient Greeks did, that people need to take responsibility for their own health and well-being.

4. Broadening the concept of well-being

The multidimensional nature of well-being was recognized in 2007 in the 'common understanding', developed in UK Government departments, of what wellbeing means in a policy context, which also acknowledged the importance for an individual of having a sense of control and autonomy (Newton, 2007):

'Well-being is a positive physical, social and mental state; it is not just the absence of pain, discomfort and incapacity. It requires that basic needs are met, that individuals have a sense of purpose, that they feel able to achieve important personal goals and participate in society.

It is enhanced by conditions that include supportive personal relationships, strong and inclusive communities, good health, financial and personal security, rewarding employment, and a healthy and attractive environment.

Government's role is to enable people to have a fair access now and in the future to the social, economic and environmental resources needed to achieve wellbeing. An understanding of the effect of policies on the way people experience their lives is important for designing and prioritising them.' (http://archive.defra.gov.uk/sustainable/government/what/priority/wellbeing/common-understanding.htm)

In New Zealand as noted earlier, local authorities have been required to address well-being, taking a sustainable development approach, since the Local Government Act, 2002 which cites four components of well-being: '*environmental*', '*social*', '*cultural*' and '*economic*'. The Act reflects the ancient New Zealand Maori view of health and well-being which: '*incorporates all aspects of a person's internal and external worlds. It assumes health in the spheres of physical, psychological, spiritual and family well-being and a balance among the individual, their environment and those around them*' (St George, 2004). It also endorses the view that environmental values, economic well-being and personal health are interdependent (Handszuh, 1991)

4.1 Well-being and the natural environment

As noted above in exploring how CAM therapies work, closely related to the benefits to well-being provided by complementary therapies and art are the sensations derived from our aesthetic experiences of the natural environment. As the artist, Paul Cezanne noted: "*Art is a harmony parallel to nature*" (Denton, 1993).

The relationship of body, mind and environment is recognized in the WHO European Charter on Environment and Health (WHO,1989), which states that: '*good health and well-being require a clean and harmonious environment in which physical, psychological, social and aesthetic factors are all given their due importance*'.

The word *aesthetic*, is defined in the Oxford Dictionary as '*having an appreciation of the sense of beauty in accordance with the principles of good taste*', but the aesthetic response also involves emotions that include being '*uplifted*', '*moved*', '*exhilarated*', and '*entranced*' (Eaton, 1995), implying the presence of qualities that are pleasing to the senses (Philipp, 2001b). The 'aesthetic quality of an environment' has been defined as: "*the extent to which an external factor or combination of factors evokes a pleasurable emotional response from the stimulation of our five bodily senses of sight, sound, smell, taste and touch. This response establishes a resonance within ourselves and with the external factors responsible for that stimulation. Resonance helps to promote positive affirmation of ourselves, enhances our well-being and encourages positive identity with the causal environmental factors*" (Philipp et al, 1999a). It has been suggested too that since nature surrounds the viewer, (s)he cannot avoid being involved and is '*likely to experience not only the landscape but perhaps also himself in an unusual and vivid way*' (Porteous, 1996)

The mechanisms behind such responses to the natural environment are believed to be the same as in many CAM therapies, with external sensory stimuli releasing natural opiates, the endorphins and enkephalins, in localised areas of the brain (Denton, 1993). Research cited in a recent overview of well-being and the natural environment (Newton, 2007) has suggested that pleasurable stimuli from nature operate as reciprocal inhibitors of depression (Burns, 2006), facilitate recovery from stress (Mace et al., 1999) and can improve mental alertness, attention and cognitive performance (Cimprich, 1993, 2003; Hartig et al., 1991; Tennessen and Cimprich 1995, as cited in Newton, 2007). This 'natural health service' is explored in the report '*Natural Thinking*' (Bird, 2007) which investigates the links between the natural environment, biodiversity and mental health. The report considers the evidence for the three main hypotheses concerning the restorative effect for humans of the sounds and sights in nature:

- **Biophilia (Wilson, 1984)** which believes affiliation to nature is innate, and that we are programmed through evolution to respond to environments where we feel safe;
- **Attention Restoration Theory (Kaplan and Kaplan, 1989)** which proposes that a natural environment provides the necessary qualities to enable a person to 'be away' from the things which routinely require direct attention, and the effort that that entails, because our effortless involuntary attention (or fascination) is held by pleasurable stimuli; and
- **Psycho-physiological Stress Recovery Theory (Ulrich, 1983)** which is derived from the involuntary physiological responses to nature which have been observed, such as lowered blood pressure, reduced muscle tension and slower pulse rate, which are associated with the limbic system (Bird, 2007).

The aesthetic dimensions of nature and art produce similar responses and have often been combined in the literary and visual arts and have been extensively made use of in arts and health programmes. Two terms have been introduced to describe aspects of psychological and emotional support to be gained from people identifying with roles of the arts for the imagery of place and purpose. They are '*tootling*', and '*doodling*'.

The English word '*tootle*', is defined in the Oxford Dictionary as "to move casually along". It describes the pleasure to be had from using environments of high aesthetic quality to enhance personal experience. '*Tootling*' can be seen as an activity '*in which there is environmental opportunity of sufficient aesthetic quality to be able to enjoy oneself, reflect, daydream and forget the pressures of daily living, abandon oneself to the pleasures of rhythm and exercise and resonate with the beauty of what surrounds one's being*' (Philipp, 2001b). Children for example are encouraged to develop this sort of environmental understanding with '*sensory walks*' during which they are alerted to underfoot sidewalk texture, pedestrian choreography, smells, sounds, weather, clothes, trees, colours and art, and experience running, dawdling, and asking the way; one of the goals is to increase awareness and provide a foundation for personal growth (Porteous, 1996).

The word '*doodling*' is related to tootling. It is defined in the Oxford Dictionary as "drawing or scrawling absent-mindedly". It is an activity undertaken by artists and derived from similar opportunities to tootling. Doodling can be thought of as a creative endeavour with '*the free and spontaneous expression of what the mind is experiencing from its connections of thoughts, feelings and emotions and when allowed to meander gently without specific purpose or intent*' (Philipp, 2001b). It encompasses activities such as sketching, drawing, painting, sculpting, photography, composing music, writing poetry and dance.

Tootling and doodling can be seen as benefitting psychological well-being and emotional resilience by helping to:

- replenish the spirit;
- nourish the soul;
- stimulate the mind, and;
- fuel the imagination.

These effects are consequent of certain patterns of movement and sound experienced through the five bodily senses and influencing the limbic system. They can evoke a resonance or positive feeling within oneself that imparts a sense of emotional well-being (Philipp & Sheridan, 2003). This effect is illustrated in the poem, With All My Senses (Philipp, 1995):

In the eye of the storm
Bare to the waist
and for an hour
I jogged the shore.

Under my feet I heard the pebbles scrunch
Above my head the roar of wind
The cries of gulls
and all around the raging sea.

I watched the fury of an ocean swell
The foam curl
Waves crash
and clouds scud by.

I felt it on my skin
The gusts of wind
The sheets of rain
and the lash of spray.

I tasted with my tongue
Salt on my lips
Smelled the freshness
and breathed the air.

It was delicious and a precious hour
In which I moved my limbs and cleared my mind
and enjoyed with all my senses
What it is to live and come alive. R.P.

Many of us, at a very fundamental, personal level, also have a special place where we like to be, that has special meaning for us in our lives and as such enhances our sense of well-being, and which has its own '*reality*' we wish to preserve. Being there resonates within us and can give us a deep feeling of contentment and peace. Even when away from our special place, reflecting on this resonance can give us a strong sense of belonging and pleasure. This feeling is emotionally enriching and can help to renew, restore and replenish our sense of enjoyment, direction and purpose in life. It can also encourage us, each in our own ways, to be active and involved, and to strive to help in a constructive, positive way with what is going on around us in our world. Our resonance with this imagery of a special place and a sense of purpose nourishes our sense of psychological health and emotional well-being. As an example of this feeling, the '*art of being*' can expressed as:

Back Here

What it is to be
Back here in the sun
Lying on my back;

Back to the land
Touched by the grass
Kissed by the sky;

Absorbed with the clouds
Hearing the crickets
Tuned to the birds;

Breathing the air
Floating my thoughts
Stilling my mind;

It is here for me
Inspired warmed
Renewed refreshed;

Relaxed content
Again I connect
Living my dreams. R.P.

4.2 The benefits of nature in the urban environment

Environmental psychologists, architects, developers, urban planners and public health consultants have used the recognised psychological benefits of imagery of place to good purpose for residents, tourists and other visitors. Protection of the environment can therefore be seen as a CAM. For example, in the UK, '*town planning*' has been defined as: "*the art and the science of ordering the land-uses and siting the building of communication routes so as to secure the maximum level of economy, convenience and beauty*" (Potter, 1997). The importance of incorporating '*beauty*' in support of well-being is embodied within:

- increasing recognition that living in walking distance of parks and green spaces increases the life expectancy of city dwellers and that the health status of people living on social housing estates is determined largely by the quality of their immediate surroundings rather than their housing conditions (Randall, 2004);
- awareness, reported by WHO that: "*What people see when they open their front door has a profound effect on their health*", and that social behaviour can be influenced by the environment, including perceptions of crime and security, and levels of stress, depression and general irritation (Randall, 2004);
- better understanding that environmental enrichment can be gained from the sensitive incorporation of aesthetic sensory qualities such as the balance of spatial arrangement, unity, variety, pattern, line, form, shape, colour, tone and harmony (Philipp, 2003);
- recognition of the role of '*environmental corridors*' as connecting passages and in themselves places between two or more other places, and which have their own qualities of identity and purpose, imagery and expression, such that passing through or being in them evokes an emotional response of either positive feelings of resonance, enjoyment, pleasure and a sense of well-being, or negative feelings of displeasure and discomfort in being there (Philipp, 2001b);
- uses of art and water features like fountains in public parks, squares, streets and buildings such as hospitals, libraries, schools, shopping centres and office buildings, to

open up spaces, provide landmarks for wayfinding and to give opportunities for expression, comment, humour, enjoyment, contemplation and reflection (Philipp, 2003);
- commissioning art works for display in the Metro transport systems of cities such as Brussels, Amsterdam, Toronto, Munich, Prague and Stockholm (Petherbridge, 1987);
- placing poems with thoughtful, warm, resonating, uplifting, short, readily understood and thematic qualities in public places such as, in the UK, in General Practice surgeries and the London Underground mass transport system, and in Moscow in the Moskovsky Metropoliten, to help soothe the temperament of visitors (Philipp, 2001b);
- the incorporation of '*Quiet Rooms*' in public buildings such as hospitals, airports and other large transport terminals, for rest and in support of the WHO Healthy Settings approach (Philipp, 2003);
- the use of virtual reality touch screens for people to access different forms of music in health care seclusion rooms and in support of their vulnerability and insecurity when facing uncertainty and unfamiliar settings, and so as to help reduce their pulse rate, blood pressure and stress associated with heightened alertness in such situations;
- the introduction of a '*dark skies*' policy by some supermarkets in which their car parks have downward-facing lighting to reduce light pollution and so that the stars are rendered more visible (Advertisement, 2004);
- introduction of Japanese and Zen gardens in open courtyards of factories, theatres, concert halls, shopping malls, libraries, hospitals, public and office buildings, to increase the feelings of viewscapes, space and light, and to integrate an indoor-outdoor quality with a natural environment, tranquil, restful theme;

In addition to the benefits to mental health, the interdependence of environmental values and well-being also has physical, social and cultural aspects, often acting synergistically. For example, the beneficial effects of green spaces for physical health, and the opportunities they offer for social cohesion have been well documented (Marks et al., 2006; Newton, 2007; Philipp, 2006). Green spaces are particularly relevant in the present climate of threats to the natural environment, an increasingly urbanized society and rising levels of stress and mental illness, and evidence of the benefits they provide has implications for policy makers (Newton, 2007).

Well-being and environmental issues are particularly relevant in the present age of consumerism, and the need for sustainable development is a global issue. The UK's sustainable development strategy, Securing the future (2005) states that '*the goal of sustainable development is to enable all people throughout the world to satisfy their basic needs and to enjoy a better quality of life, without compromising the quality of life of future generations*'. The sustainable development indicators include a section on well-being which covers subjective well-being measures of life satisfaction as well as other factors known to affect well-being such as poverty and education (Defra, 2010).

In view of the cost to the economy of depression and anxiety, and the accumulating evidence of the restorative effects of the natural environment, it has been suggested that a monetary value could be attributed to green spaces (Newton, 2007). A report published in June 2011 by the UK Government, assesses the economic, health and social benefits of environmental ecosystems in monetary terms (UK National Ecosystem Assessment, 2011). For example, living with a view of a green space is estimated to create UK£300 in health benefits per person per year (http://www.defra.gov.uk/news/2011/06/02/hidden-value-of-nature-revealed/). New evidence gathered for this report indicates that people also benefit economically if their homes are in favourable environmental settings, with substantial amenity value attached to domestic gardens, local green spaces and rivers, proximity to National Parks or National Trust land, or to habitats such as woodland, farmland or freshwater. Such amenities are statistically significant factors contributing to higher house prices. Analysis of the report's well-being survey revealed higher life-satisfaction amongst those who spent time in their own gardens at least once a week and those who visited urban parks or green spaces at least once a month, compared to those who did not do this (op.cit.). Users of domestic gardens and local green spaces at least once a month also reported better health in terms of physical functioning and emotional well-being, compared to those who did not. By valuing natural resources in this way, the report aims to improve decision making for a sustainable future in which natural resources are harnessed for wealth and well-being. The Green Gym programme has evolved together with these findings. It aims "*to provide people with a way to enhance their fitness and health while taking action to improve the outdoor environment*" (Wikipedia, 2011).

The United Nations Environment Programme (UNEP) has also developed further the worth of investing in this sort of 'green' viewpoint. It has just published an evidence-based approach to the wider economic gains for society (UNEP, 2011). In it, the UNEP defines a green economy as one that results in "*improved human well-being and social equity, while significantly reducing environmental risks and ecological scarcities*. Greening the economy, the UNEP reports, "*can generate consistent and positive outcomes for increased wealth, growth in economic output, decent employment, and reduced poverty*" (UNEP, 2011).

4.3 Investing in well-being with social and cultural capital

A '*value*' has been defined as: '*a set of principles which are consistent and inform and direct our thought, actions and activities*' (McGettrick, 2004). This set of principles implies that empathy, rapport and intuition are fundamental to the basis of human values (Philipp et al., 1999c). Being intuitive to the needs, wishes, aspirations, hopes and desires of others and supportive of them is also fundamental to human development (Editorial, 2002; Philipp & Dodwell, 2005). What as individuals and societies we 'value' and how we undertake our 'valuing' are therefore key issues for attempts, in support of well-being, to build both 'social capital' and cultural capital (Philipp, 2002; Philipp & Dodwell, 2005).

To help improve opportunities for enjoyment and personal growth, better understanding of the needs and welfare of other people is required (Philipp, 2006). An important part of a community's well-being comes from its social capital. This important resource encompasses human factors of talent, capability, creativity, innovation and knowledge (op.cit.). The arts and '*an artistic way*' of looking at the world are increasingly being used, not only to improve individual emotional resilience (Eames, 2003), but to help strengthen social capital by addressing cultural and social problems in society such as alienation, frustration, anger, disruption, humiliation and dislocation, and marginalisation from employment (Eames, 2003).

The protective effects of high levels of social capital are found in communities where there are high levels of trust, participation in civic life and social support (Abbott, 2002; Philipp & Dodwell, 2005). They support collective efforts in society for 'cultural well-being' and the strengthening of 'cultural capital and 'social capital' for which frameworks have been published (Eames, 2006). It has after all, been noted that: *'feeling comfortable in your own culture is essential for a healthy lifestyle and general well-being'* (Eames, 2003). Economists have found that social capital correlates closely with subjective well-being and define it as: *'the ties that bind families, neighbourhoods, workplaces, communities and religious groups together'* (Delamothe, 2005).

The United Nations Education, Scientific and Cultural Organisation (UNESCO) has defined culture as: 'the set of distinctive spiritual, material, intellectual and emotional features of society or a social group' that 'encompasses, in addition to art and literature, lifestyles, ways of living together, value system, traditions and beliefs' (Eames, 2003); in support of this, cultural capital has been defined as: 'the wealth created through celebrating and investing in cultural histories, values, ideologies, rituals and programmes' (Eames, 2006).

Greater awareness and understanding of these values and the gains of investing in social and cultural capital would benefit personal and community well-being.

4.4 Culture and heritage issues as CAMs in support of well-being

The European Charter on Environment and Health (WHO, 1989) states that every individual is entitled to an environment conducive to the highest attainable level of health and well-being, but also points out that every individual has a responsibility to contribute to the protection of the environment, in the interests of his or her own health and the health of others (Philipp and Hodgkinson, 1994). In addition, it is recognized that: *'It is also in our environment where we find recreation, health and solace, and in which our culture finds its roots and sense of place'* (John Selbourne, Foreword, in (UK National Ecosystem Assessment, 2011).

Many of the things which are valued in an environment are concerned with culture and heritage. These culture and heritage factors can therefore be considered as relevant contributors to well-being: As such and in their own right, they become CAMs.

In support of this role for culture and heritage factors, an anthropological framework for the basis of human values has been developed with the WHO, Nuffield Trust and Office of International Health Cooperation and Development of the Italian Red Cross (Philipp, 2006, 2007). It has four core components of relevance to well-being:

- appreciation of different civilisations, cultures, customs and societies;
- awareness of tools a society develops for its sense of place, purpose and security;
- knowing what influences thinking and perceptions among members of a group;
- linking within ourselves external experiences and internal feelings.

A wider understanding of the interaction of the above factors in emotional investment, and better appreciation of the enrichment to society of cultural diversity, would it has been suggested help communities to build and strengthen social and cultural capital. (Philipp & Thorne, 2011). The word 'capital' refers to money and assets and the way that they are used for economic gain (Eames, 2006), and the concept of 'cultural capital' recognizes that in order to build the economic base of any community, ideas of 'creativity, imagination, innovation, ideologies, history, values and ritual' need to be included (op cit). Heritage is an important part of a community's culture. It includes:

- **natural heritage:** an inheritance of fauna and flora, geology, landscape, landforms and other natural resources;
- **industrial heritage:** monuments, buildings,
- **cultural heritage:** the legacy of physical artefacts and intangible attributes of a group or society
- **artefacts:** heritage items such as tools, utensils, archaeological findings
- **tradition:** customs and practices inherited from ancestors (Philipp & Thorne, 2011)

These assets are used to economic effect in the increasingly popular forms of tourism (Philipp & Thorne, 2011):

- **ecotourism** with travel to areas of outstanding beauty, bird, nature, wild animal and marine reserves, national parks, and wilderness areas;
- **cultural tourism** with opportunities to explore the lifestyle of local people, their history, art, architecture, religion(s), social customs, archaeological sites, museums, public reserves, art galleries and UNESCO World Heritage Sites;
- **heritage tourism** defined by the National Trust for Historic Preservation in the United States as: "*travelling to experience the places and activities that authentically represent the stories and people of the past*"(www.wikipedia.org).

In addition to the revenue brought by visitors, a local community benefits from such tourism by a reinforced sense of identity and greater appreciation of cultural background, which can facilitate social cohesion. It also encourages conservation which is beneficial to society generally, both now and in the future.

As a starting point for organisations and authorities wishing to assess the environmental, social, cultural and economic components of well-being in their locality, and to evaluate needs, representative populations living in or visiting a locality have been asked to identify the characteristics and qualities, associations and imagery which give them a sense of belonging, or being part of something which enhances their well-being (Philipp, 2006). In this way the 'spirit of a place' can be captured (Philipp, 2006) and its contributing features nurtured and maintained for future generations. In a study following an approach for assessing environmental quality which was outlined in a recent report for the WHO (Philipp & Thorne, 2007), children's artwork, in the form of drawings, poems and photographs, was used to identify met or unmet local environmental and educational needs for well-being and sustainability in their home towns in Waikanae, New Zealand, and Bristol, UK. (unpublished data, 2009). In support of this research method, it is recognised that up to the age of 10 years, children's views tend to be spontaneous, enthusiastic, imaginative and creative (Philipp et al, 1984; Philipp et al, 1986). An awareness and understanding of children's views is therefore important in the contexts of community well-being and environmental health and sustainability. Adults are after all entrusted with stewardship of the world for younger and future generations (Philipp, 2006) and research suggests that the natural environment has a positive role in the physical and emotional well-being of children and young people (Huby & Bradshaw, 2006; Lester & Maudsley 2006; as cited in Newton, 2007). As well as identifying the qualities and characteristics, local icons, environmental and heritage features that are valued by young children and should accordingly be preserved, the study helped to engender interest in local environmental issues amongst the participants and local inhabitants and in support of their well-being (personal communication).

5. Healthy outlooks: A single framework for well-being

The likelihood of avoiding lifestyle health problems and of improved overall well-being can be influenced greatly by an increased sense of personal responsibility and individual accountability, heightened awareness of the importance of balancing personal freedom and collective responsibility, and by wider appreciation of the personal enjoyment that can be attained from having a greater sense of citizenship (Philipp, 2006). In support of this view, as well as stating that every individual is *entitled* to an environment conducive to the highest attainable level of health and well-being, the European Charter on Environment and Health notes the *responsibility* that every individual has to contribute to the protection of the environment, in the interests of his or her own health and the health of others (Philipp & Hodgkinson, 1994).

In conjunction with these points, it has been reasoned that in support of citizenship, the need for improved understanding of individual accountability and personal responsibility, and how they relate to values in society, the relationships can be addressed by greater attention to the interdependence and importance of:

- improved understanding of how our personal attitudes, outlook and behaviour are influenced by a combination of our actual (external), and perceived (internal) experiences with qualities of our surrounding natural and built environments;
- the roles of creative endeavour and aesthetic appreciation in mental health and emotional well-being;
- the aesthetic component of '*health*' which is included in the WHO European Charter on Environment and Health, developed and promulgated by the Ministers of Health and Ministers of the Environment in Europe (WHO, 1989);
- heightened awareness of the factors needed for sustainable, economic development of society and within this, the increasing importance for wider, on-going investment in social capital and emotional economics (Philipp, 2001b, 2003).

In addressing these points, as part of the *Health for All initiative*, the Ottawa Charter defined health promotion as: '*the process of enabling people to increase control over, and to improve, their health*'. In order to achieve complete physical, mental and social well-being, the Charter suggests that individuals or groups must be able '*to identify and to realize aspirations, to satisfy needs, and to change or cope with the environment*'. It further states that: '*Health is created and lived by people within the settings of their everyday life; where they learn, work, play and love*'. (WHO, 1986). This statement formed the basis of the 'healthy settings' approach to health promotion, which began with the WHO's Healthy Cities initiative in 1986. The healthy settings approach applies 'whole systems thinking' in order to integrate a commitment to health into the culture, structure and processes of life in a particular setting (Doherty & Dooris, 2006) with all who are part of that setting being involved in the assessment of needs and setting of targets. Another key principle is the development of networking and partnership building between organizations and settings. Following on from 'Healthy Cities', further national, Government supported initiatives have applied the settings approach in organizations such as schools, prisons, colleges and hospitals.

It has been proposed recently that a single framework for well-being – Healthy Outlooks – could now sit alongside the WHO's healthy settings model (Philipp, 2010). It could bring together many of the initiatives developed under a CAMs approach. With the help of the Philipp Family Foundation, a charitable trust based in New Zealand, an international programme of work is evolving to further develop the concept. The 'healthy outlooks' approach encompasses the areas of conservation, preservation, culture and heritage, alongside programmes to help the personal development of individuals in society. It is hoped that by linking with other groups and individuals who are interested in this field, a mosaic of research, practical programmes, education and learning opportunities and self-help resources can be established. A 'Road Map for Global Citizenship' is envisaged, which people could access readily. It would include self-help resources for building emotional resilience and coping skills and resources to strengthen social capital by promoting community engagement, particularly in support of those who find themselves disenfranchised or at the margins of society (Philipp et al, 2011).

6. Conclusions

The way we look outwards at the world influences our perception of it, our values of what we believe is truly important in it, and what we do with our lives in this world we inhabit. In this we each have a responsibility to help encourage human understanding and ensure that environmental values and opportunities are sustained. We can after all, it has been recognized, "*consciously alter our behaviour by changing our values and attitudes to regain the spirituality and ecological awareness we have lost*" (Capra, 1983).

The identified public health needs and findings of recent studies including the worth to society and industry of investment in social capital, justify steps that should now be taken to ensure health and well being and the prevention of ill health. Improved education is in the interests of both sustainable development and to help ensure people can lead happier, healthier, and more enjoyable lives. The arts as Complementary and Alternative Medicines (CAMs) have an important role in this aim. They encompass a broad range of approaches. With more appreciation of the philosophical view that '*everything in life is connected*' and by linking the different approaches to a Healthy Outlooks framework and clinical audit of methods and programmes that are utilized, it could help to improve wider awareness and understanding of their place and worth. The resultant outcome is then likely to be more widespread gains to well-being among individuals and within different communities.

A coordinated, sustained approach to fostering the art of well-being, with appropriate clinical audit of the CAMs used, would help more people to identify ways they could derive greater enjoyment in life and living. After all, without enjoyment, as TS Eliot noted in his poem, '*Chorus from the Rock*':

Where is the life we have lost in living?

Where is the wisdom we have lost in knowledge?

Where is the knowledge we have lost in information?

7. References

Abbott S (2002). Prescribing welfare benefits advice in primary care: is it a health intervention and if so, what sort? *Journal of Public Health Medicine*; Vol.24: 307-312.

Advertisement (2004). 100 things that make Waitrose, Waitrose. *The Sunday Times*; June 13: Sect.1:8.

Bass MM and Llabre M (2010). The effects of Equine Assisted Activities on the social functioning of children with autism. http://www.horsesandhumans.org/HHRF_Final_Report.pdf

Baum M (2006). Use of 'alternative medicine' in the NHS. *Times Online*, May 23, 2006

Bax M (1989). Doctor and poet. *The Lancet*; 4:611.

Bird W (2007). Natural Thinking. Investigating the links between the Natural Environment, Biodiversity and Mental Health. www.rspb.org.uk/policy/health

Black, Dame Carol (2008). Review of the health of Britain's working age population. *Working for a healthier tomorrow*. Presented to the Secretary of State for Health and the Secretary of State for Work and Pensions 17th March 2008 London: TSO

Boorman S (2009). *NHS Health and Well-being. Final Report.* London: Department of Health.

Burns G (2006). Naturally happy, naturally healthy: the role of the natural environment in wellbeing. *The science of wellbeing*, Oxford: Oxford University Press: 405-431.

CAM Research Methodology Conference, April 1995 Panel on Definition and Description. Defining and describing complementary and alternative medicine. *Altern Ther Health Med.* 1997;3(2):49-57

Capra F (1983). *The Turning Point: Science, Society and the Rising Culture.* pub. Flamingo, London; 516pp.

Carter CS (2003). Biological Perspectives on Social Attachment and Bonding. In CS Carter, L Arnhert, KE Grossmann et al. (Eds). *Attachment and Bonding: a New Synthesis.* From the 92nd Dahlem Workshop Report, MIT Press.

Cooke H (Ed) (2003). *The Bristol Approach to living with cancer.* London: Robinson.

Daruna JH (2004). *Introduction to Psychoneuroimmunology.* Boston: Elsevier Academic Press.

Defra (2005). *Securing the Future*: UK Government Sustainable Development Strategy.

Defra (2010). *Measuring progress: sustainable development indicators* 2010. SD Statistics, Defra.

Delamothe T (2005). Happiness. *British Medical Journal*; Vol. 331: 1489-1490.

Denton D (1993). *The Pinnacle of Life: Consciousness and Self-awareness in Humans and Animals.* Australia: Allen and Unwin; 250pp.

DoH (2004). HM Government White Paper, '*Choosing Health: Making Healthy Choices Easier*'. Department of Health.

DoH, DWP, HSE (2005). *Health, work and well-being - Caring for our future: A strategy for the health and well-being of working age people.* London: HM Government.

Doherty S and Dooris M (2006). The health settings approach: the growing interest within colleges and universities. *Education and Health*, Vol.24, No.3, 42-3.

Eames P (2003). *Creative Solutions and Social Inclusion: Culture and the Community.* Wellington: Steele Roberts Ltd., [details at: www.artsaccessinternatial.org]

Eames P (2006). *Cultural Well-being and Cultural Capital.* Pub. PSE Consultancy: 65pp. [available from www.artsaccessinternational.org]

Eaton MM (1995). The social construction of aesthetic response. *British Journal of Aesthetics*; 35(2): 95-107.

Editorial. (2002). Hierarchy of needs. [www.businessballs.com]

Editorial (2004). The Brighton Declaration - we are all responsible for the developing world. *Public Health News* 26 April: 4.

Editorial. (2011a). What is health? *British Medical Journal* 343:d4817.

Editorial (2011b). Another reason to keep moving in old age. *British Medical Journal* 343: 232.

Engel GL (1977). The need for a new medical model: a challenge for biomedicine. *Science,* 196(4286), 129-136.

Engsberg JR and Shurtleff TL (2007). Update. Available from http://www.horsesandhumans.org/New_Info/shurtleffDecember_update.pdf

Ernst E and Terry R (2009). NICE Guidelines on Complementary/Alternative Medicine: more consistency and rigour are needed. *Br J Gen Pract,* 59(566): 695.

Esch T, Guarna M, Bianchi E, Zhu W, Stefano GB (2004). Commonalities in the central nervous system's involvement with complementary medical therapies: limbic morphinergic processes. *Medical Science Monitor.* 10(6):MS6-17.

Esch T and Stefano GB (2005). The Neurobiology of Love. *Neuroendocrinology Letters,* 3(26); 175-192.

Fingret A (2000). Occupational mental health: a brief history. *Occup Med;* 50: 289-293.

French J, Caplan R and Harrison V (1982). *The Mechanisms of Job Stress and Strain.* Chichester: Wiley.

Genders N (2006). *Fundamental Aspects of Complementary Therapies for Health Professionals.* London: Quay Books.

Gold J (1985). Cartesian dualism and the current crisis in medicine – a plea or a philosophical approach. *Journal of the Royal Society of Medicine,* 78: 663-666

Handszuh H (1991). Tourism trends and patterns. Pp.8-9. In: *Travel Medicine* 2. Eds. Lobel, H.O., Steffen, R., and Kozarsky, P.E. pub. International Society of Travel Medicine, Georgia, USA; 347pp.

Health and Safety Executive (HSE) (2005). *Case study: Establishing the business case for investing in stress prevention activities and evaluating their impact on sickness absence levels.* London: HSE.

Herman PM, D'Huyvetter K, Mohler MJ (2006). Are health services research methods a match for CAM? *Alternative Therapies,* May/June;12(3): 78-82.

Howe GM and Lorraine JA (1973). *Environmental Medicine.* London: Heinemann; 320pp

Huber M et al.(2011). Health: How should we define it? *British Medical Journal;* 343: 235-237.

Isaacson R (2009). *The Horse Boy: A Father's Miraculous Journey to Heal his Son.* London: Viking.

Kafka GJ and Kozma A (2002). The construct validity of Ryff's scales of psychological well-being (SPwb) and their relationship to measures of subjective well-being. *Social Indicators Research,* 57(2), 171-190.

Kaplan R and Kaplan S (1989). The *Experience of Nature: A Psychological Perspective.* New York: Cambridge University Press.

Karasek R (1979). Job demands, job decision latitude and mental strain: implications for job redesign. *Administrative Science Quarterly;* 24: 285-308.

Keating M (2005). More focus on individual stress management. Letter. *Occup Health,* Jun/Jul:37.

Kenny A and Kenny C (2006). *Life, Liberty and the Pursuit of Utility. Happiness in philosophical and economic thought.* In J

Laycock T (2003). Letters page, *Lapidus;* Issue 5: 29.

Litchfield P (2007). At the forefront of wellbeing at work. *Society Guardian*, 14th November.

Lundeberg T, Lund I, Naslund J (2007). Acupuncture, self appraisal and the reward system. *Acupuncture in Medicine, 25(3):87-99.*

Mace B, Bell P and Loomis R (1999). Aesthetic, affective, and cognitive effects of noise on natural landscape assessment. *Society and Natural Resources*, 12(3): 225-242.

Manheimer, E., Berman, B., Dubnick, H., Beckner, W (2004). *Cochrane reviews of complementary and alternative therapies: evaluating the strength of the evidence* [P094]. www.imbi.uni-freiburg.de/OJS/cca/index.php/cca/issue/view/35

Marks N, Thompson S, Eckersley R, Jackson T, Kasser T (2006). *Sustainable development and well-being: relationships, challenges and policy implications*. DEFRA Project 3b. nef.

Maslow AH (1943). A Theory of Human Motivation. *Psychological Review* 50(4):370-96.

Mathiasen H, and Alpert JS (1980). Medicine and literature in the medical curriculum. *Journal of the American Medical Association*; 244:1491.

McGettrick BJ (2004). Dean. Faculty of Education, University of Glasgow. www.creativecommunities.org.uk

Morrison ML (2007). Health Benefits of Animal Assisted Interventions. *Complementary Health Practice Review*, January 2007; 12: 51-62.

National Cancer Peer Review Programme. *Manual for Cancer Services 2008: Complementary Therapy (Safeguarding Practice) Measures*. NHS National Cancer Action Team.

Newton J (2007). Well being and the Natural Environment: a brief overview of the evidence. Available from: http://www3.surrey.ac.uk/resolve/seminars/Julie%20Newton%20Paper.pdf

Noyes J, Popay J, Pearson A, Hannes K, Booth A (2008). Chapter 20: Qualitative research and Cochrane reviews. In: Higgins JPT, Green S (eds). *Cochrane Handbook for Systematic Reviews of Interventions*. Version 5.0.1 [updated September 2008]. The Cochrane Collaboration. Available from www.cochrane-handbook.org.

Office for National Statistics (2011). Measuring National Well-Being: Conceptual Frameworks. www.ons.gov.uk/well-being

Ottawa Charter for Health Promotion. First International Conference on Health Promotion, Ottawa, 21 November, 1986 –WHO/HPR/HEP/95.1

Petherbridge, D. (1987). *Art for Architecture: A handbook on Commissioning*. Pub. London. Her Majesty's Stationery Office; 133pp.

Philipp R (1995). Try the rhythm method: With all my senses. *University of Bristol Newsletter*; 25: 4.

Philipp R (1997). Evaluating the effectiveness of the arts in health care. In: Kaye, C., and Blee, T. eds. *The Arts in Health Care: A palette of Possibilities*. London: Jessica Kingsley, 1997; 250-261

Philipp R (2001a). A poem to benefit health. *British Medical Journal*, Vol. 323: 576

Philipp R (2001b). Aesthetic quality of the built and natural environment: why does it matter? In: Pasini W. and Rusticali F. (Eds.) *Green Cities: Blue Cities of Europe*. WHO Collaborating Centre for Tourist Health and Travel Medicine, Rimini, Italy, with the WHO Regional Office for Europe; 265pp. available at. www.artsaccessinternational.org/discussionpapers

Philipp R (2002). *Arts, Health, and Well-Being: From the Windsor I Conference to a Nuffield Forum for the Medical Humanities*. Pub. The Nuffield Trust. 114pp.

Philipp R (2003). An Ecological Sense of Healthy Place and Purpose (AESOHP). In: Pasini, W. ed. *Travel and Epidemics: Proceedings of the Third European Conference on Travel Medicine (ECTM3)*. pub. Rimini: WHO Collaborating Centre for Tourist health and Travel Medicine, 289-306. available at. www.artsaccessinternational.org/discussionpapers

Philipp R (2006). Psychological Health and Emotional Well-being When Abroad. *Proceedings of the 5th European Conference on Travel Medicine*, Venice, Italy, March, WHO Collaborating Centre for Tourist Health and Travel Medicine; available at. www.artsaccessinternational.org/discussionpapers .

Philipp R (2007). The Anthropology of Humanitarian Aid: all the unwritten rules. Pp.103-118. In: Pacifici, L.E., and Riccardo, F. *Technology and Communication for a New Humanitarian Revolution: Experimenting with the website Cholera Café*. Pub. FrancoAngeli. 232pp.

Philipp R (2010). Making sense of well-being. *Perspectives in Public Health*; 130: 58.

Philipp R, and Dodwell P (2005). Improved communication between doctors and with managers would benefit professional integrity and reduce the occupational medicine workload. *Occupational Medicine*; 55: 40-47.

Philipp R, Gibbons N, Thorne P, Wiltshire L, Burrough J, and Easterby J (2011). Evaluation of a community arts installation event in support of the public health. In press: Perspectives in Public Health.

Philipp R and Hodgkinson G. (1994). The Management of Health and Safety Hazards in Tourist Resorts. *International Journal of Occupational Medicine and Environmental Health*, Vol. 7: 207-219.

Philipp R, Pond K, Rees G, and Bartram J (1999a). The association of tourist health with aesthetic quality and environmental values. pp.195-199. In: *Mobility & Health: From Hominid Migration To Mass Tourism*. Proceedings of European Conference on Travel Medicine, Venice, 25-27 March 1998. pub. WHO Collaborating Centre for Tourist Health and Travel Medicine, and Regione Veneto; 381pp.

Philipp R, Baum M, Mawson A and Calman K (1999b). *Humanities in Medicine: Beyond the Millennium*. pub. The Nuffield Trust, London; Nuffield Trust Series No.10: 164pp.,

Philipp R, Philipp E, Pendered L, Barnard C and Hall M (1986). Can children's paintings of their family doctor be interpreted? *Journal of the Royal College of General Practitioners*; 36: 325-327.

Philipp R, Philipp E, Polton S and Graham A (1984). Interpreting children's paintings of their doctors. *New Zealand FamilyPhysician*; 11: 23-24.

Philipp R, Philipp E, and Thorne P (1999c). The importance of intuition in the occupational medicine consultation.*Occupational Medicine Clinical*; 49: 37-41.

Philipp R and Robertson I (1996). Poetry helps healing. *The Lancet*; 347: 332-333.

Philipp R, and Sheridan, A (2003). Where poetry and health combine. *New Zealand Doctor*; March 12:24.

Philipp R and Thorne P (2007). *The Assessment, Prevention and Control of Health Risks in Tourist Establishments in theMediterranean: a Working Document for the Mediterranean Pollution Action Programme (Med-Pol)*, WHO-UNEP, January 2007; pp.90. available at www.artsaccessinternational.org/discussionpapers

Philipp R, Thorne P (2008). Would Complementary and Alternative Medicine in the Workplace be Welcomed? *Public Health*,122:1124-1127.

Philipp R and Thorne P (2011). *Guidelines for Implementing the Plan of Action on Environmental Health Risks in Tourist Establishments. A Working Document for the Mediterranean Pollution Action Programme (Med-Pol)*, WHO-UNEP, March 2011. pp.47.

Porteous JD (1996). *Environmental Aesthetics: Ideas, Politics and Planning*. pub. Routledge, London; 290pp

Potter J (1997). More on the street scene. *The Environmentalist*; 17: 1-3.

PricewaterhouseCoopers (2008). *Building the case for wellness*. Report for the Department of Work and Pensions. PwC LLP, February 2008.

Puttock D. (2000). Dance as a base for the arts in therapy. The Galatea Trust, London: Newsletter No.10: 1-3.

Randall B (2004). Access to green space prolongs life. *Public Health News*: 1 March: 6.

Ray TC, King LJ and Grandin T (1988). The effectiveness of self-initiated vestibular stimulation in producing speech sounds.*Journal Occupational Therapy Research* 8:186-190.

Rothschild FS (1994). *Creation and Evolution: A Biosemiotic Approach*. pub. Bouvier, Germany; 360pp.

Royal College of Physicians (2005). Report of a Working Party of the Royal College of Physicians, December. *ClinicalMedicine*; Vol.5 (6): 18.

Ryan RM and Deci EL (2001). On Happiness and Human Potentials: a review of research on hedonic and eudaimonic well-being. *Annual Review of Psychology*, 52, 141-166.

Ryff CD (1989). Happiness is everything, or is it? Explorations on the meaning of psychological well-being. *Journal of Personality and Social Psychology*, 57, 1069-1081.

Santayana G (1988). The Sense of Beauty. Critical Edition Vol.2. Eds. Saatkamp, H.J., and Holzberger, W.G. pub. MIT Press; 248pp. The

Seligman MEP (2000). Positive Psychology. An Introduction. American Psychologist, 55:5-14.

Seligman MEP (2002). *Pleasure, Meaning and Eudaimonia.* www.authentichappiness.sas.upenn.edu

Shah P and Mountain D (2007). The medical model is dead – long live the medical model. *British Journal of Psychiatry*, 191: 375-377.

Snider L, Korner-Bitensky N, Kammann C, Warner S, Saleh M (2007). Horseback Riding as Therapy for Children with Cerebral Palsy: Is There Evidence of its Effectiveness? *Physical andOccupational Therapy in Pediatrics*, 27(2):5-23.

Sterba JA (2007).Does horseback riding therapy or therapist-directed hippotherapy rehabilitate children with cerebral palsy?*Developmental Medicine and Child Neurology*, 49(1):68-73.

St. George I. (2004). Ed. *Cole's Medical Practice in New Zealand*; pub. Medical Council of New Zealand: pp.46-47.

Stress and Health at Work Study (SHAW) .www.hse.gov.uk/statistics/causdis/stress.htm

Storr A (1997). *Music and the Mind*. London: Harper Collins.

Tait F (2008). The contribution of complementary and alternative medicine on symptoms and quality of life for people with multiple sclerosis. *Way Ahead*;12(1):6-7

Tegner I, Fox J, Philipp R, and Thorne P (2009). Evaluating the use of poetry to improve well-being and emotional resilience in cancer patients. Journal of Poetry Therapy: 22; 121-131.

Tennant R, Hiller L, Fishwick R, Platt S, Joseph S, Weich S, Parkinson J, Secker J and Stewart-Brown SL (2007). The Warwick-Edinburgh Mental Well-being Scale (WEMWBS) : development and UK validation. *Health and Quality of Life Outcomes,* Vol.5 (No.63).

UK National Ecosystem Assessment (2011). *UK National Ecosystem Assessment: Synthesis of the key findings.* UNEP-WCMC, Cambridge.

Ulrich RS (1983). Aesthetic and affective response to natural environment in Altman I and Wohlwill JF (Eds) *Behaviour and the Natural Environment.* New York:Plenum, pp85 125.

UNEP, (2011). *Towards a Green Economy: Pathways to Sustainable Development and Poverty Eradication: A Synthesis for Policy Makers.* Pub. United Nations Environment Programme, pp52. http://bit.ly/e7Brja

Wade DT (2009). *Holistic healthcare and the NHS. What is it and how can we achieve it?* Third Michael Benson lecture at the

Nuffield Orthopaedic Centre, 17th September 2009. http://www.noc.nhs.uk/oce/research-education/holistic-health-care.aspx

Walter S (1999). Holistic Health. In *The Illustrated Encyclopedia of Body-Mind Disciplines,* Rosen Publishing Group. Availableon: http://ahha.org/rosen.htm

Westra L and Robinson TM (1997). *The Greeks and the Environment.* pub. Rowman and Littlefield Inc., Oxford; pp.230.

WHO (1986). *The Ottawa Charter for Health Promotion.* www.who.int/healthpromotion/conferences/previous/ottawa/en/

WHO (1989). *European Charter on the Environment and Health.* ICP/RUD 113/Conf. Doc/1. Rev. 2, 2803r, pp7.

WHO (1995). Field Trial WHOQOL-100, February 1995. Geneva: Division of Mental Health, WHO. Available from: http://www.who.int/mental_health/who_qol_field_trial_1995.pdf

WHO (1997). Report of the Inter-regional Consultation on Environmental Health, Bilthoven, Netherlands, 14-17 July 1997.pub. WHO Geneva: WHO/EHG/EXD/97.16.

WHO (2006). Constitution of the World Health Organization. www.who.int/governance/eb/who_constitution_en.pdf

Wieland S and Manheimer E (2009). [P06-16] Issues in improving the quality and increasing the size of the Cochrane Complementary and Alternative Medicine (CAM) Field specialized register. www.imbi.uni-freiburg.de/OJS/cca/index.php/cca/issue/view/35

Wikipedia, (2011). *The Green Gym.* http://en.wikipedia.org/wiki/Green_Gym

Wilson EO (1984). *Biophilia: The Human Bond with Other Species.* Cambridge: Harvard University Press.

Wright SG (2005). *Reflections on Spirituality and Health.* London & Philadelphia: Whurr Publishers.

2

The Role of CAM (Complementary and Alternative Medicine): The Different Perspectives of Patients, Oncology Professionals and CAM Practitioners

Patricia Fox, Michelle Butler and Barbara Coughlan
UCD School of Nursing, Midwifery & Health Systems,
University College Dublin,
Ireland

1. Introduction

The purpose of this chapter is to describe the different perspectives of women with breast cancer, oncology professionals and CAM practitioners regarding the role of CAM[1] in the cancer setting. While all three stakeholder groups considered CAM as supportive, perspectives differed among oncology professionals and CAM practitioners regarding the manner in which this was so.

1.1 Methods

Semi-structured interviews were undertaken with 31 women with breast cancer, 20 oncology professionals (13 oncology nurses and 7 oncologists) and 20 CAM practitioners[2]. Interviews were analysed using a thematic networks technique (Attride-Stirling, 2001). Thematic analysis is the recognition of themes through a thorough reading and rereading of the transcripts (Ezzy, 2002, Liamputtong & Ezzy, 2005). For this study, thematic analysis was supported by and presented as thematic networks: "web-like illustrations (networks) that summarize the main themes constituting a piece of text" (Attride-Stirling 2001, p. 386).

---

[1] The definition of CAM was based on definition advanced by the "Use of Complementary/Alternative Therapies Survey" (UCATS) instrument (Lengacher *et al.*, 2003) which was used in an earlier phase of this study to survey CAM use in 406 Irish women with breast cancer.

[2] The CAM categories represented included TCM (Traditional Chinese Medicine), homeopathy, reflexology, massage therapy, counselling, nutritional therapy, and phytobiophysics. In the interest of maintaining confidentiality, the actual numbers representing each group are not identified. Most of the practitioners also had qualifications in other areas of CAM; however, the assigned titles reflect their primary specialty. Half the participants had a background in conventional medicine; eight were registered nurses and two were medical doctors. Two of the participants were cancer survivors. Five of the participants were based in CSCs, while the remaining practitioners worked in private practice.

2. The role of CAM in patients with cancer: The perspectives of women with breast cancer

Of the 31 women interviewed, approximately 75% had used some form of relaxation and/or psychological therapy while 45% had used some form of biologically based therapy (health supplements, herbal supplements or antioxidants) for their breast cancer. Essentially, participants perceived that CAM can play a supportive role in the care of women with breast cancer by facilitating respite and psychological support while complementing conventional cancer treatment (see Figure 1.1). These three themes are discussed and corroborated in the following sections.

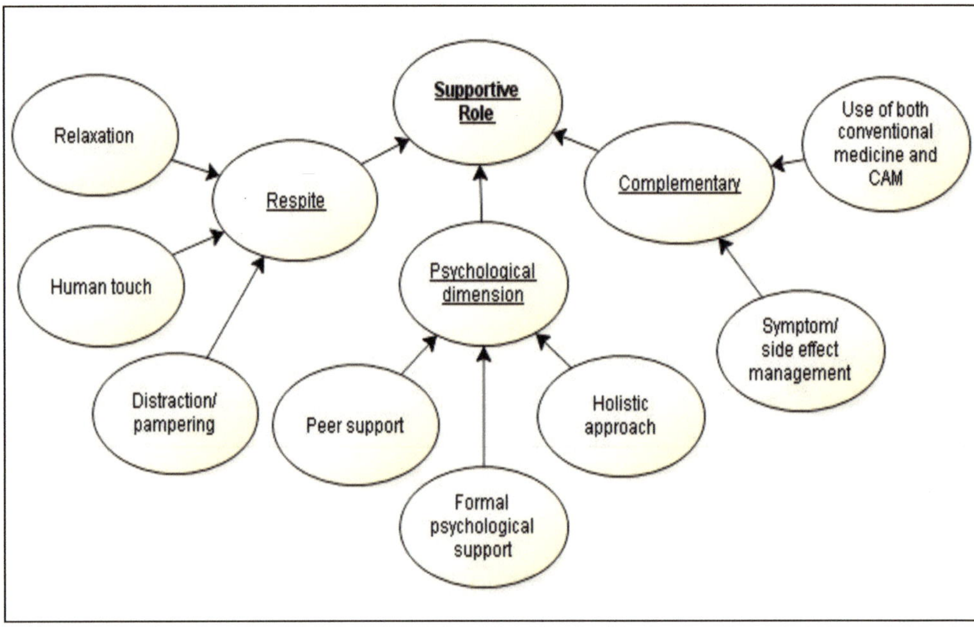

Fig. 1.1. The Supportive Role of CAM: perceptions of women with breast cancer

2.1 Respite

In terms of respite, participants underlined the importance of relaxation, human touch, distraction and pampering as they negotiated their cancer journey. The main therapies that were valued for inducing relaxation were massage, reflexology and yoga.

Participants discussed the value of different relaxation therapies to assist with coping and for stress reduction

Relaxation therapies were considered particularly valuable for newly diagnosed patients and for patients who had just had surgery.

... because it helps you get your head around it [cancer diagnosis] ... because when you are told your head is so full, it's so full (Participant 10)

... well I actually kind of relaxed a lot [following massage], ... you [are] uptight after the operation, naturally ... (Participant 18)

For one participant, relaxation therapy was instrumental in enabling her to engage with the conventional treatment plan. Following her diagnosis, her anxiety level was such that it interfered with processing the important information imparted at the outset of treatment in relation to the anticipated effects and side effects of treatment. She stated that she was unable to concentrate or read the booklets given to her until she had had a "healing" massage done.

The benefits of relaxation therapies for dealing with stress were highlighted. One participant described herself as a relaxed person; however, she noted that she had become more anxious following her diagnosis and found that CAM therapies such as reflexology "were great at making me relax". Other therapies considered beneficial for alleviating stress included yoga and acupuncture.

In discussing CAM therapies that provided respite following their breast cancer diagnosis, some of the participants also noted the significance of human touch and there was a sense that it was associated with "healing".

... touch is very healing anyway and it's something about that close contact even for a half an hour ... I think all those things help people to heal (Participant 5)

For one participant, who described conventional treatment as "a living nightmare ... a living hell", CAM therapy and human touch clearly represented a respite from the treatment. Describing the Cancer Support Centre (CSC) as a "lovely space to be in", she stated that she availed of different hands-on therapies. Human touch in the form of massage was particularly significant for one participant who perceived that some people had an irrational fear of cancer. According to this participant, she sensed that certain people were afraid that if they touched her they would develop cancer.

Further evidence to support the concept of CAM as a form of respite comes from the references to distraction and pampering. One participant spoke about the value of introducing art therapy as a distraction into one of the chemotherapy day wards. A second participant had painted throughout her life and she acknowledged the distracting nature of the therapy following her cancer diagnosis. According to a third participant, the entire experience in the CSC was a positive one from the feeling of being pampered to the ambiance of the setting. For this participant, access to more therapies would have been appreciated.

... and again like that it was a beautiful room and lovely music and soft towels and soft pillows and to be pampered ... it's just ... I think that it is so important (Participant 3)

While another participant also referred to the pampering aspects of reflexology and massage, other more substantial outcomes such as improvements in sleep were also noted.

As outlined above, certain CAM therapies were embraced because they provided a diversion and a sense of pampering for some participants during their treatment. In summary, for women with breast cancer, the elements of CAM which contributed to a sense of respite included relaxation, human touch, and distraction/pampering. Participants' views on CAM from a psychological perspective are now examined.

2.2 Psychological dimension

Fundamental to the perceived supportive role of CAM were its psychological dimensions. The psychological elements of CAM were central to coping for many participants and the merits of informal (peer support) and formal support (counselling/CBT) were highlighted in particular. Moreover, a holistic approach to care was appealing for some participants who highlighted the importance of treating both mind and body as they regarded physical and psychological states as being interdependent.

A number of the participants underlined the importance of meeting other women who were diagnosed with cancer and such meetings often took the form of support groups in the CSCs. According to the participants, the benefits included engaging with others who truly understood their situation having endured a similar experience, being able to discuss their disease openly without being fearful of engendering discomfort in others or worrying family members, and the provision of hope and practical advice. For one participant, being diagnosed with cancer was similar to grieving in that one needed "to have lost somebody to understand that horrible pain". She stated that she could not talk to her husband as he could not understand what she was going through when he did not have cancer himself.

... [patients] need to be with people [who] have had cancer to understand the pain and the anguish and the hurt ... like with like, they understand exactly ... (Participant 7)

This sense of a common bond was also described by other participants who attended support groups in the CSCs.

... there's a common bond there, it's like a member's only club ... (Participant 3)

One participant noted that it was liberating to be able to engage in an open and frank discussion about one's illness without feeling conscious of causing distress in others who do not have cancer and are therefore "quite afraid they might say the wrong thing". Other participants endeavored to protect their family and peer support enabled them to do so without having to compromise the expression of concerns for self. One participant also stated that while she initially discussed her illness with friends, as time went on she just said "I'm doing fine" because she did not want to be constantly talking about her health. She pointed to the "huge support" from her husband but noted that "there are still things that you can't say". While a second participant did discuss her illness with her family, she did not discuss it "in depth" so as not to worry them. Attending a support group and listening to another patient talk about life after her diagnosis many years before afforded some insight into life after diagnosis for one woman. She found it "unbelievable" that some patients had forgotten some details relating to their original diagnosis.

... it was incredible and at that stage I couldn't perceive a life ... but she [other patient] was talking about having a boat on X river ... (Participant 27)

For one younger participant, being linked in with other patients closer to her age was helpful on a practical level as it enabled her to discuss issues such as the cosmetic effects of treatment.

For some participants, formal psychological support in the form of counselling was central to their recovery as it also enabled participants to discuss their fears openly. Receiving practical tips and feeling listened to were particularly helpful for one participant as she was a young woman who was fearful that she would have a recurrence. She described how she had counselling in the CSC and also at another facility. If she had not had this counselling it would have made "the whole battle with the illness very, very difficult".

... just to be able to talk about you know your fears, your anxieties, what if my cancer has spread, what if I'm going to die, how will I deal with this ... (Participant 3)

One participant also noted the importance of being able to talk "out your fears" while for another counselling "helped me hugely". For another participant, counselling was so essential that it should be offered to all patients "immediately after the diagnosis". Moreover, this participant asserted that while the nurses were very supportive, it was necessary to have fully trained counsellors. Similar to views regarding the sense of ease experienced in discussing a cancer diagnosis with other cancer survivors, a key beneficial feature of counselling for one participant was the freedom from feeling she was going to cause "pain and hurt" to family and friends in the process. One participant relapsed fairly soon after her initial treatment and for this reason she actively sought out psychological support. She had counselling initially which she did not find helpful. Importantly, however, she was keen to avoid taking anti-depressants and went on to receive cognitive behavioural therapy (CBT) which she found "really, really helpful". One participant who did not attend a CSC had concerns about "reliving it again" rather than "putting it behind you". Of note, this participant did belong to a support group for another condition.

Consistent with the perspectives regarding the value of peer and formal psychological support noted previously, the importance of a holistic approach to care was highlighted by a number of women who had availed of CAM therapies. One participant gravitated towards Traditional Chinese Medicine (TCM) and homeopathy because the concept of looking at the "whole body" rather than being symptom focused appealed to her.

... I like homeopathy for the same reason, its, it's a whole body thing and symptoms are symptoms, they're not the first and only things that you look at (Participant 22)

For one participant, a holistic focus was wanting in one of the larger hospitals where she was treated. While acknowledging that she was medically well cared for, she was concerned that there was "no time for anything else"

... and you're not just a body you're a whole person so all of that is important you know like talking to people ... (Participant 14)

One participant contended that the tendency of CAM practitioners to listen and devote time to all of their patients concerns conveyed a sense of greater interest in patients, which for her was consistent with a more holistic approach in general. According to this participant, this approach contrasted with conventional hospitals which were focused on one aspect only. However, for two other participants, the provision of emotional support was not the responsibility of the medical staff as their duty is "the care of the patient and the medical side of it". While not overtly making reference to a holistic approach, other participants also pointed to the benefits of therapies which considered mind and body. According to one participant, mindfulness-integrated cognitive behaviour therapy (MiCBT) was "absolutely terrific" because it allowed one to access "what you're thinking, what you are feeling, physiologically". In addition, it was asserted that yoga meditation has an "extraordinary effect of relaxation" on the body and mind which "has to be therapeutic". For the same participant, the CSCs constituted a type of holistic refuge for patients who are recovering from their treatment and it was her contention that such Centres were "terrific really" for mind and body.

In summary, informal support in the form of cancer support groups clearly afforded a refuge for a number of the participants in their cancer journey in particular because they provided a facility whereby anxieties and fears could be openly expressed among peers. Additionally, formal psychological support in the form of counselling was credited with helping some participants cope with their illness. Counselling was also valued for reasons not dissimilar to those of peer support, that is, for enabling the discussion of concerns openly without feeling the need to hold back for the sake of others. In addition, for one participant who had relapsed, CBT was described as being very helpful. Finally, some of the participants articulated their interest in a holistic approach to care over the more specialty oriented approach of modern medicine. Consideration of the whole person addressing issues of both mind and body was considered desirable by a number of women who had availed of CAM therapies. For some of the participants, insufficient attention was directed toward a holistic approach in the larger conventional hospitals, while others did not see the provision of emotional support a necessary part of the doctors' role.

This section has provided evidence of the importance attributed to the psychological dimensions of CAM from the perspective of the participants who had availed of psychologically-based therapies. Finally, perceptions on the complementary nature of CAM are explored under the global theme of Supportive Role.

2.3 Complementing conventional treatment

Central to the notion that CAM plays a supportive role in the cancer setting was the perception that CAM is complementary to and therefore should operate in conjunction with conventional cancer treatment as opposed to instead of conventional treatment. The basic themes which provide support for this notion of CAM as "complementary" to conventional medicine include reports of patients' use of both conventional and CAM treatments and their use of CAM for symptom/side effect management as opposed to for curative intent.

Participants discussed their use both of conventional and CAM treatments and for some, integration of CAM and conventional treatment was a desirable goal.

I think working with both ... I don't think somebody should go over totally to alternative ... both together, but not one without the other ... (Participant 7)

One participant actively sought out herbal supplements for the treatment of hot flashes that resulted from conventional treatment as she wanted to avoid taking prescription medicine. For this participant also, it was important that conventional treatment and CAM should not be mutually exclusive. Another participant also spoke of her use of both systems. She sought out "natural remedies" but remained engaged with her conventional treatment. Similarly, for a third participant, CAM therapies were "just complementary ... it's not, a cure or anything like that". Of note, the idea of CAM being complementary is particularly exemplified in the case of one participant who did admit that historically she tended to gravitate more toward homeopathy and TCM rather than conventional medicine. However, when it came to treatment of her cancer she opted for conventional treatment as the primary treatment modality and used CAM as "an adjunct". This decision appeared to be motivated by a fear of the consequences that could result in forgoing conventional treatment. Likewise, although she had availed of CAM for other conditions, another participant also spoke of her fear of the consequences if she did not use conventional treatment for her breast cancer. She conceded that she preferred "to do other things" however, there appeared to be a paucity of information available regarding the efficacy of CAM in cancer treatment. Other participants expressed a desire for integration of CAM and conventional treatment with a view to combining "their skills and expertise" rather than "discount ... that whole spectrum of knowledge [in CAM]".

It is clear then that use of both systems (conventional and CAM) did feature for some participants following their cancer diagnosis. The importance of both conventional and CAM treatment was articulated. More specifically, there was a sense that conventional treatment should be the primary modality for treating cancer and it is likely that the life-threatening nature of cancer may override the philosophical preferences of some individuals who may otherwise opt to avail of CAM. However, for some participants, there was a sense that a greater effort should be made to learn from ancient medical systems such as TCM. To further illustrate the point that CAM was used more to support participants through treatment than to treat the disease itself, use for symptoms/side effects is now discussed.

One participant described how she used TCM to "support my body to get through the chemo and the radiation". Homeopathy was used by another participant "for the sickness" while a third participant used it "to aid wound healing". One participant used a Bach flower remedy for anxiety when she was first diagnosed and later took an herbal supplement (black cohosh) for hot flashes. Other participants also noted the use of biologically based CAM therapies to alleviate the side effects of treatment induced menopause while Udo's Oil was used for joint stiffness which was attributed to an aromatase inhibitor. As outlined above, herbal and health food supplements were primarily used to alleviate and/or prevent side effects of conventional treatment. In essence, CAM was used to complement and support conventional treatment rather than to replace it. Of note, other participants were reluctant to take any herbal supplements while receiving conventional treatment; concern about interactions and the fact that they were already taking enough medications were the reasons advanced for this position.

The purpose of this section was to identify the role of CAM in the cancer setting as perceived by women with breast cancer. Notwithstanding the complex nature of CAM, and drawing on the various themes emerging from the data, in the main, women with breast cancer perceived CAM as playing a supportive role in the cancer setting. The evidence for this conclusion is derived from the perceived importance of CAM in terms of respite and psychological care tempered with the recognition that that conventional treatment should be the primary modality for cancer treatment. Having elicited the perspectives of women with breast cancer regarding the role of CAM in the cancer setting, the perceptions of oncology professionals are now explored.

3. The role of CAM in patients with cancer: The perspectives of oncology professionals

Oncology professionals perceived CAM use along a continuum in relation to the inherent benefits and risks of the therapies and whether or not they should be used in addition to or instead of conventional treatment. Therapies such as relaxation treatments and psychological support occupied one end of this continuum; according to all of the participants, there is a role for these therapies in the management of patients with cancer. More specifically, participants recognised a role for CAM therapies in providing support for patients on their cancer journey. Other CAM therapies which were used as a substitute for conventional treatment were at the opposite end of the continuum and considerable concern was expressed with respect to these therapies. Finally, certain approaches such as biologically based CAM therapies and acupuncture occupied a more intermediate position on the continuum and a more guarded approach was adopted in relation to these therapies; however, this was context-sensitive, for example, certain therapies were considered acceptable in some circumstances but not in others. The themes that emerged in interviews with oncology professionals (Figure 1.2) are explored in more detail in the following sections.

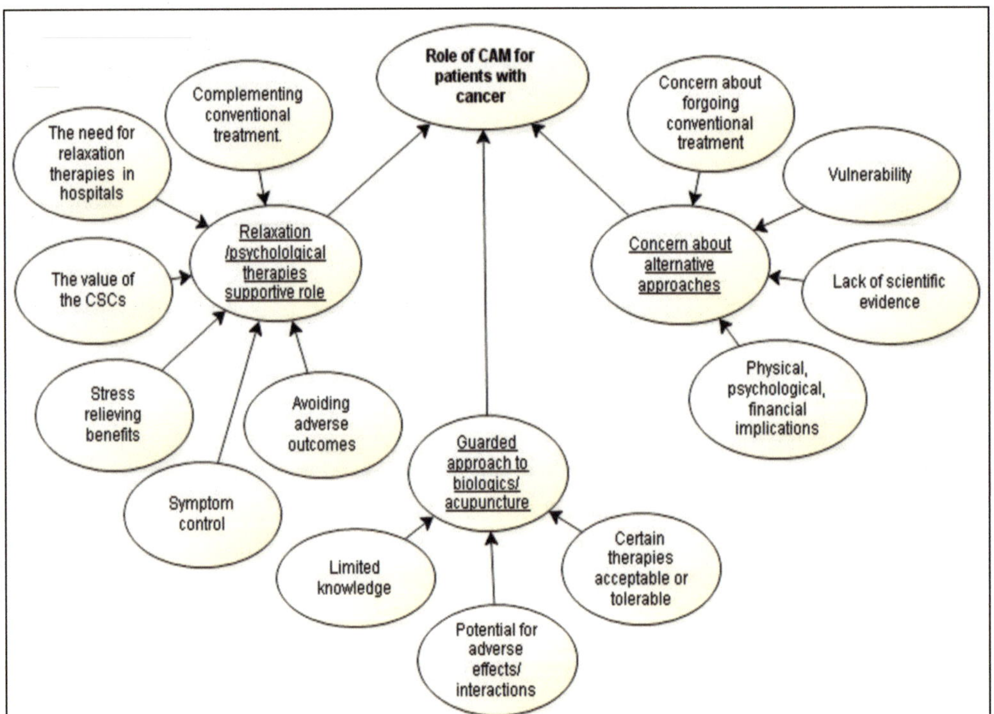

Fig. 1.2. Oncology professionals' perceptions of the role of CAM in patients with cancer

3.1 The role of relaxation/psychological-based therapies

There was a perception that relaxation and psychological therapies were important in terms of the supportive role they provide for patients with cancer. In discussing the supportive role of these therapies, oncology professionals discussed this type of CAM in relation to stress relief and such therapies were perceived as being complementary to conventional treatment. The need for more relaxation therapies in hospitals was noted; however, the value of the CSCs was clearly articulated. Although, primarily valued for their psychological benefits, relaxation therapies were also considered to benefit patients physically in some cases. While participants mainly discussed the value of relaxation/psychological based therapies, they also sounded a note of caution with respect to the potential for adverse effects.

The importance of relaxation therapies for relieving stress was highlighted with some participants placing particular emphasis on this issue for young women with families. According to one of the nurses, young women with breast cancer benefit in particular from relaxation therapies as they are dealing with the stress of the illness while trying to cope with other personal and family concerns. Another nurse also noted the "very stressful time" for young women juggling their treatments with caring for children and "school runs, all this carry on". Her endorsement of massage and reflexology was based on the positive feedback from patients on this type of CAM. According to another nurse, yoga and reiki are used by "a lot of patients" who appear to benefit from their distracting effects describing them as "a brilliant switch off mechanism" which "takes them away from the reality of the situation for a while".

In helping patients to cope with the stress of the illness and treatment, relaxation therapies were essentially seen as complementing conventional treatment.

... that they would still have the conventional treatment, the treatment that is recommended and have other treatments in conjunction with it (RN)

According to another participant, patients should be able to access any such therapies if they consider they may be helpful as long as they continue with "the general medicine". The oncologists were similarly positively disposed to relaxation/psychologically based CAM therapies as long as patients continued with their conventional treatment. Acknowledging the benefits of relaxation therapies, one of the oncologists had participated in the introduction of relaxation therapies into a hospital abroad and was investigating a similar initiative in his current workplace. While some of the nurses made reference to having a staff member in the hospital that came around on certain days, there was an interest in having a more consistent provision of CAM in the oncology day wards where patients attended for chemotherapy. For one of the nurses, this was based on her experience of having a CAM practitioner on site when she worked abroad. This participant noted that it would be beneficial to have access to massage therapists and reflexologists in her current institution to alleviate the stress for patients who were about to have their treatment. It was contended that such an approach may obviate the need to administer anxiolytics to anxious patients as is currently the practice. This notion of having certain CAM therapies available in the hospital setting was articulated by other nurses. It was maintained that such an initiative would lessen the burden for patients in terms of avoiding the inconvenience of having to go elsewhere for these therapies because they "have enough to cope with". The financial implications associated with accessing relaxation therapies privately were also noted given that patients have a lot of additional expenses because of their illness. Given that CAM services were limited or non-existent in the hospitals where the participants were based, the patients were primarily advised to attend the CSCs to avail of CAM therapies.

Although some of the participants articulated the importance of having relaxation therapies available through the hospitals, the value of the CSCs was highlighted by all of the participants. All of the nurses indicated that they encouraged patients to attend the CSCs in order to avail of those services. The tendency to recommend patients to attend the CSCs appeared to be based on the notion that they were in safe hands.

... and I suppose we all also kind of just use the safeguard 'oh go up to X CSC' (RN)

While the relaxation therapies were considered beneficial in their own right to assist with coping, the value of the extra time that accompanied some of the therapies was also noted. According to another nurse, there were "huge psychological benefits" for patients who attended the CSCs, not least because they were given "time" and were "surrounded in a non-threatening way" by knowledgeable people. Some of the therapies provided at the centres were "hugely beneficial" in assisting some patients to "get through what was a rough time" according to another nurse.

While the therapies provided in the CSCs may have some physical benefits in terms of relaxing patients or alleviating pain and/or nausea, their primary role was the provision of psychological support.

... and they may have some knock on physical effect ... but the main benefit is to help people cope psychologically with the illness (MO)

As noted, there was a perception that the benefits of relaxation/psychological therapies were primarily related to their psychological effects, however; there was also a sense that there may be benefits in terms of symptom control albeit to a lesser degree. Some of the nurses perceived that relaxation therapies such as reflexology and massage were helpful in inducing rest and sleep for patients.

In terms of restfulness and trying to sleep, I would find that they find that helps them in that respect (RN)

Massage and yoga were also considered to be beneficial for shoulder stiffness in women recovering from breast surgery which involved axillary lymph node dissection and one nurse advised her patients to visit the nearby CSC for yoga for this reason.

While there was consensus that relaxation and psychologically based CAM therapies had an important role to play for patients with cancer and were unlikely to be harmful, participants highlighted the potential for adverse outcomes in some cases. Some of the participants articulated the importance of ensuring that CAM providers possessed the requisite qualifications in order to safeguard against such adverse outcomes. Moreover, for other participants, if patients were to attend CAM practitioners outside the hospital, it was "very important" that those practitioners would have taken some formal training in treating patients with cancer and that they would be registered.

... or have done a course maybe in relation to the cancer patient (RN)

The importance of "careful selection" and "assessment" was also highlighted in order to guide patients to the therapies that may be of most benefit such as to appropriate support groups.

It is apparent then that participants were confident that relaxation/psychological therapies play an important supportive role for patients with cancer. While there was agreement regarding the supportive role of relaxation/psychological therapies in the cancer setting, a more guarded approach was adopted with regard to other CAM therapies and this is now discussed.

3.2 Guarded approach to biologically based therapies and acupuncture used in conjunction with conventional treatment

Participants were more guarded in their response to the use of biologically based therapies (health-food/herbal supplements, special anti-cancer diets) and acupuncture used in conjunction with conventional treatment. This was primarily due to limited knowledge regarding the nature of these therapies, and concern about their potential for adverse effects and interactions (with respect to supplements). This notwithstanding, not all therapies in this category were considered equal in terms of risk; in some cases, therapies were considered harmless and possibly even beneficial. In other cases, participants articulated their concerns about certain therapies but adopted a somewhat tolerant approach to their use while other therapies were considered to be problematic particularly during active conventional treatment and patients were strongly advised to avoid such therapies during that time. Of note, participants' concerns regarding some therapies were context-sensitive, that is to say, therapies that were a cause for concern in certain circumstances were considered acceptable or even beneficial in other circumstances.

Most of the participants interviewed were hesitant about herbal supplements pointing to their limited knowledge regarding the nature of this type of CAM. Highlighting the paucity of information and research available on herbal supplements, one nurse stated that when asked about herbal supplements she would advise patients to take a multivitamin only.

… I'm not knowledgeable enough about it … there's not enough information or research out there … (RN)

Limited knowledge about the nature of herbal supplements also deterred another nurse from recommending herbal supplements because "we don't know exactly what's in them". In addition to herbal supplements, in some instances anti-cancer diets were not recommended because of insufficient knowledge about them. In certain cases, where concerns existed among nurses about the nature and safety of supplements, patients' queries were referred to the oncologists. In contrast to relaxation/psychological therapies, participants appeared much less inclined to recommend biologically based therapies and there was no mention of acupuncture being recommended to patients.

One of the primary reasons for the adoption of a guarded approach to certain oral CAM therapies was concern about the potential for adverse effects and interactions with conventional treatment. Participants also expressed some general concerns about biologically based therapies regardless of the context. These concerns had to do with the potential for adverse effects relating to issues of quality control. Adulteration of herbal supplements with medications such as anticoagulants was identified as a serious issue and concern was also expressed about the potential for contamination.

… and Chinese medicines are notorious for actually having quite a lot of actual ingredients including things like steroids and goodness knows what … (MO)

For example, Chinese herbal medicines which ... are often made in vats of lead ... (MO)

Another participant noted that an unnecessary diagnostic procedure was almost performed on a patient who appeared jaundiced as a result of taking carotene supplements. Some of the oncologists also expressed concerns about the possibility of misdiagnosis if patients attended a CAM practitioner for symptom management rather than following up with the oncologist. Reservations in this context were primarily based on the likelihood of harm from recurrent or progressive disease being misdiagnosed and/or exacerbated. Osteopathy fell into this category due to concern about manipulation where there may be disease recurrence. There were similar concerns about patients with undiagnosed bone metastases seeking acupuncture for pain relief.

... that they haven't told the doctor about and that you end up with them having a pathological fracture [which] could have been treated with one single fraction of radiotherapy ... (MO)

Patients on conventional treatment were also advised against acupuncture primarily because of concerns about infection while they were immunosuppressed. In this case, concern was context-sensitive. Apart from avoiding acupuncture during immunosuppression, one oncologist who was not opposed to the therapy per se noted that it was very much on the "borderline" and practised by some GPs in the present day. Nurses' concerns about acupuncture were similarly related to the potential for complications during immunosuppression.

In addition to potential adverse effects of CAM therapies, participants were concerned about interactions with conventional treatment, particularly in relation to herbal supplements. Concerns about interactions with conventional treatment related primarily to chemotherapy; however, potential for interaction with radiotherapy was also considered.

I know there's been another case report of radiation interaction with herbal and things you know ... (MO)

Mindful of the safety implications, one oncologist asked patients to write out a list of all medications and supplements that they may be taking.

... because if somebody has an unexpected reaction to the chemotherapy, we don't know is it because they've just started taking giant hog weed extract ... (MO)

Unease was also expressed by some of the nurses with regard to the potential for drug/herb interactions. In some cases, nurses simply advised patients against taking any herbal supplements. Potential for interactions between herbal supplements and general prescription medications was also highlighted by a participant who cited the case of a patient who experienced weight loss when taking kelp while on Thyroxine.

These concerns notwithstanding, some biologically based CAM therapies were considered to be harmless and possibly even beneficial. Based on their experience, two of the nurses considered the benefits of ginger in alleviating nausea. Other supplements such as linseed and Evening Primrose Oil were also considered for their potential to alleviate menopausal symptoms. One of the oncologists indicated that he was not concerned about a lot of the supplements that patients were taking as he perceived such supplements to be harmless. As noted, other CAM therapies such as acupuncture were also considered acceptable as long as patients were not immunosuppressed. One of the oncologists suggested it would be reasonable to think about acupuncture for pain control where mainstream treatments were found to be ineffective.

Participants' views in relation to the use of some biologically based therapies also depended on the context and they were tolerated so long as there was no risk of them being taken at a time when they could interfere with conventional treatments. Participants appeared considerably more concerned about anti-cancer diets and some herbal remedies; however, there appeared to be an acceptance among participants that use of such therapies may have psychological benefits for the patients taking them. One nurse recalled her experience of caring for a patient who was undergoing conventional treatment but also taking a strict anti-cancer diet. Conscious of the obvious weight loss, this nurse expressed concern to the patient about her minimal food intake.

...and she [patient] said 'I've two young kids, its my only chance', she [said], 'this is what gets me through my day' she [said] 'when I crave for something to eat' (RN)

This nurse acknowledged that the patient appeared to benefit psychologically from this measure and admitted that if she was told she had a life-threatening illness herself it is likely that she would also explore all options. While acknowledging that it may also be disease-related, another participant spoke of her own distress on witnessing a "very sick" patient lose a significant amount of weight while on a restrictive anti-cancer diet during the palliative stage of his illness. There was recognition again that hope was the driving force behind this approach which was being encouraged by the patient's wife. Similarly, there appeared to be a degree of internal conflict for another nurse as she grappled with supporting a patient in his endeavors although she was unconvinced about the herbal supplement he was taking. According to this participant, it was particularly "difficult" because the patient frequently asked the nurses for their views on the supplement in question. Unease was also expressed by other nurses about the potential for some biologically based CAM therapies to induce nausea in patients; however, they did not appear to actively dissuade patients from taking these therapies. One nurse expressed such disquiet with respect to some of the "herbal concoctions" taken. However, again there appeared to be an attempt to strike a balance between facilitating hope and avoiding harm. Likewise, one of the oncologists asserted that he did not actively attempt to dissuade his patients from taking certain biologically based therapies. For this oncologist, there was "no point arguing about it" as patients benefited psychologically from assuming some control over their health in this manner.

As noted then, while participants had concerns about certain CAM therapies on a number of levels, not all therapies were considered equal in terms of risk. Moreover, the context-sensitive nature of some concerns added to the complexity of the situation. Participants were considerably more wary about other CAM therapies which were perceived to be harmful for various reasons and these are discussed in the next section.

3.3 Concern regarding more alternative approaches

Participants articulated considerable concern regarding the use of alternative approaches which may be substituted for conventional treatment. In addition, participants discussed issues such as vulnerability, lack of scientific evidence and the physical, psychological and financial implications of using such therapies.

Considerable concern was expressed about patients who forgo conventional cancer treatment for alternative treatments. However, it was acknowledged that this represented a very small proportion of patients and that the trend appeared to be downward.

I have seen patients pursuing alternative therapies run into serious trouble and die ... when they have refused standard care and, and ... gone an alternative route (MO)

One nurse was apprehensive about patients seeking alternative treatment on the basis of her experience with one young patient. This patient had a potentially curable colorectal cancer and subsequently developed metastatic disease having opted to undergo alternative treatment instead of chemotherapy. According to this participant, the patient had travelled to another country to receive the alternative treatment and had discontinued her conventional treatment.

In discussing their concerns about patients attending alternative practitioners, the vast majority of the oncologists alluded to the vulnerable position of patients with cancer. Pointing to patients who are exposed to the "charlatan cure" on the Internet, one oncologist stated that he encourages his patients to bring along any such information that they may wish to discuss.

... I emphasise that 'you are vulnerable, don't waste your money; these people are charlatans and you've got to be careful' (MO)

The primary concern was that in their vulnerable state, patients were open to all possibilities for treating their cancer including "unproven" treatments. The use of anecdotal reports rather than scientific evidence to promote certain treatments was identified as a particular problem and was highlighted by all of the oncologists. Perceiving that they were being deceived, one oncologist endeavoured to dissuade his patients from attending alternative practitioners who were offering treatments based on "anecdotal responses".

In discussing the issue of a lack of scientific evidence associated with certain treatments, one oncologist spoke of the importance of conducting randomized controlled trials (RCTs) to evaluate conventional treatments adding that similar "ethics" do not apply for the "charlatan cure". Some of the oncologists were "open-minded" about certain CAM therapies such as TCM; however, according to one, any use of these therapies in the future would need to employ scientific methods. Similarly, there was a suggestion that if scientific methods were employed to explore the nature of herbal supplements, they may have a role in the future. Although somewhat less vocal about the lack of scientific merit, the importance of a scientific approach to evaluating CAM therapies was also important for some of the nurses.

... but maybe some sort of scientific clinical trial; evidence might make people swing a little bit more towards it (RN)

While forgoing conventional treatment appeared to be of primary concern for participants, there was also considerable unease with regard to adverse effects resulting from the use of some CAM therapies regardless of whether they were used in addition to or instead of conventional treatment. One of the oncologists explicitly advised his patients against some therapies.

… any of the more vigorous or … intensive approaches like enemas and that type of thing, obviously I don't condone and, and advise against (MO)

One of the nurses considered a possible adverse effect from a psychological perspective in that she perceived that some patients who opted for alternative treatment may agonize over the prudence of their decision. She recalled the case of one patient who subsequently appeared more "irritable" having chosen alternative treatment instead of chemotherapy. Concern was also expressed about the cost to patients in terms of "time". There was a perception that time spent pursuing some CAM therapies was a waste of the "limited" time that was left for patients who were in the palliative stage of illness. One of the oncologists referred to patients who travel to countries such as Mexico for "unproven treatments" as an example of this.

… spend … the limited time that they have they spend it away from their family on a wild goose chase and I think that's where it has an negative impact (MO)

Participants also considered adverse effects in terms of financial implications for patients who were availing of certain types of CAM. One of the oncologists endeavored to caution his patients against spending large amounts of money and patients' vulnerability was again highlighted. Other participants also expressed their concerns about the "major cost implications" for their patients.

The person was administering completely unproven therapies to patients and charging them a fortune (MO)

Some of the nurses were also robust in their criticism of certain practitioners who were treating patients with cancer outside of the conventional setting and taking "mega money" from them.

… I've huge concerns [about] people not in a hospital setting putting up IVs [intravenous infusions] what are they putting up in them, absolutely, I think they should be arrested (RN)

The costs of travel alone were highlighted as in the case of one patient with advanced disease who was considering travelling to a faith healer in Brazil. According to the participant, the patient was paying thousands of Euros simply juts to travel there.

As outlined, oncology professionals expressed considerable concern about therapies that were used as a substitute for conventional cancer treatment. It is likely that participants were particularly emphatic in their opposition to these therapies due to their perception that patients were adversely affecting their chances of survival and/or control of cancer by forgoing scientifically tested treatments for treatments that have not been put through such rigorous tests. Adding to their concern was the fact that patients were vulnerable and that in addition to the health implications there may also be financial implications for patients in this context.

In summary then, participants' attitudes to CAM are a reflection of the complexity of the subject. Certain CAM therapies such as relaxation and psychological therapies were perceived as having an important supportive role in the care of patients with cancer. Conversely, alternative therapies did not have any place in the cancer setting while other biologically based therapies/acupuncture were seen to occupy a more intermediate position with participants adopting a guarded approach to these therapies.

4. The role of CAM in patients with cancer: The perspectives of CAM practitioners

In the main, CAM was perceived by CAM practitioners as providing a supportive role for patients with cancer (Figure 1.3). According to the CAM practitioners, a holistic approach was adopted in order to assist the patients in their cancer journey. The primary emphasis was on addressing patients' physical (symptom/side effects) and psychological needs although the importance of "mental" and spiritual concerns was also underlined by some participants. Participants also described CAM as being complementary to conventional treatment although there were different perspectives in this regard.

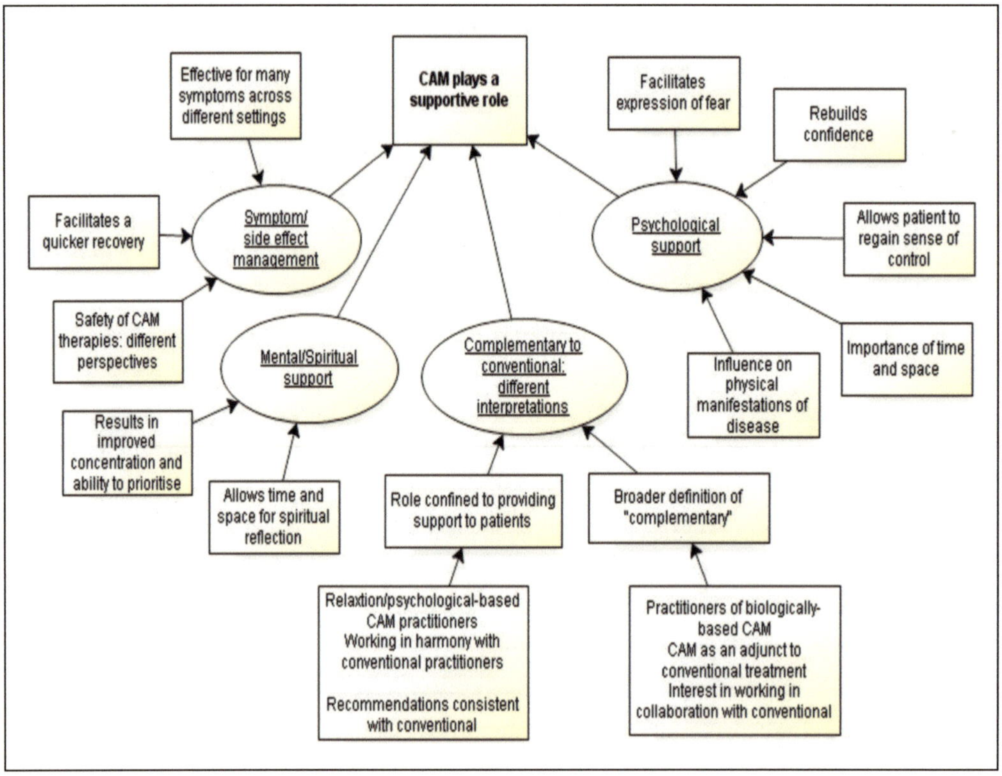

Fig. 1.3. CAM practitioners' perceptions of the role of CAM in patients with cancer

4.1 Symptom/side effect management

Although they employed different CAM therapies, all of the CAM practitioners identified the value of CAM for alleviating patients' symptoms and the side effects of conventional treatment. According to the participants, CAM facilitates a quicker recovery from side effects of conventional treatment, and it is effective for many side effects across different settings, however there were different perspectives regarding the safety of certain CAM therapies.

The TCM practitioners perceived an important role for CAM in addressing the side effects of conventional treatment. For some, CAM enabled a quicker recovery for patients.

... so that their bodies can recover maybe more quickly after they've had their chemo or radiation with less side effects (TCM).

While acknowledging the role of conventional medicine in cancer treatment, another TCM practitioner highlighted the value of CAM in strengthening patients following this treatment. According to this practitioner, patients who have received herbal medicine while undergoing chemotherapy recover more quickly than those who have not received herbal medicine.

Chinese medicine comes in, and keeps their body strong, builds their blood, their white cell count up, keeps them from vomiting ... (TCM)

Similarly, for another TCM practitioner, CAM had a role in strengthening the patients' immune system following conventional treatment which "biomedicine cancer treatment overwhelms". Another participant identified a role for phytobiophysics in addressing bone marrow suppression following chemotherapy and one of the nutritional therapists also asserted that nutrition could play a role in assisting the body to recover following chemotherapy.

The CAM practitioners also discussed the use of CAM to treat numerous side effects and symptoms in different settings. Most of the TCM practitioners identified the use of TCM for side effects such as nausea and vomiting and bone marrow suppression. However, one TCM practitioner also pointed to the use of herbal medicine for alopecia, while another highlighted its use for treating pain and fatigue. Another TCM practitioner treated women with breast cancer for relief of menopausal symptoms. According to the same practitioner, acupuncture and herbal medicine can be used to support patients with cancer in the curative setting "control of local swelling post-operatively" and in the palliative setting for "nausea and vomiting".

Relaxation therapies such as reflexology were also perceived to have a role in managing different symptoms and side effects; reflexology was beneficial for the treatment of fatigue, low energy and sleeplessness according to one of the reflexologists. It was also claimed that reflexology can alleviate other symptoms such as nausea and constipation.

A duty of one participant was to explain the different therapies that were available to patients attending the CSC. While acknowledging the benefits of reflexology in terms of relaxation and improved energy levels, this participant asserted that they were cautious about ascribing any claims to the therapy: "all we say is 'look, at times people can come back and say they feel better, or they have more energy or they feel better in themselves'". According to another reflexologist, in her experience lymphoedema in women with breast cancer can also improve with reflexology. Homeopathy was also employed to "support the system" and "build up their own immune system" while patients were receiving conventional treatment. Referring to treatment of patients in the hospice, one homeopath was keen to point out that homeopathy is appropriate for patients at all stages of cancer including those who are dying.

While there appeared to be little doubt among the participants that various CAM therapies were effective for symptom/side effect management, some difference of opinion emerged in relation to certain CAM therapies employed.

All of the CAM practitioners discussed the value of their respective CAM therapies for symptom/side effect management. However, some held considerably different views regarding the safety of certain CAM therapies which were practised and valued by other practitioners. One participant was "wary" about the use of antioxidants and of boosting the immune system fearing they may be counterproductive.

... antioxidants ... still [not clear] whether they're a good thing or a bad thing ... because is the ... tumour using them ... to protect themselves? (Nutritional Therapist)

Having practised reflexology in the past, one of the TCM practitioners expressed some concern about this therapy "because you're stimulating all these areas and you don't really know what you're doing, really, whereas the acupuncture is really pin point". Conversely, one of the reflexologists had some reservations about the use of massage unless the practitioners were "qualified or dealing with cancer patients a lot". According to one of the massage therapists, acupuncture may not be appropriate for patients who were undergoing chemotherapy due to their immunosuppressed state. This participant was also somewhat equivocal about the use of "herbs even vitamins"; acknowledging that there are practitioners who can use them to complement conventional treatment, she concluded that one would have to be "very iffy around them". In addition, most (but not all) of the TCM practitioners appeared to favour the use of acupuncture over herbal medicine perceiving that there was less risk involved with this approach.

I'd always use acupuncture because its to play it safer, it's incredibly effective anyway, so you can avoid and you're going to have no interactions with anything else anyone else is doing, so it's really, really safe (TCM)

Clearly then, symptom/side effect management was one of the key reasons identified by CAM practitioners for CAM use when supporting patients with cancer. In addition to symptom/side effect management, participants also described the supportive role of CAM in terms of psychological support and this is now discussed.

4.2 Psychological support

According to the participants, the supportive role of CAM was also concerned with the provision of psychological support to patients with cancer. In particular, it was considered essential to address patients' psychological concerns given the fear associated with cancer. The use of different CAM approaches was discussed with a view to facilitating patients to express their fears, rebuild confidence and regain a sense of control. The importance of time and space was emphasised. Moreover, there was a sense that up until recently psychological support has not been to the forefront of care for cancer patients in the conventional setting. Some of the participants perceived that patients who received greater psychological support were more likely to have improved outcomes with respect to the cancer itself.

Participants discussed the importance of enabling patients to express their "inner fears" given the fear that surrounds a cancer diagnosis.

... people feel fragile, feel vulnerable, where their questions are about the whole meaning or coping or dealing with fear (Counsellor)

One homeopath indicated that the emphasis in the conventional setting has traditionally been on the physical dimensions of cancer with less focus on psychological outcomes. Another participant suggested that while chemotherapy works to eliminate the cancer, CAM focuses on the psychological dimensions of the illness and "acknowledges" patients in a way that no longer occurs in the conventional setting. This development was blamed on "the system".

... CAM can work to kind of heal the psychological aspects of the soul, the spirit ... that was all part of our training (health professional) but its just gone out the window ... so I think in theory you all believe in it, the system doesn't allow for that ... (Massage Therapist)

One of the participants (cancer survivor) alluded to the fact that the CSCs are now redressing the balance by placing a priority on psychological support. According to this participant, prior to the CSCs there was "no support" for patients who had just completed treatment whereas patients received support from the nurses and fellow patients while on treatment. This recent focus on psychological care was also noted by one of the CSC-based practitioners who spoke of a patient describing her (the patient's) experience at a CSC three years previously as life-saving.

Acknowledging the fear that surrounds a cancer diagnosis, CAM practitioners endeavoured to attend to the psychological impact of cancer on patients with a view to facilitating expression of fear. One of the homeopaths spoke about the importance of "getting people emotionally stronger" while another used an initiative developed by Dr Rosy Daniel entitled "The Health Creation Programme" to assist patients to set priorities when "shell shocked" on receiving their diagnosis at the outset. While acknowledging that it is not counselling, one of the reflexologists suggested that reflexology may encourage patients to "open up" to a greater extent by removing any pressure to engage in a discussion while simultaneously facilitating a supportive environment should they wish to do so.

Certain CAM therapies were also considered beneficial in terms of helping patients to rebuild their confidence. According to one of the participants, hydrotherapy was very beneficial for patients in this way. Having observed the use of this treatment in the hospice setting, this participant determined that the water provided a degree of "freedom" which assisted patients who may feel "very restricted, very tight". The same participant also found that yoga released patients from being "stuck and protective" following surgery. According to another participant, in her experience "touch therapies" were particularly valuable in the terms of encouraging women who were dealing with "altered body image" to embrace themselves again.

... it can be very helpful in actually in terms of coming to terms with that and embracing, literally embracing themselves (Massage Therapist)

Of note, other participants highlighted the value of reflexology in the context of "altered body image". The impression was that all patients could benefit from touch therapies including those who were not feeling confident due to a change in their body image. One of the reflexologists contended that this therapy may be a more appropriate than massage for certain patients such as those post-mastectomy for this reason.

The value of CAM in assisting patients to regain a sense of control was highlighted across the different specialties.

... everybody's doing things for them ... now 'this is a choice that I'm making myself, because I can do something to help myself' (Reflexologist)

According to one of the CSC-based practitioners, the approach in the CSCs was to point out the different services available thereby enabling patients to take control and choose therapies on the basis of their needs. One of the massage therapists endeavoured to give patients a choice in choosing the aromatherapy oils before a massage.

In addition, participants across the different specialties discussed the importance of "time and space" in the context of providing psychological support to patients with cancer. According to one of the TCM practitioners, patients "appreciate the time that they are given, to be listened to" while another noted that "in TCM and indeed most CAM therapies they are treated as a unique individual" and are given "plenty of time to tell their story and to ask questions". One of the homeopaths stated that she would spend one hour with each patient and even two hours with a new patient in order to undertake a complete history from childhood onward while one of the reflexologists stated that she endeavored to provide time and space to facilitate patients to express their emotions. Similarly, the importance of "time and space" was also highlighted by a phytobiophysics practitioner. This practitioner also practised reiki, a therapy which was identified as being particularly valuable for patients "own healing within" regardless of their prognosis. There was a sense that a lack of time in the conventional setting precluded patients from discussing their fears about the illness.

... their doctor is not getting the time to really sit down and talk to them about their fears (TCM)

According to another TCM practitioner, conventional practitioners are "shooting themselves in the foot" by not allocating time for patients to discuss their fears. This practitioner highlighted the dissatisfaction resulting from this situation as another "negative thing" for patients. Similarly, one of the massage therapists, stated that nurses and doctors are so busy in hospitals in the present day that caring albeit time-consuming measures such as "long bed baths" are no longer undertaken and patients are being "lost in the whole system".

Addressing patients' psychological concerns was seen to have benefits which extended beyond the immediate concerns to encompass the actual disease itself. According to one of the TCM practitioners, while acupuncture given for emotional distress may not shrink the actual tumour, it may arrest further progression by containing the patient's stress.

... because the cellular division doesn't get more intensified through, through you know stress, I don't know if stress and cancer how much they've related it in Western medicine but we see a relationship (TCM)

Similarly, one of the participants considered the potential impact of psychological support on the immune system after watching a TV programme which demonstrated "an effect biochemically" in another illness. For two of the homeopaths, improved outcomes were more evident in patients who were robust from a psychological, physical and social perspective. While participants placed most emphasis on supporting patients symptomatically and psychologically, some also the highlighted the importance of providing mental and spiritual support to patients.

4.3 Mental concentration and spiritual support

A holistic approach to care also required that patients' "mental" and spiritual needs were attended to.

The homeopath … treats the whole person this means on an emotional, mental, physical and spiritual level (Homeopath)

One of the TCM practitioners contrasted their approach to care with conventional practice where she contended that the focus was only on surgically removing the tumour while there was less attention being paid to the "internal, mental, emotional". Some of the participants highlighted the value of certain therapies in terms of attaining mental clarity. It was asserted that acupuncture can improve concentration and the ability to prioritise tasks. Similarly, one of the reflexologists claimed that reflexology assisted patients to prioritise; "it clears the wool from the brain". Yoga required patients to concentrate on breathing and movement during the class so "they are not as caught up in their thoughts" according to one of the Massage Therapists.

The concepts of time and space were again considered in relation to spiritual support. During reflexology sessions, one of the reflexologists endeavored to allow "time and space" to facilitate spiritual reflection. One of the CSC-based counsellors contended that a "holistic complementary service" was "integral to the cancer journey".

because I have yet to meet somebody who … who just wants to know what is happening next and who's able to move on with life … and it touches into so many other areas of their lives, relationships, communication, goals, sense of meaning, existential questions … (Counsellor)

A spiritual approach to care was also alluded to by one of the homeopaths who spoke of the importance of viewing cancer as a challenge which could afford an opportunity for patients to make changes to their lives.

As outlined, participants indicated that CAM can provide a supportive role for patients with cancer by utilising a holistic approach to addressing their physical, psychological, mental and spiritual needs. The role of CAM in relation to conventional medicine was also considered and this is now briefly described.

4.4 Complementary to conventional medicine: Different Interpretations

While it was clear that participants were in agreement that the primary role of CAM was to support patients through their cancer journey, their views regarding the position of CAM with respect to conventional treatment were less cohesive. Essentially, most of the practitioners of relaxation/psychological therapies emphasised their role as one confined to assisting patients as they received their primary treatment in the conventional setting. In essence, they distanced themselves from suggestions that CAM therapies could be an alternative to conventional treatment. Their views differed from those of practitioners of biologically based therapies who considered a broader role for CAM which also incorporated cancer treatment and prevention. Of interest, the term "complementary" was used with respect to both views suggesting that it may have a different meaning for the different groups.

Practitioners of relaxation/psychological therapies were more inclined to refer to the "complementary" role of CAM in the context of providing assistance to patients as they received conventional treatment and negotiated their way through the cancer journey. In essence, the impression given by practitioners of relaxation/psychological-based therapies was that they were working in harmony with conventional practitioners. That is, conventional practitioners managed the actual disease while they supported the patient through the process.

...because it, cancer is a medical condition; it needs to be worked through the medical field, then yeah we are the complementary one to assist them along that journey (Reflexologist)

According to another participant, the role of CAM in the management of cancer may not be as central as that of conventional treatment; nonetheless, it complements conventional treatment by considering the psychological dimensions thereby facilitating a more holistic approach to care. Some of the participants were also keen to emphasise that the CAM provided in the CSCs was "complementary" in nature as distinct from "alternative".

First of all I consider what I do as complementary and I don't consider it alternative therapy so what I do complements orthodox treatments (Reflexologist)

It was evident then that CSC-based practitioners considered that they worked in harmony with the conventional providers. Consistent with this perspective, there was little to suggest that these participants encouraged patients to consider any treatments outside of those prescribed by their doctors.

When asked about herbal supplements by patients, one such participant stated that she advised patients against taking any biologically based therapies that the conventional practitioners had not prescribed.

I wouldn't recommend, taking any medication that the medical don't know about because you can't be sure of, you know, content or interactions ok, so that would be my standard line (Counsellor)

Another CSC-based practitioner also avoided making any recommendations regarding herbal supplements to patients attending the CSC stating that she was not qualified to do so and that CSC policy precludes the provision of such advice. According to one of the reflexologists, there is a general awareness that some CAM practitioners have been giving advice "which they shouldn't have been" and she advised her reflexology students accordingly.

... 'you don't diagnose, you don't tell people to change their medicine, you don't, you don't go off, that's not your role' (Reflexologist)

Conversely, while practitioners of biologically based therapies also discussed the "complementary" role of CAM, their understanding of the term appeared to include the use of CAM to impact more directly on the cancer itself in terms of treatment and prevention. The role of CAM in cancer treatment was highlighted by the TCM practitioners in particular. According to one of these practitioners, acupuncture and herbal medicine can be used as an adjunct to conventional treatment.

... to aid in tumour reduction itself, potentially reducing the length of time the patient needs to receive radiation and/or chemotherapy (TCM)

While other TCM practitioners described their use of CAM to primarily support patients rather than to directly treat the cancer, they also pointed to the value of TCM as a treatment in its own right and the benefits of using it in conjunction with conventional treatment. One practitioner highlighted the use of TCM in addition to chemotherapy and radiotherapy in China; however, she did state that her practice was focused more on supporting the patient and that she was not going to "pretend" she was treating the cancer although "it shouldn't be just one way". Similarly, another TCM practitioner maintained that she would be in favour of people using conventional treatment as their "first line" and did not agree with CAM being used as "stand alone therapy" in cancer treatment. Nonetheless, she also underlined the more dominant position of TCM in China whereby Western diagnostic procedures are used but treatment involves the use of herbal medicine and acupuncture.

Ok, in the West we will use ourselves as complementary practitioners but you know in Asia we are stand alone (TCM)

One of the TCM practitioners contended that there was "no infrastructural backup" in Ireland to enable practitioners to treat cancer directly. This being the case, he treated patients primarily for side effects of conventional treatments. Nonetheless, he did express an interest in a system whereby herbal medicine would be offered in a cancer hospital which would allow patients to choose between CAM and conventional treatment.

that they are given a choice between the two (TCM)

The role of diet in controlling cancer was also considered. According to one of the nutritional therapists, addressing conditions such as food intolerances and allergies may release the immune system to deal with other problems such as cancer cell growth. Another participant highlighted the use of TCM in the management of early cancers. However, this participant admitted to adopting a conservative approach to the treatment of patients with cancer due to fear of repercussions if patients were to subsequently develop problems due to interactions with conventional treatment.

... not when they're in treatment, you don't cross over treatments ... we've got to be very wary insurance-wise because you know if something happens you know because you're the, you're the first point of call if there's something wrong (TCM)

One of the nutritional therapists also expressed similar concerns. Mindful of the potential consequences if there was an interaction with conventional treatment, this practitioner avoided giving supplements to patients once they started on conventional treatment.

Given the concerns about interactions with conventional treatment and the potential repercussions, it is not surprising then that most of the practitioners of biologically based therapies expressed an interest in working in collaboration with conventional providers.

... I don't want to take a risk ... of maybe just it's brushing over the medical side and say I go just only complementary but I know that the complementary side of medicine has a huge big place and it's ... not replaceable (Homeopath)

One of the TCM practitioners indicated that some patients with advanced disease opted to use TCM over conventional cancer treatment. While this practitioner spoke of having seen some "incredible results" with TCM alone, she also indicated that she would only treat patients in this way when they had discussed the issue with their oncologists because "you know the odd person comes in and it completely helps them but that doesn't mean it's going to do it for everybody."

Other practitioners also indicated that they encouraged patients to remain involved with their conventional practitioners.

... [on] no occasion do we say don't go to a doctor, quite the opposite, a good responsible homeopath, professional homeopath will say look check it out with your GP if you think you have a serious problem a cancer, growth, tumour whatever by all accounts (Homeopath)

... they might initially not tell you that they've decided to drop their conventional treatment, which I would always tell them not to (TCM)

Acknowledging that it is rare, another homeopath also stated that patients sometimes wish to use homeopathy as an alternative to conventional treatment. However, this participant stated that he discourages his patients from adopting this approach, underlining the fact that he wants them to have a "conventional diagnosis" as he does not have the diagnostic equipment necessary for assessing the extent of disease. The legal implications were also acknowledged.

An interest in collaboration was also expressed by others. Another homeopath stated that he would "love" to work with "surgeons and other doctors" who would acknowledge his role as a practitioner who would "strengthen" and "prepare" patients undergoing conventional treatment. The "ideal" for one of the phytobiotherapists was a "medical centre" where both sides would adopt a multidisciplinary approach to patient care. Other participants discussed the concept in terms of integration. For one of the nutritional therapists, integration was "key" and it was important for CAM not to be "completely out on your own" and adopting the notion that conventional medicine is undesirable.

According to one of the massage therapists (also a trained herbalist), an integrated health care system would be "wonderful". However, she was particularly emphatic that such an integrated system should not be based on the notion that complementary therapies were harmless but unlikely to be effective, a concept articulated by some "very intelligent personnel" and "so there needs to be a huge amount of learning".

In addition to cancer treatment, a role for CAM in cancer prevention was also highlighted by certain participants.

According to one of the nutritionists, CAM was there to "complement what orthodox medicine has to offer"; however, prevention was major focus for this practitioner. Referring to those with a family history of breast cancer, it was noted that referring them to a nutritionist may "get them sorted" so that cancer never develops. Other practitioners also highlighted the role of CAM in cancer prevention.

One of the most effective roles that TCM can fulfill is to help re-establish an underlying balance in the individual, and to unravel the complex patterns inherent in the body which can, if left untreated, lead to the development of cancer (TCM)

One of the homeopaths described the use of homeopathy in persons with a family history of cancer "to try and stimulate a vital or innate response in the system that the predisposition could be lessened".

It is clear then that the term "complementary" had a somewhat different meaning for the different practitioners. Practitioners of relaxation/psychological therapies discussed the "complementary" role of CAM in terms of supporting patients as they coped with the disease and conventional treatment. Conversely, the practitioners of biologically based therapies also considered a role for CAM in the treatment and prevention of cancer. However, the term "complementary" in this context also considered the use of CAM with respect to impacting more directly on the cancer itself in terms of treatment and prevention. In particular, the existence of TCM as a "stand-alone" system was highlighted. However, identifying the limitations of CAM as a single modality treatment, some of the practitioners were not comfortable in using CAM by itself to treat cancer. Moreover, the potential for interaction with conventional treatment also resulted in some practitioners adopting a somewhat cautious position. For these reasons, most of the participants expressed an interest in working in collaboration with conventional medicine alluding to the risks inherent in operating separately. In the absence of such collaboration, it appears likely that many practitioners opted to concentrate on supporting patients through treatment as they considered the limitations of CAM as a primary modality. In addition, there was a perception that the "infrastructure" did not exist in Ireland at this time to facilitate a greater role for CAM in the treatment of cancer.

In summary then, the participants described CAM as providing a supportive role for patients with cancer. Patients were supported using a holistic approach to care according to the participants. That is, there was an emphasis on addressing the physical, psychological, mental and spiritual needs of patients and participants perceived that CAM was complementary to conventional treatment.

5. Discussion

Prior to this research, a literature search found no qualitative research specifically addressing the role of CAM in the cancer setting from the perspectives of patients, oncology professionals or CAM practitioners. However, reasons for CAM use and attitudes toward CAM use in the cancer setting have been examined in other studies and these are now discussed in light of the findings of this study.

In this study, women with breast cancer perceived that CAM plays a supportive role for patients with cancer and this is consistent with the findings of international studies which have identified symptom/side effect relief (Cui et al., 2004, Hann et al., 2005, Lengacher et al., 2006, Molassiotis et al., 2006), psychological stress relief (Hann et al., 2005; Henderson & Donatelle, 2004; Lengacher et al., 2006) and a desire for greater control (Chen et al., 2008; Cui et al., 2004; Hann et al., 2005, Henderson & Donatelle, 2004,) as the primary reasons for CAM use among women with breast cancer. Importantly, in allowing patients to provide greater detail regarding their experience of CAM therapies and their perceptions of the role of CAM, this study has allowed greater insight into the significance of CAM for patients. More specifically, it is less likely that a patient survey could capture for example the importance of human touch for patients with cancer. The value placed on the CSCs by study participants across the different stakeholder groups is also an important finding as there appears to be a dearth of literature in this particular area.

The descriptions of relaxation therapies in this study resonate with the findings of Billhult & Dahlberg (2001) and Billhult et al., (2007) regarding the notion that such therapies provide a respite from conventional treatment. Billhult et al., (2007) identified five themes following their interviews with ten breast cancer patients who had received massage during conventional treatment. These included distraction from a frightening experience, a change from negative to positive, a sense of relaxation, a reinforcement of caring and a sense of feeling good. While acknowledging that their study was small (n=63), Pruthi et al., (2009) pointed to the likelihood that massage may help patients with breast cancer to relax and feel better overall. Similar to our study, Gottlieb & Wachala (2007) observed high levels of consumer satisfaction in their critical review of 44 studies of professionally led cancer support groups. This level of satisfaction may be related to feeling happier and more at ease, receiving practical and emotional support and experiencing a sense of comfort and camaraderie (Hoey et al., 2008).

The finding that some patients would welcome a greater emphasis on CAM in the cancer setting is also consistent with Balneaves et al., (2007) study which found that some patients were disappointed by their interactions with conventional providers on the subject of CAM. In addition, these authors noted that women who engaged in a "bringing it all together" decision-making process favoured healthcare that was tailored to them as individuals focusing not only on their cancer but also on their overall wellbeing (p.980). All of these women were prior CAM users and were highly committed to using CAM throughout their cancer journey. While perceiving their cancer as serious but "beatable" with conventional treatment, these women also believed that CAM was essential to enhancing their physical, psychosocial and spiritual health and as such they employed a variety of CAM therapies to help them cope with their changed circumstances post treatment and to prevent a recurrence (p.980). However, Balneaves et al., (2007) also noted that a certain cohort of patients whom they identified as the "playing it safe group" appeared to be less committed to incorporating oral CAM therapies into their overall treatment plan (p.979) as they were concerned about risks such as potential interactions with conventional treatments, a concern also echoed by some of our study participants.

Undoubtedly, informed by patients' expressed desire for a more holistic and patient-centred approach (Fitch, 2005; Kendall *et al.*, 2006; Liu *et al.*, 2006, Turton & Cooke, 2000), the Institute of Medicine (IOM) (2007) issued a report designed to address the needs of the "whole" person with cancer. According to the report, all cancer care should enable the provision of appropriate psychosocial support by facilitating effective communication between patients and health professionals and by identifying each patient's psychosocial health needs. Moreover, where the need existed, patients should be linked up with psychosocial services and their physical and psychosocial care should be co-ordinated. All cancer care should endeavor to engage and support patients in managing their disease and treatment and finally, it would be necessary to ensure systematic follow-up, re-evaluation, and modification of care as required (IOM 2007). Similarly, a position paper by the European Society of Mastology (EUSOMA) (Baum *et al.*, 2006) has identified the importance of providing psychosocial and spiritual support to women with breast cancer.

With regard to oncology professionals' perceptions of the role of CAM in the cancer setting, the results of this study are broadly reflective of international studies which have explored oncology professionals' attitudes toward CAM use in general among their patients. In particular, for the most part, there is consistency regarding oncology professionals' response to and support for relaxation/psychological therapies (Bourgeault , 1996; Cindy Wang & Yates, 2006; Hessig et al., 2004; Newell & Sanson-Fisher, 2000; Risberg et al., 2004; Roberts et al., 2005; Salmenperä et al., 2003; Tovey & Broom, 2007) versus their response to and concerns regarding biologically based therapies (Bourgeault, 1996; Cindy Wang & Yates, 2006; Hyodo et al., 2003; Newell & Sanson-Fisher, 2000; Salmenperä et al., 2003). However, in a more recent study (Zanini et al., 2008), approximately one fifth of oncology nurses were interested in attending training courses about TCM while almost one third were interested in training courses on homeopathy. Those interested in attending courses on progressive relaxation and massage was approaching 50% (Zanini et al., 2008). According to Fitch et al., (1999), without exception, oncology nurses endorsed the notion that patients have a right to information, that information is essential for decision-making and that ultimately decisions concerning health are up to the individual. As such, these nurses envisioned their role as one concerned with providing information, facilitating access to information and assisting patients to filter the information acquired. Moreover, they expressed an interest in engaging patients in discussions about CAM rather than avoiding the subject.

As noted above, a new finding from this study concerns oncology professionals' perceptions of the CSCs. It is also interesting to note the challenges faced by oncology professionals who endeavour to achieve a balance between supporting patients who may wish to avail of CAM therapies that they (oncology professionals) have concerns about whilst simultaneously seeking to ensure that patients avoid harm from such therapies.

Literature on CAM practitioners' perceptions of the role of CAM in the cancer setting is sparse; however, one study (Gray et al., 1999), pointed to CAM practitioners' interest in playing a role in caring for patients with cancer. In addition, CAM practitioners consider that there is strong or very strong evidence to support various CAM therapies in cancer treatment and/or symptom/side effect management (Lee et al., 2009). According to Mackereth et al., (2009), factors influencing individuals to work as complementary therapists in the cancer/palliative care settings included the desire to provide individualised treatment while adopting a patient-centered caring approach.

The research literature on CAM practitioners in general (including but not exclusive to the area of cancer) points to certain trends: for the most part, CAM practitioners articulate a general sense of respect and goodwill toward conventional practitioners (Barrett et al., 2004), desire closer communication (Klimenko et al., 2006, Klimenko et al., 2007) and greater collaboration with mainstream medicine (Barrett et al., 2004, Ben-Arye et al., 2007). Of note, Barrett et al., (2004) also pointed to practitioners' contentions that major differences and barriers existed between CAM and mainstream medicine. Moreover, they indicated concern about accessibility issues in healthcare and asserted that attitudes and beliefs were often greater barriers to integration than economic or scientific issues. This study has also highlighted significantly different views between oncology professionals and CAM practitioners particularly with respect to the use of biologically based therapies while patients are receiving conventional treatment.

Although integrative healthcare (IHC) has developed in some settings (White 2002), the degree of integration may be less than that envisioned due to the continued existence of dominant biomedical patterns of professional interaction (Hollenberg, 2006; Soklaridis et al.,

2009). The purported limited evidence base for CAM therapies (Ernst, 2009; Gerber et al., 2006) is likely to be a major contributing factor in this context; moreover, given the challenges faced by CAM practitioners in the design and conduct of CAM research in the general (Ben-Arye et al., 2004; Coulter, 2007) and oncology settings (Gerhard et al., 2004, Richardson et al., 1998) it is unlikely that the problem of CAM research will be easily resolved. However, Vickers (2001) argues that there are no good reasons to suggest that evidence-based medicine (EBM) and CAM are incompatible as the former provides CAM with an opportunity to find an "appropriate and just place in health care" (p.1). This assumes, however, that CAM practitioners have expertise in research methods which according to a study (n=65) by Hadley et al., (2009) the majority do not, given their inadequate training in research methods and evidence-based practice.

Our study has provided some insight into the role of CAM in the cancer setting as perceived by Irish CAM practitioners. The sector is currently undergoing a process of self regulation, a position supported by the Irish Government in 2006 following the launch of a report (National Working Group on the Regulation of Complementary Therapists 2005) which was commissioned to examine regulatory issues in the area. Importantly, this study also reflects the difficulties associated with using the term CAM to describe all practitioners who are not currently working in the conventional setting including those whose perspectives may be more aligned with those of conventional practitioners than with those of CAM practitioners.

6. Conclusion

While all three stakeholder groups considered CAM as supportive, perspectives differed among oncology professionals and CAM practitioners regarding the manner in which this was so. In general, there was consistency among all three groups with respect to the supportive nature of relaxation-based therapies and psychological therapies. However, oncology professionals and CAM practitioners' perspectives differed significantly with respect to the role of biologically based therapies in the cancer setting. These converging and diverging perspectives most likely reflect the complexity of the subject whereby CAM encompasses many different approaches, therapies and practitioners. Given this situation, it seems prudent that continued efforts should be made to engage with all patients with cancer with a view to ascertaining their perspectives on CAM and endeavouring to meet their needs where it appears safe to do so. Engaging with patients in this way should ensure that patients are referred to CSCs and/or accredited community-based practitioners for relaxation/psychological therapies should they wish to avail of these therapies. Such an engagement should also facilitate a discussion regarding patients' intentions to consume biologically based therapies while receiving conventional therapy thereby decreasing risks associated with interactions between these treatments and/or adverse effects apart from such interactions.

7. References

Attride-Stirling, J. (2001) Thematic networks: an analytic tool for qualitative research. *Qualitative Research,* Vol. 1, pp. 385-405.

Barrett, B; Marchand, L; Scheder, J; Appelbaum, D; Plane, M.B; Blustein, J., Maberry, R. & Capperino, C. (2004) What complementary and alternative medicine practitioners say about health and health care. *Ann Fam Med.* Vol. 2, No. 3, pp. 253-259.

Balneaves, L.G; Truant, T.L; Kelly, M; Verhoef, M.J. & Davison, B.J. (2007) Bridging the gap: decision-making processes of women with breast cancer using complementary and alternative medicine (CAM). *Support Care Cancer.* Vol, 15, No. 8, pp. 973-983.

Baum, M; Cassileth, B.R; Daniel, R; Ernst, E; Filshie, J; Nagel, G.A; Horneber, M; Kohn, M; Lejeune, S; Maher J; Terje R. & Smith, W.B. (2006) The role of complementary and alternative medicine in the management of early breast cancer: recommendations of the European Society of Mastology (EUSOMA). *Eur J Cancer.* Vol 42, No. 12, pp. 1711-1714.

Ben-Arye, E; Frenkel, M. & Margalit, R.S. (2004) Approaching complementary and alternative medicine use in patients with cancer: questions and challenges. *J Ambul Care Manage.* Vol 27, No. 1, pp. 53-62.

Ben-Arye, E; Scharf M. & Frenkel M. (2007) How should complementary practitioners and physicians communicate? A cross-sectional study from Israel. *J Am Board Fam Med.* Vol 20, No. 6, pp. 565-571.

Billhult, A. & Dahlberg, K. (2001) A meaningful relief from suffering: experiences of massage in cancer care. *Cancer Nurs* Vol 24, pp. 180–184.

Billhult, A., Stener-Victorin, E. & Bergbom, I. (2007) The experience of massage during chemotherapy treatment in breast cancer patients. *Clin Nurs Res.* Vol 16, No. 2, pp. 85-99.

Bourgeault, I. L. (1996) Physicians" attitudes toward patients' use of alternative cancer therapies. *Canadian Medical Association Journal,* Vol 155, No. 12, pp. 1679-1685.

Chen, Z; Gu, K; Zheng, Y; Zheng, W; Lu, W. & Shu, X.O. (2008) The use of complementary and alternative medicine among Chinese women with breast cancer. *J Altern Complement Med.* Vol 14, No. 8, pp, 1049-1055.

Cindy Wang, S.Y. & Yates, P. (2006) Nurses' responses to people with cancer who use complementary and alternative medicine. *Int J Nurs Pract.* Vol. 12, No. 5, pp. 288-294.

Coulter, I.D. (2007) Evidence-based complementary and alternative medicine: promises and problems. *Forsch Komplementmed.* Vol 14, No. 2, pp. 102-108.

Cui, Y; Shu, X.O; Gao, Y; Wen, W; Ruan, Z.X; Jin, F. & Zheng, W. (2004) Use of complementary and alternative medicine by Chinese women with breast cancer. *Breast Cancer Res Treat.* Vol. 85, No. 3, pp. 263-270.

Department of Health and Children (2006) National Working Group on the Regulation of Complementary Therapists, *Report of the National Working Group on the Regulation of Complementary Therapists to the Minister for Health and Children.* The Stationary Office, Dublin.

Department of Health and Children (2006) Press Release: Launch of Report of the National Working Group on the Regulation of Complementary Therapists (2006). Available at: http//www.dohc.ie (accessed October 24th 2009).

Ernst, E. (2009) How Much of CAM is Based on Research Evidence? *Evid Based Complement Alternat Med.* May 21. PMID: 19465405.

Ezzy, D. (2002) Qualitative Analysis: Practice and Innovation. Routledge, London.

Fitch, M. I. (2005) Needs of patients living with advanced disease. *Can Oncol Nurs J.* Vol 15, No. 4, pp. 230-242.

Fitch, M.I; Gray, R.E; Greenberg, M; Douglas, M.S; Labrecque, M; Pavlin, P; Gabel, N. & Freedhoff S. (1999) Oncology nurses' perspectives on unconventional therapies. *Cancer Nurs.* Vol 22, No. 1, pp. 90-96.

Gerber, B; Scholz, C; Reimer, T; Briese, V. & Janni, W. (2006) Complementary and alternative therapeutic approaches in patients with early breast cancer: a systematic review. *Breast Cancer Research and Treatment,* Vol 95, pp. 109-209.

Gerhard, I; Abel, U; Loewe-Mesch, A; Huppmann, S. & Kuehn, J.J. (2004) Problems of randomized studies in complementary medicine demonstrated in a study on mistletoe treatment of patients with breast cancer. *Forsch Komplementarmed Klass Naturheilkd.* Vol, 11, No. 3, pp. 150-157.

Gottlieb, B.H. & Wachala, E.D. (2007) Cancer support groups: a critical review of empirical studies. *Psychooncology* Vol, 16, No. 5, pp. 379-400.

Gray, R.E; Fitch, M; Saunders, P.R; Wilkinson, A; Ross, C.P; Franssen, E. & Caverhill K. (1999) Complementary health practitioners' attitudes, practices and knowledge related to women's cancers. *Cancer Prev Control.* Vol 3, No. 1, pp. 77-82.

Hadley, J; Hassan, I. & Khan, K.S. (2008) Knowledge and beliefs concerning evidence-based practice amongst complementary and alternative medicine health care practitioners and allied health care professionals: a questionnaire survey. *BMC Complement Altern Med.* Vol. 23, No. 8:45.

Hann, D; Baker, F; Denniston, M; Entrekin, N. (2005) Long-term breast cancer survivors" use of complementary therapies: perceived impact on recovery and prevention of recurrence. *Integr Cancer Ther.* Vol. 4, No. 1, pp. 14-20.

Henderson , J.W. & Donatelle , R.J. (2004) Complementary and alternative medicine use by women after completion of allopathic treatment for breast cancer. *Altern Ther Health Med.* Vol. 10, No. 1, pp. 52-57.

Hessig, R.E; Arcand, L.L. & Frost M.H. (2004) The effects of an educational intervention on oncology nurses' attitude, perceived knowledge, and self-reported application of complementary therapies. *Oncol Nurs Forum,* Vol. 31, No. 1, pp. 71-78.

Hoey, L.M; Leropoli, S.C; White, V.M & Jefford, M. (2008) Systematic review of peer-support programs for people with cancer. *Patient Education and Counseling,* Vol. 70, No. 3, pp. 315-337.

Hollenberg, D. (2006) Uncharted ground: patterns of professional interaction among complementary/alternative and biomedical practitioners in integrative health care settings. *Soc Sci Med.* Vol. 62, No. 3, pp. 731-744.

Hyodo, I; Eguchi, K; Nishina, T; Endo, H; Tanimizu, M; Mikami, I; Takashima, S. & Imanishi, J. (2003) Perceptions and attitudes of clinical oncologists on complementary and alternative medicine: a nationwide survey in Japan. *Cancer,* Vol 97, No. 11, pp. 2861-2868.

Institute of Medicine (2007) Cancer care for the whole patient: meeting psychosocial health needs. Available from: http://www.iom.edu. (Accessed April 22nd 2010).

Kendall, M; Boyd, K; Campbell, C; Cormie, P; Fife, S; Thomas, K; Weller, D. & Murray, S.A. (2006) How do people with cancer wish to be cared for in primary care? Serial discussion groups of patients and carers. *Fam Practice,* Vol. 23, No. 6, pp. 644-650.

Klimenko, E. & Julliard, K. (2007) Communication between CAM and mainstream medicine: Delphi panel perspectives. *Complement Ther Clin Pract.* Vol 13, No. 1, pp. 46-52.

Klimenko, E; Julliard, K; Lu, S.H & Song, H. (2006) Models of health: a survey of practitioners. *Complement Ther Clin Pract.* Vol. 12, No. 4, pp. 258-267.

Lee, C.D; Zia, F; Olaku, O; Michie, J. & White, J.D. (2009) Survey of complementary and alternative medicine practitioners regarding cancer management and research. *J Soc Integr Oncol.* Vol. 17, No. 1, 26-34.

Lengacher, C.A;, Bennett, M.P; Kip, K.E; Gonzalez, L; Jacobsen, P. & Cox, C.E. (2006) Relief of symptoms, side effects, and psychological distress through use of complementary and alternative medicine in women with breast cancer. *Oncol Nurs Forum*, Vol. 33, No. 1, pp. 97-104.

Liamputtong, P. & Ezzy, D. (2005) *Qualitative Research Methods.* Oxford University Press, South Melbourne.

Liu, J.E; Mok, E. & Wong, T. (2006) Caring in nursing: investigating the meaning of caring from the perspective of cancer patients in Beijing, China. *J Clin Nurs.* Vol. 15, No. 2, pp. 188-196.

Mackereth, P; Carter, A; Parkin, S; Stringer, J; Roberts, D; Todd, C; Long, A. & Caress, A. (2009b) Complementary therapists' motivation to work in cancer/supportive and palliative care: a multi-centre case study. *Complement Ther Clin Pract.* Vol. 15, No. 3, pp. 161-165.

Molassiotis, A; Scott, J.A; Kearney, N; Pud, D; Magri, M; Selvekerova, S; Bruyns, I; Fernadez-Ortega, P; Panteli, V; Margulies, A; Gudmundsdottir, G; Milovics, L; Ozden, G; Platin, N. & Patiraki, E. (2006) Complementary and alternative medicine use in breast cancer patients in Europe. *Support Care Cancer,* Vol. 14, No. 3, pp. 260-267.

National Working Group on the Regulation of Complementary Therapists, *Report of the National Working Group on the Regulation of Complementary Therapists to the Minister for Health and Children.* The Stationary Office, Dublin (2005).

Newell, S. & Sanson-Fisher, R.W. (2000) Australian oncologists' self-reported knowledge and attitudes about nontraditional therapies used by cancer patients. *Med J Aust.* Vol. 172, pp. 110-113.

Pruthi, S; Degnim, A.C; Bauer, B.A; DePompolo, R.W. & Nayar, V. (2009) Value of massage therapy for patients in a breast clinic. *Clin J Oncol Nurs.* Vol. 13, No. 4, 422-425.

Richardson, M.A; Post-White, J; Singletary, S.E. & Justice, B. (1998) Recruitment for complementary/alternative medicine trials: who participates after breast cancer. *Ann Behav Med.* Vol. 20, No. 3, pp. 190-198.

Risberg, T; Kolstad, A; Bremnes, Y; Holte, H; Wist, E.A; Mella, O; Klepp, O; Wilsgaard, T. & Cassileth, B.R. (2004) Knowledge of and attitudes toward complementary and alternative therapies: a national multicentre study of oncology professionals in Norway. *European Journal of Cancer,* Vol. 40, No. 4, pp. 529-535.

Roberts, C.S; Baker, F; Hann, D; Runfola, J; Witt, C; McDonald, J; Livingston, M.L; Ruiterman, J; Ampela, R; Kaw, O.C. & Blanchard, C. (2005) Patient-physician communication regarding use of complementary therapies during cancer treatment. *J Psychosoc Oncol.* Vol. 23, No. 4, 35-60.

Salmenperä, L; Suominen, T. & Vertio, H. (2003) Physicians' attitudes towards the use of complementary therapies (CTs) by cancer patients in Finland. *Eur J Cancer Care* (Engl). Vol. 12, No. 4, pp. 358-364.

Soklaridis, S; Kelner, M; Love, R.L. & Cassidy, J.D. (2009) Integrative health care in a hospital setting: communication patterns between CAM and biomedical practitioners. *J Interprof Care*, Vol. 23, No. 6, pp. 655-667.

Tovey, P. & Broom, A. (2007) Oncologists' and specialist cancer nurses' approaches to complementary and alternative medicine and their impact on patient action. *Soc Sci Med.* Vol. 64, No. 12, pp. 2550-2564.

Turton, P. & Cooke, H. (2000) Meeting the needs of people with cancer for support and self-management. *Complement Ther Nurs Midwifery*, Vol. 6, No. 3, pp. 130-137

White, J.D. (2002) The National Cancer Institute's perspective and agenda for promoting awareness and research on alternative therapies for cancer. *J Altern Complement Med.* Vol. 8, No. 5, pp. 545-550.

Zanini, A; Quattrin, R; Goi, D; Frassinelli, B; Panariti, M; Carpanelli, I. & Brusaferro, S. (2008) Italian oncology nurses' knowledge of complementary and alternative therapies. *JAN*, Vol. 62, No. 4, pp. 451–456.

3

Alternative and Traditional Medicines Systems in Pakistan: History, Regulation, Trends, Usefulness, Challenges, Prospects and Limitations

Shahzad Hussain[1], Farnaz Malik[1], Nadeem Khalid[2], Muhammad Abdul Qayyum[2] and Humayun Riaz[3]

[1]*Drugs Control and Traditional Medicines Division, National Institute of Health, Islamabad*

[2]*PTPMA, Karachi,*

[3]*School of Pharmacy, Sargodha University, Islamic Republic of Pakistan*

1. Introduction

The Islamic Republic of Pakistan, with an area of 796095 Km^2 is the sixth largest country of the world and has population of 160 million. Of these 43.2% are less than 15 years, 53.4% from 15-64 and 3.4% 65 plus, with a per capita income of US$ 492. 33 percent of the population lives in the urban areas and 67.0% lives in the rural areas. Its population growth rate is 2.06% (NIPS, 2003).

Over the last few decades, there has been a considerable interest worldwide in Traditional medicine/Complementary and Alternative Medicine (TCAM) particularly in herbal products. The World Health Organization also advocates the important role of alternative and traditional medicines in preventive, promotive and curative health, especially in developing countries and encourages member states to support traditional medicines to and plan for, formulation of policies with appropriate regulations (WHO, 2001).

Major categories of Traditional/Complementary and alternative medicines (TCAM) in vogue in the developing and developed countries are categorized as: whole body systems (Ayurveda, homeopathy, Unani, and Traditional Chinese Medicine); mind-body medicine (meditation, prayer, mental healing); biologically based therapies (use of natural substances, such as herbs, foods, vitamins, dietary supplements, herbal products); manipulative and body-based practices (massage); and energy medicine (Reiki) (Shaikh *et al.*, 2009). In Pakistan traditional medicines have been a strong part of our cultural heritage and playing a significant role in providing health care to a large part of the population. However, there has been lack of concerted efforts for proper utilization of traditional medicines in the health care system. Primarily three categories i.e. Tibb-e-Unani, Ayurveda and Homoeopathy are in vogue whereas Chinese Traditional System, Reiki, Acupuncture and aromatherapy has been introduced in certain parts of the country in the last few years (Malik *et al.*, 2006).

The Government of Pakistan in the last two decades for providing a comprehensive, universal and equitable health care to all Pakistani nationals in line with WHO's goal i.e. " Health for all by 2000" has declared its official policy on TRM as part of National Health Policy. This goal cannot be achieved without utilizing the Traditional and/Complementary and alternative medicines (TCAM) (WHO, 1978). The National Policy of Health, 1997 suggested developing a new curriculum, prerequisite for admissions in Tibba/Homoeopathic Colleges has been changed from Matric (Grade 10) to FSc (Pre-medical i.e. Grade 12) for which the colleges needs affiliation with universities, enactment of a law to cover manufacturing of traditional medicines, strengthening the roles of National Council for Tibb and Homoeopathy and supporting research and development. The policy suggested regulation of traditional medicines practice and education, establishment of pharmaceutical laboratory at federal level and conducting training courses for the collection of medicinal plants. The National Health Policy of 2001 also suggested amendments of Unani, Ayurvedic and Homoeopathic (UAH) Act, 1965 to incorporate degree and post graduate level courses (NHP, 97, 2001) which have now been implemented.

1.1 Tibb-e-Unani

According to basic principles of Tibb-e-Unani (Greco-Arab) body is made up of the four basic elements, which are "earth", "air", "water" and "fire" with different "temperaments" i.e. cold, hot, wet and dry. The body organs get their nourishment through four "humors" i.e. Blood, Phlegm, Yellow Bile and Black Bile. Concept of health in Tibb-e-Unani is a state of body in which there is equilibrium in the "humors" and functions of the body are normal in accordance with its own temperament and the environment. When the equilibrium of the "humors" is disturbed and the functions of body are abnormal, that state is called disease. It takes a holistic approach towards prevention of diseases, cure and promotion of health and relies on drugs made from medicinal plants, herbs, minerals, metallic and animal origin for the treatment of diseases.

Unani system of medicine has its origin in Greece. It is believed to have been established by the great physician and philosopher- Hippocrates (460-377 BC). The Arabian scholars and physicians under the patronage of Islamic rulers of many Arabian countries have played great role in the development of this system. Many disciplines like chemistry, pharmaceutical procedures like distillation, sublimation, calcinations and fermentation were developed and refined by them. The most influential historical figure in this golden era of Unani medicine was Avicenna (980-1037 A.D). His most important medical work was "The cannons of medicine" Al-Qunoon. The present form of Unani medicines greatly owes to him. His book Al-qanoon or (The canon of medicine) was an internationally acclaimed book on medicine, which was taught in European countries till the 17th century. Many physician of Arab descent in Spain have also contributed to the development of the system. Some of the important names are-Abul Qasim Zohravi (Abulcasus 946 – 1036 AD) and he is the author of the famous book on surgery "Al Tasreef"-(http://www.indianmedicine.nac.in).

The Arabs were instrumental in introducing Unani medicine in sub-continent in around 1350 AD. The first known Hakim (Physician) was Zia Mohd Masood Rasheed Zangi. Some of the renowned physicians who were instrumental in development of the system are-Akbar Mohd Akbar Arzani (around 1721 AD)- the author of the books- Qarabadin Qadri and Tibb-e- Akbar; Hakim M. Shareef Khan (1725-1807)- a renowned physician well-known for his book Ilaj ul Amraz. Hakim Ajmal Khan (1864-1927) a great name among the 20th Century Unani physicians. He was a multifaceted personality besides being a physician he was a scientist, politician and a freedom fighter. He was instrumental in the establishment of Unani and Ayurvedic College at Karol Bagh, Delhi. He was a keen researcher and has supervised many studies on Rauwolfia serpentina- the source plant for many well-known alkaloids like reserpine, Ajamaloon etc. Another great contributor is Hakim Kabeeruddin (1894-1976) and had translated 88 Unani books of Arabic and Persian languages into Urdu. The first institution of Unani medicine was established in 1872 as Oriental College at Lahore in the undivided India. Thereafter many institutions came into existence. Practically, Unani medicine is innovative in that it has accepted the challenges like professional practice-patient relations, forms of intervention and disease conceptualization itself. Unani medicine has maintained its popularity in a number of South Asian countries and it account for more than 30% of the total medicinal consumption (Jabin, 2011, Ravishankar and Shukla, 2007, Siddiqui, 2004).

1.2 Homeopathy

Homoeopathy means treating diseases with remedies, prescribed in minute doses, which are capable of producing symptoms similar to the disease when taken by healthy people. It is based on the natural law of healing-" Similia Similibus Curantur " which means " likes are cured by likes". Dr. Samuel Hahnemann (1755-1843) gave it a scientific basis in the early 19th century. Homoeopathic system of medicine was introduced to this part of the subcontinent a little over a century ago and has blended well with the traditional concepts. It has gained tremendous popularity in Islamic Republic of Pakistan. The City of Lahore in Pakistan has the privilege of being the first city of undivided India, where Homoeopathy was introduced by Dr. J. M. Honigberger, a German Physician. The first homoeopathic college of the Punjab was opened in Lahore in early 1920. It was started by an American Missionary, Dr. Freeburn and Maj. Dr. Sadiq Ali. This institution, the Central Homoeopathic Medical College, produced many eminent homoeopaths of Subcontinent. (*www.nchpakistan.com*)

2. Regulation of traditional/complementary and alternative medicines

Traditional/Complementary medicines practiced in Pakistan are regulated under Unani, Ayurvedic and Homoeopathic (UAH) Act of 1965 which has been amended to recognize the degrees Course. The practitioners of these systems have to be registered by their respective councils i.e. National Council for Tibb (NCT) and National Council for Homoeopathy (NCH).

National Council for Tibb (NCT): It is responsible for developing curriculum, education and examination of Tibb-e-Unani and Ayurvedic system of medicine and for registration of Tabibs who have passed the examination. Out of total 22 council members 14 are elected through a process of postal ballot and remaining are nominations from the federal and provincial government, term of members is 5 years. The council members elect the president from amongst themselves. There are approx. 45,799 Hakims / Tabibs and 537 Vaids registered with NCT and about 28 recognized Tibbia colleges (Malik *et al.*, 2005). There are two Universities who are imparting five years BEMS degree along with M. Phil and PhD degrees.

National Council for Homoeopathy (NCH): Like NCT, National Council for Homoeopathy is responsible for developing curriculum, education, examination of Homoeopathic system of medicine and registration of homoeopathic doctors. The council members are elected through the same process as with National Council for Tibb. There are about 118,000 homeopaths registered with NCH and 135 recognized Homeopathic colleges in Pakistan (Malik *et al.*, 2005). There are three Universities who are imparting five years BHMS degree along with M. Phil and PhD degrees.

The bill to regulate the manufacture, storage, import and export of Tibb-e-Unani, Ayurvedic, Homoeopathic, Herbal and Non-allopathic medicines 2010 has been prepared in consultation with the stakeholders of the TRM Sector and is with National Assembly of Pakistan for final enactation very soon. Till today manufacturing is not regulated by any Government body. However manufacturers are self regulating by adopting cGMP (current good manufacturing practices) to ensure safety and quality of their products. The abuse of allopathic medicines by the practitioners or manufacturers is being trialled under Drugs Act of 1976.

3. Trends in use of traditional/complementary and alternative medicines

Traditional/Complementary and Alternative medicines have been practiced in many countries for centuries, including parts of the world where biomedical healthcare is readily available. According to one estimate, around 75-90% of the developing world's population and about half of the industrialized world's population still depend on the complementary and alternative systems of medicine (Robinson and Zhang, 2011). The studies showed that 42% of Americans, 52% of Australians, and between 20% and 65% of Europeans use some form of CAM (Zollman and Vicker, 1999, Maclennan *et al.*, 2004, Ernst, 2000). Estimates of CAM use in Western countries range from about one third to half of the general population (Menniti-ippoliti *et al.*, 2002, Gianelli *et al.*, 2004). In Italy, the proportion has almost doubled during the last decade (14) although it still remains far below the estimates reported in many European countries and the United States. The analysis of data collected in 1999–2000 among the general population by the Italian National Institute for Statistics showed that in Tuscany, 13.6% of adults had made use of CAM in the previous year (Maclennan *et al.*, 1996). In African and other developing countries, up to 80% of the population depends on CAM, including herbal remedies, for health maintenance and therapeutic management of disease (WHO, 2001). The persuasive appeal of CAM is premised on the fundamental assumptions and principles by which the system operates. These include the presumption that CAM modalities are "natural," provide the user with a connection to life-supporting forces (vitalism), have a "scientific basis," and promote "spirituality" as well (Kaptchuk and Eisenberg, 1998). In Pakistan, alternative system of medicines has been considered to be the first line of treatment in rural areas where 80% of the country's population lives.

The overall trend in Pakistan shows that 51.7% chose Traditional and complementary and alternative medicine (TCAM) while 48.3% chose biomedicine. Of those who chose CAM, 20% also used biomedicine as well; 16% homeopathy, 12.4% Unani medicine, 2.1% mind-body medicine (faith healing), 0.9% biologically based practices (home remedies, diet and nutrition) 0.05% energy medicine (Reiki), 0.05% Traditional Chinese Medicine, and 0.02% aromatherapy. About half of the studied population used TCAM. The population estimates of use of TCAM are within the range reported elsewhere. It reflects an increasing popularity of CAM in Pakistan as well. Combined use of biomedicine with TCAM was common and often patients did not reveal the use of TCAM to the biomedicine practitioners (Shaikh *et al.*, 2009).

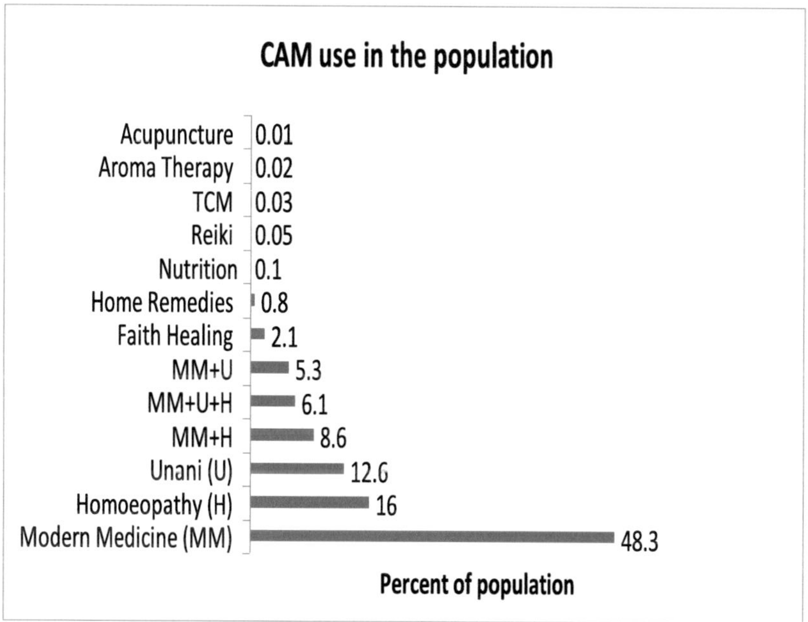

Fig. 1. Source: Shaikh *et al.*, 2009

4. Research and development in traditional/complementary and alternative medicines sector

Pakistan has not been able to develop a coordinated institutional infrastructure and human resource to add value to the medicinal plants resources for its sustainable use of floral wealth. Major research activities on medicinal plant research in Pakistan are on the documenting level. The research is being conducted mainly in universities and that too as ethno-botanical listing of resources. Recently the work on various medicinal plants were carried out in various institutes to establish their antimicrobial, antiplatelet and acetyl-cholinesterase, inhibitory constituents, inflammatory, analgesic, gut modulatory, anti-diarroeal effects and constipation effects (Malik *et al.*, 2010, 2011, Ghayur *et al.*, 2011, Ahmad and Gilani, 2011, Khan *et al.*, 2011, Bashir *et al.*, 2011, Mahmood *et al.*, 2011).

Some of the institutions involved in research of various aspects of medical plants are as follows,

Taxonomy, collection, herbarium

i. Pakistan Forest Institute, Peshawar
ii. National Agriculture and Research Council, Islamabad.
iii. Quaid-i-Azam University, Islamabad.
iv. Pakistan Museum of Natural History, Islamabad.
v. National Institute of Health, Islamabad.

vi. Herbarium, University of Karachi, Karachi.
vii. Hamdard University, Bait-ul-Hikmah, Karachi
viii. Botany Department of Various Universities of Pakistan

Phyto-chemistry

i. International Center for Chemical Research, Institute of Chemistry, University of Karachi;
ii. Pakistan Council for Scientific and Industrial Laboratories, Peshawar
iii. Chemistry and Pharmacology Departments of various Universities of Pakistan

Pharmacology

i. National Institute of Health, Islamabad.
ii. HEJ Research Institute, University of Karachi, Karachi
iii. The Aga Khan Medical University, Karachi.
iv. Hamdard University, Karachi.
v. University of Agriculture, Faisalabad.
vi. University of Veterinary and Animal Sciences, Lahore.
vii. University of Agriculture, Peshawar.
viii. Pharmacology and Pharmacognosy Departments of various Universities of Pakistan.
ix. Al-Majeed College of Eastern Medicines, Hamdard University, Karachi

Ethno-Botany Data Base

i. Pakistan Forest Institute, Peshawar, KPK
ii. Botany Departments of various Universities of Pakistan
iii. Hamdard University, Karachi

Standardization, Quality Control and Safety Assurance

i. National Institute of Health, Islamabad.
ii. Hamdard University, Karachi
iii. Pharmacognosy Department, University of Karachi, Karachi.
iv. HEJ Research Institute, University of Karachi, Karachi.

Medicinal Plants Cultivation, Tissue Culture

i. Hamdard University Karachi.
ii. National Institute of Health, Islamabad.
iii. Qarshi Industries, Hattar.
iv. University of Malakand, KPK.
v. PMNH, Islamabad.
vi. Hamdard Laboratories, Karachi.
vii. PARC, Islamabad
viii. NARC, Islamabad

Propagation

i. University of Malakand, KPK
ii. NARC, Islamabad.
iii. NIBGE, Faisalabad.

iv. NIAB, Faisalabad.
v. PCSIR laboratories, Karachi

Conservation

i. Forest Department, Peshawar, KPK.
ii. MACP, Pakistan
iii. WWF, Pakistan
iv. IUCN, Pakistan
v. SDC/IC, Pakistan
vi. AKRSP, Pakistan
vii. Palas Conservation and Development Project (PCDP) Kohistan, KPK, Pakistan

5. Intellectual property rights and protection of indigenous knowledge

Intellectual property (IP) has been considered a fundamental human right for all people since the adoption of the Universal Declaration of Human Rights (UDHR) in 1948. Article 27 of the Declaration states that everyone has the right "to the protection of the moral and material interests resulting from any scientific, literary or artistic production of which he is the author." Since 1948, many international human rights instruments and documents have reinforced the importance of IP as a human right. The importance of TCAM in developing countries cannot be overemphasized, as indigenous people cannot survive or exercise their fundamental human rights as distinct nations, societies and people without the ability to conserve, revive, develop and teach the wisdom they have inherited from their ancestors.

Natural resources are open to exploitation from within and outside the country. Thus commercial activities may lead to problems of access to medicine, loss of biodiversity, extinction of the endangered species and destruction of natural habitats and resources. If TRM are patented and fall into private ownership, people would be deprived of the only accessible and affordable source of medicine needed to protect health. Already patenting of some of the material indigenous to this subcontinent has been patented in the West endangering accessibility to this lifesaving material to the native population. The Trade Related Intellectual Property Rights (TRIPS) agreement does not adequately safeguard against such misuse of indigenous resources of the country in a foreign country. This is thus a critical issue for developing country where a large population still relies heavily on the TCAM. Unjustified patent protection can result in affordability problem for the people mainly due to higher prices which obviously would be the outcome. In various WHO workshops participants have urged countries to investigate all available ways and means of protecting such knowledge and TCAM products from abuse. Documentation, national legislation and bilateral agreements are some of the safeguards. However, collection, compilation for documentation of traditional knowledge and products and their wide publication is the most effective way of preventing their misuse by not allowing their patents for not having fulfilled the patentability criteria.

Thus under the implications of WTO/TRIPS protection of indigenous knowledge of traditional medicines is extremely vital for Pakistan in order to ensure continued availability of traditional medicine resources at affordable cost. Pakistan's patent ordinance does not allow patenting of plant materials, but this may not be enough to address the threat from outside. There is still lack of awareness in government and public sector about TRIPS Agreement and its implications. Stake holder's needs to be educated about mechanisms for patenting their products and awareness about protection of indigenous knowledge. Hussain and Malik (2006, 2009, and 2010) from time to time have proposed various strategies in order to obtain following objectives;

- Protection of indigenous knowledge and medicinal plant resources in Pakistan.
- Continued availability of cost effective traditional medicine products and services.
- Awareness about Trade Related Intellectual Property Rights (TRIPS) Agreement and Patent Laws in all concerned.

6. Medicinal plants: Sustainable cultivation, collection and use

Pakistan has an area of 80,943 km2, lies between 60° 55′ to 75° 30′ E longitude and 23° 45′ to 36° 50′ N latitude and an altitude ranging from 0 to 8611 m. Therefore, has a variety of climatic zones and a unique biodiversity. It has about 6,000 species of higher plants. It has been reported that 600 to 700 species are used for medicinal purposes. It has also been estimated that 70% of the total species are uni-regional and about 30% are bi-or pluri-regional (Shinwari, 2010). The country has four phyto-geographical regions:

i. Irano-Turanian (45% of species)
ii. Sino-Himalayan (10%)
iii. Saharo-Sindian (9.5%)
iv. Indian element (6%).

Despite the Saharo-Sindian Region being the biggest area, the diversity of species confined to this area is lowest for any phyto-geographical region (Ali and Qaiser, 1986). The local communities of different regions of Pakistan have centuries old knowledge about traditional uses of the plants occurring in their areas. This indigenous knowledge of plants has been transferred from generation to generation. These plants are used to treat almost any kind of disease from headache to Stomachic to cut and wound (Bhardwaj and Gakhar, 2005). Some of the important plants are commercially harvested for extraction of various types of active ingredients. Though different systems of Unani, Ayurvedic (Eastern medicines) are largely based on the medicinal properties of plants, yet the precious wealth of indigenous knowledge is in danger of being lost. The use of traditional knowledge also reflects the values embedded in the traditions upheld by elders, especially with regard to medicine. Medicinal plants practitioners know that respecting Plants is often essential to the efficacy of medicines, which should not be seen as 'miracle' cures based on chemical compounds, but due to curative energy that draws its medicinal qualities founded on a relationship between the plants and the people (Juden, 2003). There are few educational institutes where they are studying practical implications of medicinal plants. Major reason of use of plants as medicines is that medicinal plants contain synergistic and/or side-effects neutralizing combinations (Gilani and Atta-ur-Rahman, 2005). There is also a concern about the harmful effects of synthetic chemicals; hence, trends are changing towards natural products. Besides the research based activities, the medicinal plants from the wild resources are also exploited for commercial purposes which lead to the endangerment of species in their respective habitats. Though these medicinal plants are also important sources of income for poor people as well as for herbal dealers, and exporters but still no cultivation practices for these medicinal plants are observed in Pakistan.

6.1 Major issues pertaining to medicinal plants cultivation and conservation

The major issues that the medicinal plants face in Pakistan, besides the prospects of cultivation and conservation are as follows;

i. Increased global demand of herbal medicines and current status

Globally, there is a rising trend to shift resources from allopathic to traditional healthcare systems. The global market estimates to surge US$ 5 trillion by 2050. Twelve percent of Pakistani flora is used in medicines and more than 300 medicinal plants are traded. Ten leading Dawakhanas (Herbal manufacturers) of Pakistan annually consume more than 2 million kg of 200 medicinal plants in 1990s while its consumption increased multifold in the last two decades. According to an estimate, 22 species of medicinal plants worth Rs.14.733 million were traded in 1990 while in 2002, this value rose to more than Rs.122 million, an eight-and-a-half times increase. In 1990, 95 species were consumed worth Rs. 36 million while in 2002, medicinal plants worth Rs. 218 million were consumed: a six-fold increase (Shinwari *et al.*, 2002). Shinwari *et al.* (2006) published a "pictorial guide of medicinal plants of Pakistan" enlisting more than 500 species of flowering plants, being used as medicine. It has also been reported that nearly 37% (266 species) of the total of 709 endangered species are endemic to Pakistan. Endemic species may also be explored for ethnobotanical, pharmacological and pharmaceutical activities (Shinwari, 2010).

Hence there is a global need to cultivate and conserve medicinal plants. In Russia 50,000 tons of medicinal plants are used annually of which, 50% are cultivated. In Lucknow (India) medicinal plants worth Rs.90 million are grown annually. European Union (EU) uses 3,000 kg of Glycerrhiza each year for which 400 tons plant roots are needed. In China, in the year 2000, the total output value of the pharmaceutical industry was 233 billion yuan (28 billion US$). By the year 2010, the share of traditional Chinese medicine in the international market of herbal medicine was projected to improve to 15% from the existing 3%. Unfortunately in Pakistan not enough emphasis has been given to the cultivation of medicinal plants (Shinwari, 2010). Recently, the Government of Pakistan through Ministry of Food Agriculture and Livestock (MINFAL) has started a project entitled as "Production of Medicinal Herbs in Collaboration with Private Sectors" (PMHPS) in July 2006 to promote the cultivation of medicinal herbs and spices plants as crop in Pakistan. The project has focused the production of medicinal herbs on commercial scale through research based technology package oriented to World Health Organization (WHO) guideline of good agriculture, collection and processing practices (Aslam, 2008).

ii. Causes of threats to existence of medicinal plants in Pakistan

The hotspots of medicinal plants in Pakistan are spread over 13 Natural Regions from alpine pastures to mangrove forest. More than 10% of the flora is endangered (Shinwari *et al.*, 2000, 2002). Reasons of endangerment includes population pressure, poverty and poor quality of the natural resource-base, breakdown of social institutions, lack of land use plans and lack of enforcement of existing rules in whatever form these are. In addition rapid infrastructural development (roads, building construction), deforestation, spread of irrigation system, pollution and to top it all, the destructive activities of the colossal influx of the Afghan refugees also contribute in threatening the medicinal plants

Over-harvesting of medicinal plants for commercial purposes and chemical analysis has also threatened their abundance, and even occurrence. Human pressure has also caused fragmentation of populations (Gilani *et al.*, 2009).

iii. Policy issues in relation to promoting large scale cultivation and conservation

Almost all the medicinal plants in Pakistan are collected from the wild. Local collectors are unaware of the best collection procedures. Medicinal plants from the sites of collection to the national and international markets pass through various middlemen. Consequently, the prices of the crude drugs increase more than 100% along the trade chain. The rapid loss of floristic and cultural diversity, and the state of absolute material poverty of 30% of people in Pakistan, makes it urgent that we should find solutions to their problems and to take active roles in making decisions about the management of natural resources and about the legal status of their traditions and knowledge.

The sustainable supply of good quality medicinal plants can only be made possible through proper collection, conservation and cultivation. The following strategies have been proposed to achieve the objectives such as to carry out mapping regarding availability of medicinal plant growth in wild for their sustainable supply, improve the quality of the source materials, this in turn would improve the quality, safety and efficacy of subsequent finished traditional medicines, encourage and support the cultivation of quality medicinal plants on commercial scale for their continued availability, promote environmental protection and conservation of medicinal plants, introducing guidelines on Good Agricultural and Field Collection Practices for medicinal plants and to promote organic agriculture for the promotion of healthy living.

7. Challenges faced by system: Global viz-a-viz Pakistan

The last few decades have seen certain national and international policies for preserving and promoting traditional medicine sector but the progress of their implementation has been rather sluggish. Furthermore, these policies fail to redress a number of concerns related to traditional medicines such as education, safety, efficacy, quality, rational use, availability, preservation and development of such health care, sustainable use of natural resources and assuring equity in transactions at various levels and so on (WHO, 2002, Bodeker *et al.*, 2007). The traditional medicines sector not only in Pakistan but also globally is confronted with challenges like recognition, uniform quality standard, education standards, evidence based research, safety and efficacy, rational use, herbal and drug interactions, inadequate understanding of socio-cultural context of their practice and usage, protection of intellectual property rights of knowledge holders, assuring sustainable natural resource use, regulation and capacity building of non-formal practitioners, developing appropriate methodologies for evaluation, resolving conflicts with mainstream medicine.

1. Recognition

It is necessary that Traditional Medicines (TRM) are recognized, respected and endorsed by governments for full actualization of their potential. The World Health Organization has defined three types of health systems to describe the degree to which TCAM is an officially recognized element of healthcare: the Integrative system, the inclusive system and the tolerant system (WHO, 2002).

Integration is currently being practiced in China, the Koreas, Viet Nam and supported by Australia (Cohen, 2004). China, India, Canada, Nigeria, Mali and UK among others, provide Governmental support to strengthen training; research and the use of TRM in their national healthcare strategies (Patwardhan *et al.*, 2005, 2006). Similar practices are also observed in other parts of the world, including the EU and the Americas. The WHO Global Atlas of TM/CAM remains an excellent information and reference resource

2. Education standards

It is becoming important to educate medical students and registered medical practitioners about TCAM therapies (Brooks, 2004). Two important dimensions have been identified in traditional medicines education. The first one is to ensure that the knowledge, qualifications and training of traditional medicines practitioners are adequate. Secondly, there should be good understanding between traditional medicines practitioners and that of conventional or biomedicine practitioners. In many developing countries informal, experiential learning by apprenticing with physicians continues to be the major trend. All of them have their own attendant issues. Little attention has been paid by allopathic students when it is integrated into their curriculum, a university level formal education for traditional medicines makes it difficult to transfer many of the experience based aspects of tradition in an institutional milieu. For example pulse diagnosis or the understanding of vital points or certain non physical methods of treatments are seldom taught today. Recently, the Traditional Medicines, Department of Health System Governance and Service Delivery, World Health Organization (WHO, 2010), Geneva, Switzerland has developed Benchmarks for training in Unani Medicines, Ayurveda, Nuad Thai, Traditional Chinese Medicines, Naturopathy and Tuina.

3. Safety, efficacy and quality standards of traditional medicines

The uniformity in the composition of the active constituents of the medicinal plants is not possible owing to different collection places of origin along with time of collection, process of storage, drying etc. It reflects inconsistent quality of the pharmacologically active secondary metabolites that is not desired. Hence efficacy of traditional medicines is a concern as sufficient scientific data is not available to support its use worldwide (WHO, 2002). There are two aspects of safety evaluations: Firstly, to ensure right quality of material and right processes; secondly to ascertain that there is no contamination, adulteration or spiking. There are reports that steroids, heavy metals and other allopathic ingredients are found in herbal preparation (Keane, 1999, Saper *et al.*, 2004). Such studies are wrongly used to limit the use of TCAM. In fact, such a QC failure should not create a bias against TCAM. Various reasons are attributed to these, such as malpractice, lack of documentation, non-appropriate policies and lack of standardized research methodologies. It is argued that modern medicine emphasizes on a scientific approach, while traditional medicine have developed rather differently with much influence by the culture and historical context in which they first evolved. Their principles, concepts and practice are quite different from those of Western biomedicine (Shankar *et al.* 2006). They generally tend to focus on a holistic approach to life, equilibrium between mind and body and environment and to adopt a preventive approach (WHO, 2002) thus making it difficult to develop appropriate methodologies without harming these unique features. Furthermore, issues such as chemical complexity of multiple plant based formulations are also challenges for developing a suitable methodology for research.

There is a general perception and understanding that herbal medicines are safe. However reports of toxicity in traditional medicines have been a matter of grave concern. Effective quality control and regulation are certainly needed without limiting public access to these preparations or resorting to restrictive trade practice, at the same time ensuring public interest (Patwardhan, 2005). Standardization of several aspects such as nomenclature of medicinal plants and other resources, their collection practices, semi processes and final processing, packaging, preservation, storage, product life, labeling and modes of distribution including clinical application are needed to ensure quality, safety and efficacy of traditional medicines.

4 Rational prescribing and use

Information, education and communication are three major pillars of rational use. Qualification and licensing of providers, proper use of products of assured quality, good communication between traditional medicines providers, allopathic practitioners as well as patients and provision of scientific information and guidance for public are some of the key challenges in assuring rational use (WHO, 2002).

5. Herbal and drug interactions

Herbal Medicines are readily available in the market from health food stores without prescriptions and are widely used in Pakistan and all over the world. According to recent survey the majority of people who use herbal medicines do not inform their physicians about their consumption that can cause abnormal test results and confusion in proper diagnosis. Drug herb interactions can results in unexpected concentration of therapeutic drug. Several herbal products interfere with immunoassays used for monitoring the concentrations of therapeutic drugs. Herbal medicines can also cause undesired effects. Therefore, the common belief that anything natural is safe is not correct. Contrary to popular belief that "natural are safe", herbal medicines can cause significant toxic effects, drug interaction and even morbidity or mortality (Pamer, 2005). Some of the reported drug-herbal medicines interactions are as follows;

a. Ginseng and Warfarin may decrease effectiveness
b. Ginseng and Thenelzine produce toxic symptoms e.g. headache insomnia and irritability,
c. St. John's Wort and Paroxetine hydrochloride produce Lethargy, Nausea
d. St. John's Wort and Theophylline lower concentration and efficacy
e. St. John's Wort and Indinavir lower concentration and may cause treatment failure in HIV patients.
f. Ginkgo Biloba and Aspirin produce Bleeding, can inhibit PAF
g. Ginkgo Biloba and Warfarin can cause hemorrhage
h. Ginkgo-Biioba and Thiazide: Hypertension.
i. Kava and Alprazolam Addictive effects with CNS depressants.
j. Alcohol, Garlic and Warfarin can increase effectiveness of Warfarin

6. Access and cost effectiveness

In developing countries over 50% of deaths are attributed to five infectious diseases. Common communicable diseases are widely prevalent in areas where access to modern drugs is non-existent or limited (WHO, 2002). In the developing countries traditional medicines continues to be comparatively cost effective and accessible though it is feared that a technology intensive production process would make traditional medicines unaffordable.

For the health sector to improve, measures such as improving physical and economic access, preventive strategies, wellness management, promotion of best and essential practices in both communicable and chronic diseases, increased cooperation between various medical systems, sustainable natural resource use, protection of traditional medicines and knowledge, and equitable transactions are vital.

7. Evidence based medicines (EBM) or scientific evidence

The Scientific Evidence or Evidence Based Medicines (EBM) has emerged as an important dimension in modern medical care. The modernist attitude towards traditional knowledge has been as 'either modernize or disappear'. In a context where the mightiest comes to be identified with the best reason (Couze and Featherstone 2006), traditional medicine is in a challenging process of proving itself through a completely different epistemology. However public preferences are moving in a direction where science is not the starting point for health decision making (Terasawa, 2004, Janska, 2005). It is feared that imposition of EBM, research on selected aspects of traditional medicines through randomized controlled studies, and the absorption of successful practices as evidence based 'modern' medicine would result in medical absorption and finally resulting in an erosion of 'alternate' approaches to health.

8. Ecological obligation

The significance of this concern becomes evident in connection with the discussion of article 8(j) of the Convention on Biological Diversity 1992, where it is implied that medicinal plants, blood samples from indigenous people and research conducted by foreigners into indigenous ways of life, supported by indigenous possessors of traditional knowledge, have led to patentable discoveries of benefit solely to those foreign researchers, with no economic return to indigenous people themselves. The traditional medical knowledge of indigenous peoples throughout the world played an important role in identifying biological resources worthy of commercial exploitation. Knowledge about the way in which local people have used plants has always been important to collectors. Unfortunately, no international system has yet successfully designed and implemented a mechanism that provides for an effective legal protection to traditional knowledge holders' rights at the international level (UNESCO/WIPO, 1999, Burgland, 2005).

9. Value addition

The herbal materials are usually supplied in unprocessed form to the dealers. However, if the plants are processed into a consumer usable form, the value added product would fetch higher income as compared to the raw material.

10. Intercultural approach

In the promotion of traditional and complementary and alternative medicines in the contemporary context it is essential to have an intercultural approach. As mentioned earlier traditional medical knowledge in various countries have evolved within socio-cultural and historical context and their epistemic framework, principles, concepts and practice are quite different from those of modern science (WHO, 2002, Shankar *et al.*, 2007). While there is a contemporary value in applying modern science and technology tools for creating objective and verifiable standards for traditional knowledge products and concepts. Currently the approach to creating standards is one-sided, because it does not adequately consult the available qualitative TCAM standards and parameters. Furthermore, most therapies in traditional medicines involve both drug as well as non-drug interventions (Shankar *et al.*, 2007) making it complex to develop appropriate methodology.

Some additional challenges faced by Traditional Medicines System in Pakistan are as under;

- Market Demand is unknown
- Absence of regulatory environment and framework i.e., Traditional medicines Act, Policy, Strategy, Action Plan, Dwindling resources, R&D Facilities, Infrastructure and allocation of appropriate financial resources

8. Prospects and limitations of the system

8.1 Prospects

There has been significant paradigm shift at the policy level in terms of Traditional and Alternative medicines regulation in Pakistan. The Government has in place a number of organizations and initiatives aimed at strengthening the infrastructure and coordinating various aspects of the sector, supplemented by non-government organizations (NGOs) and private sector cooperation and initiatives. However, political will, stronger coordination of the sector at the national level under a long term strategic action plan has become imperative. Approximately 40539 registered Unani and 118,000 homoeopathic medical practitioners are practicing both in the public and private sector in urban and rural areas. About 360 tibb dispensaries and clinics provide free medication to the public under the control of the health departments of provincial governments (Shaikh *et al.*, 2009).

People have been consulting traditional healers for ages and they will keep on doing so for various reasons. The solution lies only in bringing these traditional medicines healers into the mainstream health infrastructure by providing them with proper training, facilities and back-up for referral. The regulatory authorities and policy makers have to play a crucial role in this scenario, in terms of recognition of traditional medicines and their role, financing and appreciating training and research in this field. The inclusion of some courses in line with WHO Guidelines, 2010 about various Traditional/ Complementary medicines into the medical curriculum of pharmacy and allopathic medical schools may be considered. A positive interaction between all stakeholders of health care providers, academicians, policy makers and researchers has to be initiated to work for a common goal to improve the health of the people. It is important to note that as the global use of healing practices outside conventional medicine is on the rise, ignorance about these practices by physicians and scientists risks broadening the communication gap between the public and the profession that serves them (Wetzel *et al.*, 1998, Chez and Jonas, 1997). The National Institute of Health, Islamabad, Pakistan has conducted many workshops in order to harmonize modern and Traditional medicines Sector in the region (Hussain and Malik, 2010).

The integration of the two systems at least in terms of evidence-based information sharing is necessary. It would also be worthwhile to emphasize that regular systematic review of traditional medicines therapies are imperative in the process of recognizing the traditional medicines sector. In order to achieve ambitious and gigantic targets in Millennium Development Goals, gross improvements in quality and efficacy of medical care would require strengthening and integration of public health programs (World Bank, 2004).

Evidence based traditional medicines should be accessible and cost-effective for the people at primary health care level of developing countries and, more importantly, the outcomes of the treatments could be very efficacious (Cooper, 2004). Moreover, financial allocation and distribution on the basis of research and evidence would be another important change to bring about in order to reduce the disease burden. Through more rigorous research, the evidence based recommendation of some traditional medicines therapies and the evidence-based rejection of others will become more definitive (Eisenberg *et al.*, 2002). Today, in the West, there is an overwhelming effort towards integration of alternative medicine with the mainstream allopathic therapeutics, Pakistan being no exception (WHO, 2001). However, before this can be done, research into traditional medicines itself needs to be recognized as a mainstay to design any public health interventions (Travis *et al.*, 2004). Guidelines for policy formulation, regulation, promotion and development of traditional medicine need to be developed. With the current state of affairs of health system utilization and health-seeking behavior in Pakistan, it is highly desirable to reduce the polarization in health system utilization by exploring more opportunities for integration of traditional and modern medicine. For instance, conservation and sustainable utilization of resources can be achieved through community participation. Non-governmental organizations need to be involved in bio-prospecting and benefit sharing (Gilani, 1992). A true partnership would make an invaluable contribution towards achieving the goals of environmental and biodiversity conservation; and an increased share of international trade in raw materials relating to medicinal plants. This would require the implementation of government policies and incentives for the exporters (Fink, 2002). A close collaboration among all stakeholders including allopathic practitioners, traditional medicine practitioners, ethno-botanists, phytochemists, pharmacologists, agricultural experts and other related disciplines would be encouraging.

8.2 Limitations

The relationship between the conventional allopathic physician and the traditional medicines provider is of rivalry and animosity, just as happens in any other part of the world (Fink, 2002). Orthodox medicine has never been in favor of traditional medicine; therefore, these practices are denounced vigorously by restricting their access, labeling them as antiscientific and imposing penalties on their practice.

Some understandable factors for this rejection include lack of education, training, regulation and the evidence base for traditional medicines practitioners. Moreover, lack of accountability in the medical profession, both modern and complementary, results in untrained quacks practicing medicine in different names, thus giving traditional medicines practitioners a bad name and lowering respect for them in the community. In terms of political economy, the allopathic system of cure is a British colonial legacy that retained influence on the entire health care system of the country. With this elite backed system, the attitude of looking down on the indigenous systems has been coupled with an established antagonism between the practitioners of the two systems (Zaidi, 1988). Current evidence, although limited, suggests that physicians may reasonably accept some traditional medicines therapies as adjuncts to conventional care and discourage others. The National health policy of Pakistan just mentions a plan to bring amendment to the existing law on tibb to recognize the post-graduate level education; however, the stance on its integration or development is unclear (NHP, 2001). Other policy documents bear certain lacunae on profit sharing, intellectual property rights, registration of herbal products and other related legislation (Gilani, 1992). The traditional medicines therapies being used have not been thoroughly researched, and by and large there is only evidence from old documents. Furthermore, indigenous people have no training in gathering and storing of medicinal plants, and hence the sustainability of such plants is threatened. The indigenous knowledge of identification and use of medicinal herbs is dying out. Deforestation and threat of extinction is also alarming because the area covered by forests is decreasing day by day due to lack of water and repeated droughts.

9. Conclusion

The health care system the world over and more so in developing countries, seems to have become more complex in the last half century, quite contrary to the astonishing advances in medical sciences and technologies. Increase of chronic diseases, awareness about limitations of modern medicine, proven efficacy of TCAM systems in selected conditions, emerging interest in holistic preventive health, integrated approach to medical education and increasing awareness among physicians are some of the reasons for renewed interest in traditional medicine. Against modern medicine, TMs may not appear much but they are like catalysts and enzymes in biological processes - small in size and amount but beacons and guides to macro-processes. It is hoped that researchers, policy makers and practitioners will see the pivotal place of TCAM in the global health-care system and use them wisely to enable the peoples to alleviate their miseries due to number of diseases.

The people of Islamic Republic of Pakistan have a great faith in TCAM, which has thousands of year's history. The practice/prescriptions are traditionally and empirically passed from generation to generations despite relatively less research in the modern era, concerted efforts have been made to revive to improve and promote the TCAM by introducing change in the education and bring reforms in the policy of sale, storage, import and export of TCAM. Commitments have been shown by the Government to bring it into main health care system in spite of numerous challenges being confronted by TCAM.

Among the measures taken to revive and promote the system are as follows;

i. Development of proposals for National Policy on Traditional Medicines
ii. Finalization of Master Plan for the implementation of National Policy on TRM
iii. An ACT named "Tibb-e-Unani, Ayurvedic, Homoeopathic, Herbal and Bio-chemic Medicines drugs 2010" to regulate the manufacture, storage, import and export of Traditional Medicines has been approved by the Federal Cabinet and Standing Committee on Health of the National assembly and will be enacted very soon.
iv. Development of standards and specifications for medicinal plants are in progress.
v. Following documents has been developed in consultation with the stakeholders;

   a. Guidelines for Good Agriculture and Field Collection Practices
   b. Manual for training of collectors for the collection of medicinal plants.
   c. Manual for sustainable cultivation, preservation, propagation and collection of medicinal plants
   d. Manual for the conduction of clinical trials on traditional medicines
   e. Manual containing GMP and QA guidelines for the Traditional Medicines.

vi. Monographs of commonly used medicinal plants vol-1
vii. Inventory of the commonly used medicinal plants in Pakistan.
viii. List of essential TRM for use at Primary Health Care level.

There is a need to foster effective collaboration between allopathic and traditional health practitioners along with research institutes, universities and close collaboration amongst traditional health practitioners associations. The creation of information network on TCAM and monitoring of emerging trends will help collection of data and subsequent analysis. The above measures will help promote the scientific and rational integration of TCAM into main health care system especially at primary health care level.

10. References

Ali SI, Qaiser M (1986). A Phytogeographical Analysis of the Phanerogames of Pakistan and Kashmir. Proc. R. Soc. Edinburg 89B: 89- 101.

Ahmed T, Gilani AH. (2011). A comparative study of curcuminoids to measure their effect on inflammatory and apoptotic gene expression in an Aβ plus ibotenic acid-infused rat model of Alzheimer's disease. Brain Res. Jul 11;1400 :1-18.

Aslam M. (2009). Annual Report (2007-2008) on Production of Medicinal Herbs in Collaboration with Private Sector (PMHPS). Ministry of Food, Agriculture and Livestock, Islamabad, Pakistan

Bashir S, Memon R, Gilani AH. (2011). Antispasmodic and Antidiarrheal Activities of Valeriana hardwickii Wall. Rhizome Are Putatively Mediated through Calcium Channel Blockade. Evid Based Complement Alternat Med. 304960. Epub 2011 Mar 3.

Bhardwaj S, Ghakar SK (2005) Ethnomedicinal plants used by the tribals of Mizoram to cure cut and wound. Indian Journal of Traditional Knowledge 4(1): 75-80.

Bodeker G., Kronenberg F., Burford G. Policy and public health perspectives in traditional, complementary and alternative medicine: An overview. In: Bodeker G., Burford G., editors. *Traditional, complementary and alternative medicine. Policy and public health perspectives.* London: Imperial College Press; 2007. pp. 9–40.

Brooks PM (2004). Undergraduate teaching of complementary medicine. Medical Journal of Australia, Vol. 181 (5), pp 274-75

Burgland M (2005). The protection of Traditional Knowledge related to Genetic resources, *SCRIPT-ed*, Vol. 2 (2), pp 243-263.

Chez I, Jonas W (1997). The challenge of complementary and alternative medicine. *Am J Obstet Gynecol* 177:1156–61.

Cohen, A. M., Stavri, P. A. & Hersh, W. R. (2004). A categorization and analysis of the criticism of evidence-based medicine. *International Journal of Medical Informatics*, 73, 35–43.

Cooper EL (2004). Complementary and alternative medicine, when rigorous, can be science. *eCAM* ;1:1–4.

Couze V and Featherstone M. (2006). Problematizing Global Knowledge and the New Encyclopaedia Project: An Introduction. Theory, Culture & Society May. 23: 1-20,

Eisenberg DM, Davis RB, Ettner SL, et al. (1998). Trends in alternative medicine use in the United States, 1990–1997: results of a follow-up national survey. *JAMA*. 280:1569–1575.

Eisenberg DM, Ted J, Kaptchuck T. (2002). Advising patients who seek complementary and alternative therapies for cancer. *Ann Intern Med*;137: 889–903.

Ernst E. (2000). The role of complementary and alternative medicine. BMJ; 321:1133–1135.

Farkhunda Jabin. (2011). A GUIDING TOOL IN UNANI TIBB FOR MAINTENANCE AND PRESERVATION OF HEALTH: A REVIEW STUDY. Afr J Tradit Complement Altern Med. 8(S):140-143 140

Fink S. (2002). International efforts spotlight traditional, complementary, and alternative medicine. *Am J Publ Health* 2002;92:1734–9.

Giannelli M, Cuttini M, Arniani S, et al. (2004). Complementary and alternative medicine in Tuscany: Attitudes and use among the general population. Epidemiol Prev. 28:27–33.

Ghayur MN, Kazim SF, Rasheed H, Khalid A, Jumani MI, Choudhary MI, Gilani AH. Zhong Xi Yi Jie He Xue Bao. (2011). Identification of antiplatelet and acetylcholinesterase inhibitory constituents in betel nut Jun; 9(6):619-25.

Gilani A. (1992). Phytotherapy—the role of natural products in modern medicine. *J Pharm Me* ; 2:111–8.

Gilani AH, Atta-ur-Rahman. (2005). Trends in ethnopharmacology. J. Ethnopharmacol. 100: 43-49.

Gilani SA, Kikuchi A, Watanabe KN. (2009). Genetic variation within and among fragmented populations of endangered medicinal plant, *Withania coagulans* (Solanaceae) from Pakistan and its implications for conservation. Afr. J. Biotech. 8: 2948-2958.

Hussain S, Malik F. (2006). Non-Traditional Forms of IP: Protection of Traditional Knowledge, Folklore and framework access to genetic resources. WIPO roundtable on formulation and implementation of National Intellectual Property Strategy, Islamabad, Pakistan 16-18 August.

Hussain S, Malik F. (2006). Protection of Traditional Medicines and Knowledge: Rationale, Access benefit sharing and prior informed consent. Seminar on "Opportunities for Pakistan's Pharmaceutical Sector under WTO regime, 13th September, Lahore, Pakistan

Hussain S, Malik F. (2009). IPRs and Traditional Medicines and Knowledge: An Overview : National Workshop to educate the stakeholders about the implications of TRIPs/WTO at NIH, Islamabad, October.

Hussain S, Malik F. (2009). Protection of Traditional Knowledge and Traditional Medicines: Consultative workshop on Laws related to Plant Genetic Resources and Seed with focus on Access Benefit Sharing (ABS) and Prior Informed Consent (PIC), 12th September Islamabad- Pakistan. Organized by SDPI in collaboration with Ministry of Environment

Hussain S, Malik F. (2010). Intellectual Property Rights: History, International Framework and Controversial Patents. National Workshop to educate the stakeholders about the implications of TRIPs/WTO, Hamdard University, Karachi, 8-9 November.

Hussain S, Malik F. (2010). Harmonization of Modern and Traditional Medicines System: An overview. National Workshop to harmonize Traditional and Modern system of medicines. National Institute of Health,Islamabad-Pakistan.

Hussain. SA, Saeed. A, Ahmed. M, Qazi. A. (2011). Contemporary role and future prospects of medicinal plants in the health care system and pharmaceutical industries of Pakistan. URL http://www.telmedpak.com/doctorsarticles. [accessed on 6/5/2011.

Janska Emilia. (2005). "What Role Should Traditional Medicine Play in Public Health Policy?" UNU-IAS Working Paper No. 142

Juden LK (2003). Spiritual link is part of traditional knowledge. Nature 421: 313.

Kaptchuk TJ, Eisenberg DM. (1998). The persuasive appeal of alternative medicine. Ann Intern Med 129:1061–1065.

Khan S, Mehmood MH, Ali AN, Ahmed FS, Dar A, Gilani AH. (2011). Studies on anti-inflammatory and analgesic activities of betel nut in rodents. J Ethnopharmacol. Jun 1;135 (3):654-61.

Khan AU, Ali F, Khan D, Gilani AH. (2011). Gut modulatory effects of Daphne oleoides are mediated through cholinergic and Ca(++) antagonist mechanisms. Pharm Biol. Aug; 49(8):821-5.

Keane FM. (1999). Analysis of Chinese herbal creams prescribed for dermatological conditions. British Medical Journal. Vol. 318, pp 563-564.

MacLennan AH, Wilson DH, Taylor AW. (2006). The continuing use of complementary and alternative medicine in South Australia: Costs and beliefs in 2004. Med J Aust. 184:27–31.

Malik F, Hussain S, Dil AS , Hannan A, Gilani AH. (2005). Islamic Republic of Pakistan. Chapter 22, In: Ong CK, Bodeker G, Grundy C, Burford G, Shein K, editors. WHO Global Atlas of Traditional, Complementary and Alternative Medicine (Map volume). Geneva : WHO. p. 275-283.

Malik F, Mirza T, Riaz H, Hameed A and Hussain S. (2010). Biological screening of seventeen medicinal plants used in the traditional systems of medicine in Pakistan for antimicrobial activities. African Journal of Pharmacy and Pharmacology Vol. 4(6), pp. 335-340, June

Malik F, Hussain S, Mirza T, Hameed A, Ahmad S, Usmanghani K. (2011). Screening for antimicrobial activity of thirty three medicinal plants used in the traditional system of medicine in Pakistan (Journal of Medicinal plants Research 18th July, 2011)

Mehmood MH, Aziz N, Ghayur MN, Gilani AH. (2011) Pharmacological basis for the medicinal use of psyllium husk (Ispaghula) in constipation and diarrhea. Dig Dis Sci. May; 56(5). 1460-71.

Menniti-Ippolito F, Gargiulo L, Bologna E, et al. (2002). Use of unconventional medicine in Italy: A nation-wide survey. Eur J Clin Pharmacol . 58:61–64.

MacLennan AH, Wilson DH, Taylor AW. (1996). Prevalence and cost of alternative medicine in Australia. Lancet;347:569–573.

Pakistan (1997). National Health Policy. The Way Forward: Agenda for Health Sector Reform. Islamabad. Government of Pakistan, Ministry of Health.

Pakistan (2001). National Health Policy. The Way Forward: Agenda for Health Sector Reform. Islamabad, Government of Pakistan, Ministry of Health.

Parmar V. (2005): Herbal Medicines: Its Toxic Effects & Drug Interactions. The Indian Anaesthetists' Forum – (www.theiaforum.org). Online ISSN 0973-0311 October

Patwardhan B., Warude D, Pushpangadan P, Bhatt N. (2005). Ayurveda and Traditional Chinese Medicine: A comparative overview. Evidence based Complementary and Alternative Medicine, Vol. 2 (4), pp 465-473.

Patwardhan B and Patwardhan A. (2006). Traditional Medicine: S and T Advancement. TECH MONITOR. Nov-Dec.

Population growth and its implications, Islamabad, National Institute of Population Studies, Pakistan, July, 2003.

Ravishankar and Shukla (2007). INDIAN SYSTEMS OF MEDICINE: A BRIEF PROFILE. Afr. J. Trad. CAM (2007) 4 (3): 319 - 337

Robinson MM, Zhang X. (2011). The World Medicines Situation. WHO/EMP/MIE/2.3. Traditional Medicines: Global Situation, Issues and Challenges, WHO, Geneva

Saper R. B., et al. (2004). Heavy metal content of Ayurvedic herbal medicinal preparations. Journal of the American Medical Association. Vol. 292 (23), pp 2868-2873.

Shahzad H. Shaikh, Farnaz Malik, Henry James, Hamid Abdul. (2009). Trends in the use of complementary and alternative medicine in Pakistan: a population-based survey. The Journal of Alternative and Complementary Medicine. May, 15(5): 545-550.

Shankar D, Unnikrishnan, PM, Venkatasubramanian P. (2007). "Need to develop Inter-cultural standards for quality,safety and efficay of traditional systems of medicines. Current Medicines. Vol. 92, Issue 2, pp, 1499-1505.

Shinwari ZK, Gilani SS, Kohjoma K, Nakaike T. (2000). Status of medicinal plants in Pakistani Hindukush Himalayas. Proceedings of Nepal - Japan Joint Symposium on Conservation and utilization of Himalayan Med. Resour. pp. 257 – 264.

Shinwari ZK, Gilani SS, Shoukat M. (2002). Ethnobotanical resources and implications for curriculum. *In:* Shinwari, Z. K., A. Hamilton and A. A. Khan (Eds.). Proceedings of workshop on curriculum development in applied ethnobotany. May, 2 – 4, Nathiagali, Abbotabad. WWF- Pakistan. pp. 21 – 34.

Shinwari ZK. (2010). Medicinal plants research in Pakistan. Journal of Medicinal Plants Research Vol. 4(3), pp. 161-176

Siddiqui MKHK. (2004). Unani Medicine in India. Central Council for research in Unani Medicine, New Delhi, May.

Terarsawa K. (2004). "Evidance based Reconstruction of Kampo Medicines" Part-1. Is Kampo CAM? eCAM Oxford University Press, Vol-1, Issue 1, pp. 10-16.

Travis P, Bennette S, Haines A. et al. (2004). Overcoming health systems constraints to achieve the Millennium Development Goals. *Lancet* 2004;364: 900–6.

UNESCO/WIPO (1999). Regional Consultations on the Protection of Traditional and Popular Culture (Folklore), UNESCO Activities, June, p. 38-39.

World Health Organization. Traditional Medicine Strategy 2002–2005. Geneva: WHO, 2001.

Wetzel M, Eisenberg. D, Kaptchuk. T. (1998). Courses involving complementary and alternative medicine at US medical schools. J Am Med Assoc. 280:784–7

WHO. (1978). Declaration of Alma-Ata, International Conference on Primary Health Care, Alma-Ata, USSR.

World Bank (2004). The Millennium Development Goals for Health: Rising to the Challenges. Washington, DC.

World Health Organization. (2001). Legal Status of Traditional Medicine and Complementary and Alternative Medicine: A World Review. Geneva: WHO.

Zaidi SA. (1988). Issues in the health sector in Pakistan. In: The Political Economy of Health Care in Pakistan. Lahore: Vanguard Books (Pvt) Ltd

Zollman C, Vicker A. (1999). ABC of complementary medicine: Users and practitioners of complementary medicine. BMJ. 319:836–838

http://www.indianmedicine.nac.in). Visited in March and April, 2011

http://www.nchpakistan.com visited in May, 2011

Part 2

Homeopathy

4

Towards a Better Understanding of Health and Disease

Arup Bhattacharya
Roswell Park Cancer Institute, Buffalo, NY, USA

1. Introduction

Health is not merely an absence of disease or infirmity but a state of complete physical, mental and social well-being [1]. What then is a 'dis-ease' and what is a considered to be a state of complete physical, social and mental well-being? Being 'healthy' is often based on a statistical norm of 'normalcy' – the basis for most diagnostic tests. Health care as a biopsychosocial model is going through a transformation as shown in Table I. In the newer model, causes, development and outcomes of an illness are not looked at in isolation but are determined by physiology, biochemistry and their interaction with psychological, social and cultural factors. Human being is not merely a physical reality but a continuum of consciousness or awareness with the physical body at one end of this awareness spectrum. In complex systems, the whole is more than the sum of its components expressing properties not seen or predicted from the individual components [2]. Many of the behavioral health factors such as freedom from physical and emotional pain, freedom from selfishness, increased adaptability, and creativity define health to a complementary and alternative or CAM practitioner [3] and are consistent with a Lorenz attractor pattern, attractors that balance entropy and provide dynamic order out of chaos. There is thus a need for a more meaningful unifying explanation for health and disease in order to better understand the role of interventions in various health care modalities.

Health care component	Old view	Evolving view
Focus	Combative	Fostering health
Emphasis	External factors	External and Internal factors
Causative agent	Germs as pathogens	Re-visiting the seed & soil hypothesis – host pathogen interaction
Role of Client/Patient	Passive recipient of Rx	Proactive and interactive
Belief system	No role	Critical role
Healer/Physician's role	Primary	Secondary – a catalyst & a collaborator in regaining balance

Table 1. Changing view of Health Care

The psychosomatic nature of most illness is but obvious today and from the recorded past. Hippocrates had mentioned: "It is better to know the patient who has the disease that it is to know the disease which the patient has". Galen made the observation that only 20% of his patients had some physical basis for their symptoms. This paradigm was reflected in a recent study which found that only 16% of complaints in general medical clinic patients could be explained by biophysical paradigm of disease [4]. Contrary to what is commonly assumed, not all victories over illness and disease were a direct result of biomedical advances or better nutrition or availability of clean water. Diseases such as measles, scarlet fever, pneumonia, tuberculosis, typhoid, diphtheria and polio were on a decline even before the advent of medical advances specifically targeting these diseases [5]. An increase in hope and a decrease in despair and hopelessness during the beginning of last century had been a critical factor underlying this improvement. Hopelessness and pessimism has been linked to risk of disease [6] and is significantly associated with mortality such as in heart disease [7].

Human being, the epitome of the evolutionary process on this planet, is a myriad complex life form that has attributes not easily mirrored by other life forms such as being capable of manifesting emotions of altruism even towards a perceived enemy that inflicts pain. Life as a dynamic system involves ongoing interactions between stimuli and the sensory apparatus. Stimuli can be both external and internal - some of which being the result of a conditioned repetitive behavior or habit patterns. 'Awareness' (a.k.a the Vital Force of homeopaths) is that part of the consciousness a total absence of which from the physical web of matter defines 'physical death' and which when sullied away from the present moment by enmeshing in a web of unmet needs of cravings and aversion gets constricted by a strong behavioral pattern seeking pleasure while avoiding pain that often leads to the initiation, progression and maintenance of a 'dis-ease' process. To be healthy means to flourish within an optimal range of functioning connoting goodness, generativity, growth, and resilience [8]. An un-constricted awareness involved in flourishing promotes and maintains sensations of well-being and promotes self-actualization.

2. Three domains of reality

Awareness can exist in three domains of reality. The Newtonian domain is our day-to-day world of interaction in the superfluous physical world of cause and effect. Underlying this is the world of quantum reality constituting mainly of space and subatomic particles. Behind these veils of external reality is the non-local phenomenon from which consciousness emanates and permeates as awareness or VF in all other dimensions including mind. A cell is a basic building block of the physical reality of the human body while the sub-atomic particles are the basic unit of the quantum world and 'awareness' is an element of the non-local self that permeates, integrates and operates the quantum and the physical body. Awareness enables the approximately thousand trillion individual cells that constitute a human being to function in synchronicity and in harmony as a 'self' or an independent functional unit. At death, it leaves the physical web of matter behind leading to its disintegration and breakdown - to be reclaimed back by mother earth. Consciousness has been described as analogous to but preceding the quantum field that has the hall mark of complementarity, non-locality, scale-invariance and undivided wholeness [9]. In the strict sense of neurological science consciousness is defined as consisting of two major compartments: arousal and awareness. Arousal refers to alertness level that is supported by the subcortical arousal systems in the brainstem, mid-brain and thalamus while awareness is generally referred to as the content of consciousness supported by the functional integrity of the cerebral cortex and its subcortical connections [10]. Awareness brings with it a source of abundant and inexhaustible energy from the non-local domains that can maintain health, cause flourishing, manifest disease and when properly harnessed will fuel the healing process back to health from a dis-ease condition. Awareness when it is undivided and sharp in its clarity and not conjoined in any conditioning, identification or judgement is in an innate state of perpetual bliss and flourishing.

3. Life as continuum of sensations

Life at the physical plane is based on the perceptions of various stimuli received through the five sensory organs and their interaction with mind and the intermingling state of emotions - leading to 'sensations'. Life can be defined as a continuum of sensations which at physical death ceases to influence the physical self. Sensations can be neutral or positive or negative. Most sensations are self-perpetuated through the default behavior pattern of 'pain' avoidance and 'pleasure' seeking learnt through the instinctive drive for need satisfaction and physical survival present within us. When a sensation is not resolved completely, it tends to perpetuate itself in the mind, emotion and the body and invests the attention of awareness. At a certain threshold, sensations become primary center of attention for the awareness which often gets identifies with the sensations and manifests, increases and maintains its' mental, emotional and physical characteristics or 'symptoms' registering it as a pain or discomfort that tends to constricts the awareness in the vice of same repetitive 'feelings'. As for pleasure, most pleasurable things in the long run tend to be a source of pain and hence this repetitive behavior pattern tends to lead one away from well-being and flourishing.

The four interacting information processing systems in humans that are critical in 'flourishing' and 'well-being' are the mind with the functioning of the brain, the endocrine systems, the nervous system and the immune system [11]. Nervous, endocrine and immune systems - the three physical information gateways – cross talk to each other via receptors present on critical cells that can receive and exchange information through messenger molecules [12; 13; 14; 15]. Sensations when they are in consonance with satisfying of our 'needs', promote a feeling of well-being or 'flourishing'. When they are in contrary to our needs it can potentially mitigate the clarity and strength of our 'awareness' by entangling it in feeling agitated, frustrated and despondent leading to a not-at-ease/dis-ease state. Once the seed of inner disturbance is formed, it can attract energy through the modus of awareness and get a life force of its own. This constricts and mitigates the original awareness affecting our mental, emotional and physical well-being and acting as an 'attractor' for generating future disturbance of the mind, emotions and body. In other words, such identification of cause a minuscule split in the original web awareness (a.k.a Vital Force) that permeates all levels of our existence including our disease states which are very much part of our'self' at a given point of time. This germination of a split in awareness from its' original wholeness culminates in a disarray of emotional and or physical unease, pain, functional imbalance that over due course of time leads to physiological, functional and pathobiological changes. An unhindered, un-constricted awareness supports the synchronicity of the trillions of individual cells that function in unison to manifest the physical 'self'. What then influences the pattern of sensations in an individual that leads to disease?

4. Critical role of belief system in fostering well being

While genetics and pathogens play a role in disease causation [16], personality [17], lifestyle [18] and environment [19] also play a critical role in manifesting disease [19]. It is known that many individuals despite being infected with a pathogen do not develop symptoms or exhibit 'dis-ease' behavior [19; 20]. Anthropological evidence suggests that beliefs and expectations not only contribute to sickness and disease but also promote healing. Our thoughts, feelings, beliefs and optimism modulate chemical and electrical activity in the brain that can coordinate biological changes. The body responds to external stimuli based on the inner constructs of belief system irrespective of whether the beliefs and ideas are imaginary or based on reality. Similarly, what is important is not so much the presence of actual coping skills the individual has or do not have but what one believes to have or do not have that is a determinant of upsetting health-related equilibrium at the onslaught of any stress [5]. Thus, the perception of a situation is seemingly more critical at times than the situation itself and as mentioned by Hans Selye: "It is not what happens that counts; it is how you take it"[21]. While an adverse incidence can lead to a consequent adverse emotion of trauma or helplessness such as in post-traumatic stress disorder, not all adverse sensations can compromise or constrict the awareness with a negative experience and in contrast may foster more strength and resilience leading in the long run to a higher feeling of well-being as seen in post-traumatic growth [22]. A belief system is what makes a difference between one or the other consequent emotional possibilities arising from an adverse incidence or stimuli. Feeling victimized by circumstance and having a belief system that reinforces this pattern, can find oneself completely traumatized by the situation while a belief system that fosters every experience as an opportunity to flourish will enable one to overcome the seemingly negative experience and become strongly grounded in well-being. A positive belief system seems to strengthen awareness and keep the individual cells in the positive loop of synchronicity or well-being. A completely open belief system is a critical factor in continuing well-being of the individual as it acts as a rudder for directing the power of awareness at maintaining, growing and reinforcing well-being. A study that followed women with early stage breast cancer for five years reported that patients with high score of helplessness at baseline were more likely to have relapsed or died during the five years [23]. A belief system that often evolves from past experiences initiates and strengthens habit patterns in an individual. As our feelings, thoughts, beliefs and hopes change, the ensuing changes in the electrical activity of the brain is changing our biology. Dr Eric Kandell, a Nobel Laureate in 2000 in Physiology/Medicine, explains that belief becomes biology through regulation of gene expressions [24]. Knowledge of the world [25], inner resources [26] made of belief, assumptions and predictions, social support in terms of interpersonal relationships [27], and, spirituality (or spiritual beliefs) [28; 29] are the four important categories of our coping skills [21]. A healthy and positive belief system is a strong defense to illness that allows for re-balancing at the face of an onslaught of stress or adverse situation. Gratitude which is being recognized by modern positive psychology as a critical component in enhancing a sense of coherence through positive reframing is an important element in nurturing a positive resilient belief system.

5. Understanding needs and human motivation

Since the initiation or continuation of any 'sensation' often arises from the process of satisfying a particular need, Maslow's hierarchy of needs is a tool that enables us to understand the underlying motivation for need satisfaction in the journey of awareness through life. As shown in figure 1, though deficiency-needs or 'D-needs' do not positively reinforce a feeling of well-being and flourishing, if not satiated to a certain degree can lead to a feeling of 'ill-being' that potentially can countermand and mitigate flourishing and well-being. If on the contrary, the needs are more than satisfied at these levels, it still does not positively promote flourishing or well-being. The journey of the human life from birth onwards involves satiety of these needs to a certain required degree for example the basic physiological needs for food, water and air - critical for our survival, if not met to a required degree will manifest as a feeling of distress and disease. On the contrary, a conditioned or tainted belief system would get the awareness stuck through unhealthy identification in one of these needs level therby seeking continuous gratification that constricts awareness in a powerful entanglement of a blind repetitive habit pattern of pain avoidance and pleasure seeking behavior at that particular need level. When this happens, the possibility of pursuing an immediately higher needs levels by awareness including those of 'Being' needs for self-actualization and flourishing gets compromised. This state fosters an inner resistance and a state of inner conflict that weakens our system allowing seeds of disease including external disease causing factors such as germs to have a better foothold in order to manifest disease and illness behavior. It is as though the awareness is restricted in a narrow constricted web of activity ceaselessly trying to satiate unresolved sensation of deprivation arising from that particular category of need. The problem often at this 'D' or deficiency need-level is that sensations that causes pleasure ends up very often causing pain and suffering in the long run – and so trying to continuously satisfy needs at a particular D-level is unlikely to lead to a feeling of long term well-being. If on the other hand, awareness does not get afflicted at the D-level which has been satiated to the healthy levels required then it is likely to be available for pursuing the 'Being' or 'B-needs' that leads onwards to self-actualization positively enhancing well-being and flourishing. The possibility of awareness to be aware of itself in its' pristine non-local element in a global way whilst being connected to everything (Universe) and yet being in the body is a highest positive state of well-being and flourishing with a corresponding higher state of psychological, neurological, immunological and endocrinological well-being that can ward of any feeling of 'disease'. Awareness in the physical body of a new born is instinctive in seeking to satisfy the physical and physiological 'D' – needs. This often sets in the age-old habit pattern of pain avoidance and pleasure seeking behavior that manifests itself as personality or ego traits. The ego is a mask that imparts a coping mechanism and a transient feeling of protection from presumed or real adverse conditions and situations. This ego or the mask when it goes through self-deprecating life experiences develops a negative belief system allowing adverse emotions such as despair and hopelessness to manifest immediately on facing a perceived adverse situation. While a positive life experience strengthens the link of the body-mind-awareness synchronicity, a negative life experience causes accumulation of sensation of discomfort in the body-mind interface that if unresolved over a period of time leads to bodily pain, discomfort and will promulgate functional, physiological and pathological dis-ease changes in the body.

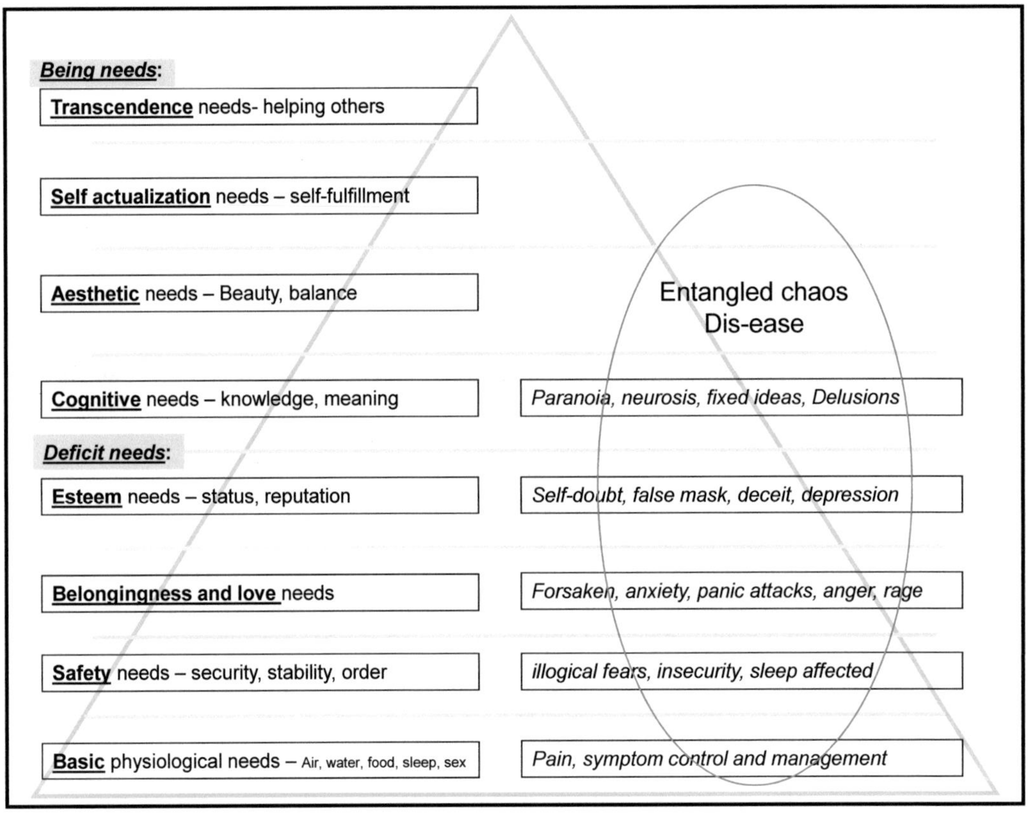

Fig. 1. Maslow's Hierarchy of Needs

6. Role of emotions

Thoughts are abstract concepts that without the interface of emotions seldom impact the body physiologically. Emotion enable us to assess a situation as beneficial or detrimental without depending on external evaluation and are a result of millions of years of evolution that often cause a default response to common experiences. Emotion produces coordinated changes in thoughts, actions and physiological response and help in one's pursuit of pleasures and satisfaction. While negative emotions narrow one's thought-action repertoires and manifest specific action tendencies (such as attack or flee), positive emotions broaden one's momentary thought action repertoires evoking a wider range of thoughts and actions (play, explore, savor, integrate) that enables flourishing [30]. One can say that negative emotion constricts and positive emotion enables maintenance or expansion of awareness that can lead to better flourishing of an individual. Positive emotion enables one to cope effectively with chronic stress, enhance psychological and physiological resilience enabling speedy recovery from disease. While perceiving threat in negative experience does have some immediate adaptive benefits, in the prolonged period this can have deleterious effects on one's psychological and physical well-being.

The subject of positive psychology that has caught up with researcher's interest is not new and can be found in ancient esoteric tradtions. For instance, the 2,000 years old Buddhist teachings embodied in 'Abhidhamma Samuccaya' had dealt with this topic quite exhaustively while laying down its' importance in physical and psychological well-being. In Buddhist doctrine, flourishing that arises from equanimity and insight into nature of reality is considered more critical for a lasting well-being than a fleeting arousal of emotion or mood though sensory and conceptual stimuli. Similarly the concept of suffering in Buddhism is not merely an unpleasant feeling but the basic vulnerability to suffering and pain consequent to misapprehending the nature of reality. Training in attention, emotional balance and mindfulness (sati) is considered important for sustained well-being that arises from learning to distinguish between the way things are as they appear to the senses and the conceptual superimpositions projected upon them. The goal is not just individual flourishing but also a feeling of universal well-being to which too belongs all other sentient beings and their flourishing [31]. It specifically lists the following eleven positive emotions as virtuous faculties that will help harness awareness into flourishing and self-actualization: faith, integrity, consideration for others, non-attachment, non-hostility, non-harmfulness, non-confusion, joyous efforts, equanimity, pliancy and conscientiousness. Similarly it lists 26 metal faculties along with its' negative emotions as afflictive constricting awareness and increasing dukkha or suffering and ill-behavior: attachment, anger, pride, ignorance/confusion, deluded pride, deluded view/outlook, wrath, non-alertness, inconsideration, vengeance, spite, de-stimulation, jealousy, excitement, dullness, pretention, distraction, complacency, destructiveness, lack of integrity, concealment, unconscionable, laziness, miserliness, lack of faith, harmfulness and forgetfulness. The three mental processes that is the basis for all dis-ease are cravings (tanha), aversion or hatred and grasping onto one's own or others' reified personal identities (ego) as real. Craving, the desire to acquire objects and situations for self, disrupts the mind as it falsely displaces the source of one's well-being from one's own mind to objects thereby disrupting the balance of mind and giving rise to anxiety, misery, fear and anger with their corresponding emotions. Cravings results in dopamine activity in the nucleus accumbens of the brain and results in reinforcement of a behavior addiction pattern that is not associated with pleasure in the long term. Similarly hatred or aversion traps the mind into the deluded belief that the source of suffering belongs entirely to an external object and constricts awareness and enables 'dis-ease' states to manifest. Since the 'self' is in a constant dynamic flux that is interdependent with other beings and environment, superimposing the concepts of permanence, singularity and autonomy onto reality is the root cause 'ill-behavior' based on craving, hatred, jealousy and arrogance [31].

7. Mindfulness and well-being

Mindfulness is paying attention in a particular way to the internal and external experiences occurring in the present moment non-judgementally in order for one to be aware of thoughts, feelings and bodily sensations without trying to modify or act on them. It enables one to learn the skills of recognizing and disengaging from self-perpetuating patterns of ruminative, negative thoughts [32]. A sustained mindfulness, introspection and meditation practice is conjoined with cultivation of attentional stability and vividness. Mindfulness-based cognitive therapies protects against relapse and recurrence of psychiatric disorders on a par with that of maintenance antidepressant pharmacotherapy [33]. Oxytocin [34], opiates and serotonin are generated in the amount required by the central nervous system as a result of meditation and mindfulness, for enhancing flourishing and a sensation of well-being [35]. Mindfulness based techniques have been shown to significantly improve various conditions: pain ratings and other medical and psychological symptoms in chronic pain patients; anxiety disorders, panic attacks, depression; binge eating; fibromyalgia, and, quality of life in cancer patients [36]. The effect of meditation on stress reduction and healing or re-balancing is been studied by researchers. It has been found to reduce plasma and salivary cortisol levels, bring the cytokine and natural killer cell activities closer to normal levels in cancer patients, increase antibody titer to influenza vaccine, lowered stress-induced increase in interleukin-6 and decreased C-reactive protein [32].

8. Healthcare modalities

As stated above, unremitted and unresolved sensations cause malaise and disease. How a treatment modality approaches to help re-balance the self into attaining well-being differs on the modality type. In conventional or allopathic medicine, a drug is administered based on the principles of 'contraria contrariis curantur' where the active ingredient opposes the onset of symptoms by blocking or cutting off one of the key element of the disease symptom manifestation biochemical pathways and thereby not allowing pain or symptoms of malaise to come up. In most cases, the drug is not curative and with the drug effect wearing away with time – the drug needs to be repeated. While this modality allows for pain amelioration, it has the following setbacks:

a. It is rarely, if at all curative and hence needs to be taken periodically on a regular basis for chronic illnesses, thus making one dependent on it - often for a life time with the consequent high cost to medical health care system;
b. Since the course of drug action becomes smaller over a period of time, the dosage often needs to be increased or the drug changed when it is found to be no longer effective in ameliorating the symptom conditions of the disease;
c. Many drugs are known to have side-effects where additional symptoms or sensations of a newer type of discomfort arise in the body-mind continuum. Approximately 6.5% of

all hospitalization in general population is as a result of adverse drug events [37] causing ~225,000 deaths annually in US alone [38];

d. Often the individual's well-being declines over time due to strengthening of the primary disease with conventional medication.

Conventional allopathic medical practitioners due to their training base are not easily able to incorporate the biopsychosocial model in their practice except occasionally in some chronic illness management. This resistance is due to an increased demand in knowledge base and time investment, besides learning a new style of patient-doctor relationship required to better understand and manage patient illness [39].

In contrast, many of the CAM modalities try an approach that is conducive with the inner sensation of 'dis-ease' reversing itself. A moot case in point is homeopathy, where the remedy is tailored to the needs of the patient based on the presenting symptom picture which includes symptoms of the mind, body and emotion. Homeopathy follows the doctrine of 'similia similibus curantur' where a substance that can cause a similar discomfort in a healthy individual is used, often, in a non-material dose. This use of a non-material dose itself is a paradox which makes it difficult to study the underlying mechanism. Classical homeopathy case taking is generally quite elaborate as it individualizes each case by determining the four quadrants of manifesting symptoms: sensations, locations, modalities and concomitants. Furthermore, symptoms other than the primary complaints are also delved into including possible past or current mental or emotional stressor that may have at least partially be responsible for the presenting disease conditions. The advantages of a CAM modality such as homeopathy are:

a. It is non-toxic, inexpensive and is not known to cause any side effects in most cases;
b. It promotes re-balance without undue suppression of symptoms through use of remedies that elicits a response from the psychoneuroimmunoendocrinological systems through making available sensation similar to that of the natural disease (corollary as in vaccination which uses the principle of same) for the system to wake up and initiate a healing process back to health and well-being, thereby promoting a complete cure where after the remedy is no longer needed;
c. Homeopathic case taking by itself has a proven positive therapeutic effect as it delves into great details in understanding the origin and maintaining factors of the disease condition;
d. Often the emotional and psychological causative factors underlying the physiological or functional or pathological condition gets resolved prior to complete cure;
e. The process encourages a proactive approach on the part of the patient. In the long term, this ensures a positive health benefit by instilling a sense of positive participation in the maintenance of one's well-being. This instills a feeling of positive empowerment and not helplessness with one's condition in chronic cases;
f. Finally and importantly, it frees awareness from entanglement with the symptom producing complex enabling it to continue its onward journey towards expansion and flourishing.

9. References

[1] D. Callahan, The WHO definition of 'health'. Stud Hastings Cent 1 (1973) 77-88.

[2] I.R. Bell, D.A. Lewis, 2nd, S.E. Lewis, A.J. Brooks, G.E. Schwartz, C.M. Baldwin, Strength of vital force in classical homeopathy: bio-psycho-social-spiritual correlates within a complex systems context. J Altern Complement Med 10 (2004) 123-131.
[3] G. Vithoulkas, The Science of Homeopathy, Grove Weidenfeld, New York, 1980.
[4] J.M. Merrill, Z. Camachao, L.F. Laux, J.I. Thornby, C. Vallbona, How medical school shapes students' orientation to patients' psychological problems. Academic Medicine 66 (1991) S4-S6.
[5] O. Ray, How the mind hurts and heals the body. Am Psychol 59 (2004) 29-40.
[6] L.D. Kubzansky, D. Sparrow, P. Vokonas, I. Kawachi, Is the glass half empty or half full? A prospective study of optimism and coronary heart disease in the normative aging study. Psychosom Med 63 (2001) 910-916.
[7] T. Maruta, R.C. Colligan, M. Malinchoc, K.P. Offord, Optimists vs pessimists: survival rate among medical patients over a 30-year period. Mayo Clin Proc 75 (2000) 140-143.
[8] B.L. Fredrickson, M.F. Losada, Positive affect and the complex dynamics of human flourishing. Am Psychol 60 (2005) 678-686.
[9] M. Kafatos, R.E. Tanzi, D. Chopra, How consciousness becomes the physical universe. The Journal of Cosmology 14 (2011).
[10] A. Demertzi, A. Vanhaudenhuyse, M.A. Bruno, C. Schnakers, M. Boly, P. Boveroux, P. Maquet, G. Moonen, S. Laureys, Is there anybody in there? Detecting awareness in disorders of consciousness. Expert Rev Neurother 8 (2008) 1719-1730.
[11] S.F. Maier, L.R. Watkins, M. Fleshner, Psychoneuroimmunology. The interface between behavior, brain, and immunity. Am Psychol 49 (1994) 1004-1017.
[12] C.L. Raison, A.H. Miller, The neuroimmunology of stress and depression. Semin Clin Neuropsychiatry 6 (2001) 277-294.
[13] A. Trautmann, E. Vivier, Immunology. Agrin--a bridge between the nervous and immune systems. Science 292 (2001) 1667-1668.
[14] P.H. Patterson, Leukemia inhibitory factor, a cytokine at the interface between neurobiology and immunology. Proc Natl Acad Sci U S A 91 (1994) 7833-7835.
[15] S. Bhowmick, A. Singh, R.A. Flavell, R.B. Clark, J. O'Rourke, R.E. Cone, The sympathetic nervous system modulates CD4(+)FoxP3(+) regulatory T cells via a TGF-beta-dependent mechanism. J Leukoc Biol 86 (2009) 1275-1283.
[16] J.A. Winkelstein, B. Childs, Why do some individuals have more infections than others? JAMA 285 (2001) 1348-1349.
[17] R. Grossarth-Maticek, H.J. Eysenck, Coca-Cola, cancers, and coronaries: personality and stress as mediating factors. Psychol Rep 68 (1991) 1083-1087.
[18] M.A. Jacobs, A. Spilken, M. Norman, Relationship of life change maladaptive aggression, and upper respiratory infection in male college students. Psychosom Med 31 (1969) 31-44.
[19] R.J. Haggerty, Life stress, illness and social supports. Dev Med Child Neurol 22 (1980) 391-400.
[20] S. Cohen, D.A. Tyrrell, A.P. Smith, Psychological stress and susceptibility to the common cold. N Engl J Med 325 (1991) 606-612.
[21] B. Justice, Critical life events and the onset of illness. Compr Ther 20 (1994) 232-238.

[22] C. Peterson, N. Park, N. Pole, W. D'Andrea, M.E. Seligman, Strengths of character and posttraumatic growth. J Trauma Stress 21 (2008) 214-217.

[23] M. Watson, J.S. Haviland, S. Greer, J. Davidson, J.M. Bliss, Influence of psychological response on survival in breast cancer: a population-based cohort study. Lancet 354 (1999) 1331-1336.

[24] E.R. Kandel, A new intellectual framework for psychiatry. Am J Psychiatry 155 (1998) 457-469.

[25] T. Pincus, R. Esther, D.A. DeWalt, L.F. Callahan, Social conditions and self-management are more powerful determinants of health than access to care. Ann Intern Med 129 (1998) 406-411.

[26] L. Kamen-Siegel, J. Rodin, M.E. Seligman, J. Dwyer, Explanatory style and cell-mediated immunity in elderly men and women. Health Psychol 10 (1991) 229-235.

[27] J.S. House, K.R. Landis, D. Umberson, Social relationships and health. Science 241 (1988) 540-545.

[28] W.R. Miller, Spirituality, treatment, and recovery. Recent Dev Alcohol 16 (2003) 391-404.

[29] W.R. Miller, C.E. Thoresen, Spirituality, religion, and health. An emerging research field. Am Psychol 58 (2003) 24-35.

[30] B.L. Fredrickson, C. Branigan, Positive emotions broaden the scope of attention and thought-action repertoires. Cogn Emot 19 (2005) 313-332.

[31] P. Ekman, R.J. Davidson, M. Ricard, B.A. Wallace, Buddhist and psychological perspectives on emotions and well-being. Current Directions in Psychological Science 14 (2005) 5.

[32] S.N. Young, Biologic effects of mindfulness meditation: growing insights into neurobiologic aspects of the prevention of depression. J Psychiatry Neurosci 36 75-77.

[33] Z.V. Segal, P. Bieling, T. Young, G. MacQueen, R. Cooke, L. Martin, R. Bloch, R.D. Levitan, Antidepressant monotherapy vs sequential pharmacotherapy and mindfulness-based cognitive therapy, or placebo, for relapse prophylaxis in recurrent depression. Arch Gen Psychiatry 67 1256-1264.

[34] K. Uvnas-Moberg, Oxytocin may mediate the benefits of positive social interaction and emotions. Psychoneuroendocrinology 23 (1998) 819-835.

[35] K. Rubia, The neurobiology of Meditation and its clinical effectiveness in psychiatric disorders. Biol Psychol 82 (2009) 1-11.

[36] R.A. Baer, Mindfulness training as a clinical intervention: a conceptual and empirical review. Clinical Psychology: Science and Practice 10 (2003) 19.

[37] M. Pirmohamed, S. James, S. Meakin, C. Green, A.K. Scott, T.J. Walley, K. Farrar, B.K. Park, A.M. Breckenridge, Adverse drug reactions as cause of admission to hospital: prospective analysis of 18 820 patients. BMJ 329 (2004) 15-19.

[38] S. Madeira, M. Melo, J. Porto, S. Monteiro, J.M. Pereira de Moura, M.B. Alexandrino, J.J. Moura, The diseases we cause: Iatrogenic illness in a department of internal medicine. Eur J Intern Med 18 (2007) 391-399.

[39] Y. Alonso, The biopsychosocial model in medical research: the evolution of the health concept over the last two decades. Patient Educ Couns 53 (2004) 239-244.

5

Homeopathy: Treatment of Cancer with the Banerji Protocols

Prasanta Banerji and Pratip Banerji
Prasanta Banerji Homeopathic Research Foundation, India

1. Introduction

Looking back into the history of mankind, one is often startled to find the emergence of some outstanding personalities at different intervals of time. Their thoughts and futuristic viewpoints revolutionized the existing perspective in the fields of science, philosophy and social order. The embodiment of such a personality in the field of medicine was Samuel Christian Friedrich Hahnemann, the father of homeopathy. He was born on the 10th April 1755 in the small town of Meissen, near Dresden in Germany. A doctor in the conventional medicine of his time, by 1790 he was recognized as one of the most distinguished physicians of his generation and was appointed physician to the king. Soon however, he became dissatisfied with contemporary medical ideas and the often cruel practices that ensued, as well as the drugs being prescribed. He realized that many of these medicines owed their pride of place in the Materia Medica due to their very biologically active nature, which could easily occasion death or produce new diseases on whomever they were applied. Disillusioned, Hahnemann renounced his practice of medicine. While engaged in translating a treatise on herbal medicine, he felt dissatisfied with the explanation given for the cure of malarial fever by giving cinchona bark. He took the drug himself in order to investigate the changes induced by it on his healthy system. Peculiarly, the symptoms of malaria made their appearance in him, one after the other, but without the chilly rigor. This reminded him of Hippocrates' aphorism, "*Similia similibus curentur,*" meaning "*Let likes be cured by likes*" (Hobhouse, 2002).

Hahnemann felt convinced that the drug, which was the best agent to cure malarial fever, produced in him the initial symptoms of that fever. He then investigated the action, on healthy human beings, of as many as 50 more drugs over a period of six years. He recorded the symptoms produced, and compared them with the symptoms of diseases against which they were used successfully.

1.1 What is homeopathy?

In 1776, Hahnemann published the results of his findings in a paper entitled "Essay on the new principle for ascertaining the curative power of drugs." In this, he postulated the most important principle of homeopathy, stating, "*Every powerful medicinal substance produces in the human body a kind of peculiar disease, the more powerful the medicine, the more particularly marked and violent the disease. We should imitate nature, which sometimes cures a chronic disease, by superadding another, and employ in the disease (especially chronic) we wish to cure, that medicine which is able to produce another very similar artificial disease, and the former will be cured similia similibus.*" In 1810, he published *The Organon of the Rational Art of Healing,* his greatest book, wherein he elucidated systematically the methods and principles of a system of medical treatment to which he had given the name of "Homeopathy" (Hahnemann, 1982).

The homeopathic approach is holistic, that is, while treating a patient a homeopath will consider not only the disease, but the whole constitution of the patient. The patient is treated as a whole. To know about homeopathy we should know what *"individualization"* and *"similimum"* mean because these two are the basic tenets on which selection of homeopathic medicines depends, as practised and taught from the time of Hahnemann.

What is *"individualization"*? Every individual person is different from the other physically, mentally, constitutionally and in their likes and dislikes. In general, we may find some persons alike, but all individuals have their own special features. *"Similimum"* means the most similar medicine as per symptoms narrated by a patient. After noting down the symptoms of a patient the physician thinks of a few medicines out of which he finds one medicine which appears to be the most similar to the symptoms narrated, considering the mental and constitutional status for that particular individual. In classical homeopathy only a single medicine is given in a single dose and then the patient is observed for his/her response.

Classical homeopathy has, therefore, no specific remedy for any disease by name, but it has specificity for each individual case of disease. A specific drug cannot be used for a specific disease. In general, when a homeopathic physician examines a patient, only a few medicines come to his mind. This small group of medicines exhibits similar symptoms when given to healthy subjects for pharmacological testing (a process called "proving.".. Finally only one is selected as a result of practical experience and this procedure requires a long and intense interrogation of the patient. In an interesting study of homeopathic diagnosis and treatment, it was shown that a typical classical homeopathic initial consultation took 117 +/- 43 minutes for each adult patient and 86 +/- 36 minutes for each child patient. Theoretically there should be only one such medicine considering the entirety of the patient (Becker-Witt, et. al., 2004).

The homeopathic drug is not administered in usual pharmacological doses, but in minute doses prepared according to certain principles. These medicines are produced using various plant extracts, salts, animal products, minerals etc. and then diluting the extracted mother tincture or the crude materials, per pharmacopoeial methods. These solutions are serially diluted and succussed (agitated) until the desired potency is produced. Greater dilution leads to greater potency of the medicine. The crude or slightly diluted extract when ingested by healthy volunteers produces symptom complexes that mimic various diseases. The symptoms produced and recorded are a result of the dynamic action of drugs on healthy volunteers or *"provers."* The symptoms produced by the drug in provers are exactly what the potentized medicine is prescribed for in the sick.

1.2 The central problem of classical homeopathy

Although classical homeopaths believe that the above-described method of selecting medicines is essential to the worth of their medical system, the central problem is, whether a correct *similimum* can be selected by such a method of individualization. The subjective symptoms elicited in the typical two-hour initial consultation are often "lost in the translation."Thus, should a patient be examined separately by different homeopaths on the same day, he will be perplexed to find that none of them seem to agree as to the so-called "*similimum.*" Then how can individualization be explained logically and used to benefit the suffering population? Do all the medicines suggested by various homeopaths for a patient behave as a *similimum* for that particular case? Obviously not! Then what is the solution to this central question of how the correct medicine should be determined? The answer is to rationalize the selection of medicines based on previous experience and experimentation and to develop routine treatment protocols following a scientific method for selecting medicines. Another practical problem may be mentioned here. If a homeopath examines six or eight cases daily, he may have to charge high fees from each individual patient for maintenance. This will put homeopathy out of reach to the suffering population who really need it. At the same time, with such a small number of patients, a homeopath hardly gets enough clinical experience to become a true physician. It is common knowledge that experience makes a doctor.

Scientific validation of the efficacy of homeopathic medicines, which are nontoxic and inexpensive - making them ideal as "the People's Medicine" - has been stalled due to the inability to conduct clinical trials using standardized treatment protocols with these medicines. The true healing potential of homeopathy, then, has been repeatedly challenged and denied by mainstream medicine because of this problem. Thus, this system of medicine is at risk of being delegated to the archives of history.

1.3 The Banerji Protocols

In the clinics of our research foundation,, we do not practice classical homeopathy. We have developed a method of treatment in which specific medicines are prescribed for specific diseases. Diseases are diagnosed using modern state of the art scientific methods. This is done because modern diagnostic approaches incorporate and help in the selection of medicines so that specific medicines can be easily prescribed for specific diseases. With the passage of time and the availability of new diagnostic tools like ultrasonography, magnetic resonance imaging, cancer biomarkers and other advanced tests, we have been able to further streamline the treatment protocols. The efficacy of this approach is reflected by the encouraging results of our new method of treatment, which we call the "Banerji Protocols." We often combine two potentized medicines and use the combination in our practice. This combination of two potentized medicines is made in a meaningful way based on years of clinical observations by us. Medicines are combined for special advantages in treatment, so that the aggravation due to the medicines can be checked, side effects of the medicines abated, and quick and uneventful recovery can be ensured in a much shorter time. We will discuss the Banerji Protocols in more depth later in this chapter.

2. The global use of homeopathy

Homeopathy currently is used in over 80 countries around the world. In several countries including India, Mexico, Brazil and the UK homeopathy is integrated into the healthcare systems. In the United States, homeopathic remedies are regulated as nonprescription drugs, which give them a unique status over other natural therapies and supplements. Homeopathy is very popular in the UK, where the Royal Family has had homeopathic physicians since the 1830s. In England, as many as 45% of conventional MDs refer patients to homeopaths and the treatment is part of the National Health Scheme (NHS). In France, 40% of the population use homeopathy. Thirty thousand French doctors use homeopathic medicines, there are twenty thousand pharmacies providing them, and 32% of French family physicians use homeopathy. In Italy, homeopathy is the most popular alternative therapy, used by 86% of the population. In Germany 25% of family physicians use homeopathy, and non-MD homeopaths are eligible for licensure and until recently were reimbursed by the National Health System. Nine million people use homeopathy in Brazil. In 1985, homeopathy was included among the therapeutic options offered at the outpatient facilities of the Brazilian public health system. Fifteen thousand Brazilian doctors practice homeopathy (Marino, 2008).

In Asia, the homeopathic medical system is very popular, especially in India, Pakistan and Sri Lanka. The epoch-making statement of Mahatma Gandhi, "*Homeopathy.... cures a larger percentage of cases than any other method of treatment and is beyond doubt safer and more economical and most complete medical science,*" added another feather to the cap of homeopathy. In India today there are 162 degree colleges teaching homeopathy and the largest pool of homeopaths in the world - over 200,000 doctors practice homeopathy. About 100 million people use homeopathy (Ghosh, 2010; Singh, 2005). This is a very conservative estimate because in the 1950ss and 1960s there were not many conventional doctors available for the treatment of the masses. In that era, most village school masters and scholars educated themselves in this economical and easy to administer treatment form. Thus homeopathy had a much further reach amongst the general population than conventional medicine. Of India's 1.16 billion population, approximately 70% live in villages and rural areas, where access to expensive conventional medical facilities is limited (World Health Organization, 2006).

3. History of homeopathy in India

Seen through the mist of years, the early history of the advent of homeopathy in India is a fascinating episode. As early as 1810, some German missionaries landed in Bengal. They used to distribute homeopathic remedies among the poor people to alleviate their sufferings. Slowly the elite of society recognized its efficacy and many civil servants and military personnel became amateur homeopaths. On the other hand, due to the efficacy and affordability of the medicines, in the rural environment many school teachers also took to reading the homeopathic materia medicas and prescribing to their village communities. In 1852 John Martin Hoenigberger, who was initiated into homeopathy by Hahnemann himself in Paris in 1835, published a book which gave a glimpse of the beginning of Indian homeopathic practice in Lahore, at the court of Maharaja Ranjit Singh. In his chronicles, he gives a vivid account of his successful treatment of Maharaja Ranjit Singh's chronic disease of partial paralysis (Hoenigberger, 1852).

During the second half of the nineteenth century some homeopathic dispensaries were opened in Bengal and in the south. The pioneer in this field in Calcutta was Rajendralal Dutta (1818-1889). He belonged to a scholarly and aristocratic family of Bengal. He engaged a French doctor, Dr. Tonnere, and placed him in charge of a homeopathic hospital and dispensary in Calcutta in 1852. Unfortunately, this venture failed. Subsequently Rajen Dutta himself took up the cudgel and started practice in homeopathy. Among his illustrious patients may be mentioned the great early social reformer Pandit Ishwarchandra Vidyasagar and Raja Radhakanta Dev Bahadur. Rajen Dutta cured Pandit Vidyasagar of a migraine which the conventional system had failed to cure. Furthermore the cure of a gangrenous ulcer of Raja Radhakanta Dev Bahadur created a sensation in Calcutta at the time.

In order to strengthen the roots of homeopathic practice in India, Dutta looked around for a suitable person of eminence. His efforts were crowned with success when he was able to persuade Dr. Mahendralal Sircar, medical doctor and skeptic of homeopathy, to test its scientific efficacy and curative potential. In his experiment, administration of homeopathic medicines became effective even when Dr. Sircar's conventional medicine failed. Thus Dr. Sircar became converted to homeopathy and carved a niche for it in the medical history of India. A number of allopathic doctors started homeopathic practice following Sircar's lead. The Calcutta Homeopathic Medical College, the first homeopathic medical college, was established in 1881. This institution took on a major role in popularizing homeopathy in India (Ghosh, 2010).

Gradually homeopathic dispensaries opened in other cities like Benares and Allahabad, and by the beginning of the twentieth century homeopathy had spread all over India. In 1973, the Government of India recognized homeopathy by setting up the Central Council of Homeopathy (CCH) to regulate its education and practice. Now, only qualified registered homeopaths can practice homeopathy in India. At present, in India, homeopathy is probably the most popular system of medicine, due to the fact of its easy administration in the home setting and its affordability.

4. Cancer and homeopathy

The role and efficacy of homeopathic medicines for treatment of malignant tumors is largely unknown and unproven so far. Homeopathic therapy is mainly used for supportive cancer care and some have suggested an integration of this therapy with conventional methods (Kassab, et al., 2009). However, in numerous studies, it has been found that orthodox medicine is not meeting the needs of some patients and that Complementary and Alternative Medicine (CAM) may wholly or partly substitute for conventional medicines. Most patients indicate that their problems improve with CAM (Ernst, 2005; Frenkel, 2010).

Cancer is a subject of great concern because there is a lack of effective treatment even in the 21st century. Along with a search for conventional solutions, researchers are actively trying to identify treatment options offered by various systems of complementary and alternative medicine, including homeopathy. We believe that the Banerji Protocols have an important role to play in this effort.

A comprehensive worldwide survey of studies of the use of complementary and alternative medicine by cancer patients concluded that its use is common and widespread. Within this broad arena of therapies, homeopathy is consistently listed as one of the systems chosen by patients with cancer (Ernst, 2000). A large descriptive survey of cancer patients in Europe found that on average 35.9% were using some form of complementary or alternative therapy. Homeopathy was the most commonly used of these therapies in Belgium and was in the top five choices in six other countries. In other European countries, it was second only to herbal medicines. In France, a recent study in an oncology department revealed that 34% of the patients were using complementary medicine and homeopathy was the most frequently used of these (Träger-Maury, 2007). Homeopathy is one of the eight most popular complementary therapies used by cancer patients in the UK (Chang, 2011).

A recently reported European study conducted a prospective one-year observational study of cancer patients comparing one cohort of 259 patients under homeopathic treatment with a matched cohort of 380 patients undergoing conventional treatment. Outcomes compared included quality of life (QOL), fatigue, and anxiety/depression. The researchers found a significant improvement in quality of life in the homeopathy group after three months and a continued improvement after twelve months. The conventionally treated group had no improvement in one QOL scale after three months and a slight improvement in the other QOL scale; at twelve months there was a slight increase in one indicator and a decrease in the other. Fatigue and anxiety/depression were not improved in the conventionally treated group; fatigue but not anxiety/depression improved in the homeopathy group (Rostock, et al., 2011). A meta-analysis of all clinical studies on cancer treatment outcomes using homeopathy (Milazzo et al., 2006) found that all studies examined were investigating the use of homeopathy for adjunctive symptom treatment, not as primary antitumor treatment.

There are a number of in vitro and in vivo studies, however, that have investigated the antitumor activity of homeopathic medicines. In India, the laboratory of Khuda-Bukhsh has reported a significant anti-tumor effect of homeopathically prepared Chelidonium and Lycopodium (Banerji, A., et al., 2010; Pathak, S. et al., 2006). In America, several studies have reported the in antitumor effect of five homeopathic remedies used for treatment of prostate cancer. There was a 23% reduction in tumor incidence, and for animals with tumors, there was a 38% reduction in tumor volume in homeopathy-treated animals versus controls (Jonas, W.B., 2006). However, in another study there were no direct cellular anticancer effects demonstrated in these researchers' in vitro and in vivo studies (Thangapazham, R.L., 2006). A third study examined *in vivo* effects on mice treated with homeopathically prepared *Sabal serrulata* and clearly demonstrated a biologic response to homeopathic treatment as manifested by cell proliferation and tumor growth. Two other homeopathic medicines tested did not show similar anti-tumor effects (MacLaughlin, B.W., 2006). Another study done in India reported that homeopathic drugs retarded liver tumor growth in mice and reduced the incidence of chemically-induced sarcomas and also increased the life span of mice harboring these tumors (Kumar, K.B., 2007). What we see in this review of laboratory research of homeopathy is consistent reports of its effectiveness in slowing tumor growth in mice without a clear mechanism of action being demonstrated.

Our own studies done in collaboration with American researchers at the M.D. Anderson Cancer Center, University of Texas must be mentioned at this point, for they have demonstrated plausible biological mechanisms for the antitumor effects of the homeopathic medicines tested. In one report we described 15 patients diagnosed with documented intracranial tumors who were treated exclusively with the homeopathic remedies *Ruta graveolens 6c* and *Calcarea phosphorica 3X* without additional chemotherapy or radiation. Of these 15 patients, six of the seven who had glioma showed complete regression of the tumors. In this study we also reported that these medicines stimulated induction of survival-signaling pathways in normal lymphocytes and induction of death-signaling pathways in brain cancer cells. Cancer cell death was initiated by telomere erosion and completed through mitotic catastrophe events (Pathak, S., 2003). More recently we reported a study of four homeopathic remedies that we use for treating breast cancer against two human breast adenocarcinoma cell lines (MCF-7 and MDA-MB-231) and a cell line derived from immortalized normal human mammary epithelial cells. The remedies exerted preferential cytotoxic effects against the two breast cancer cell lines, causing cell cycle delay/arrest and apoptosis. These effects were accompanied by altered expression of the cell cycle regulatory proteins, including downregulation of phosphorylated Rb and upregulation of the CDK inhibitor p27, which were likely responsible for the cell cycle delay/arrest as well as induction of the apoptotic cascade that manifested in the activation of caspase 7 and cleavage of PARP in the treated cells (Frenkel, et al., 2010).

5. Evolution of the Banerji Protocols

Research in homeopathy and the introduction of Homeopathic medicinal mixtures in India are due to the late Dr. Pareshnath Banerji, nephew of illustrious Pandit Ishwarchandra Vidyasagar, who himself happened to be an ardent follower of homeopathy after his above-described cure. Dr. Banerji started his charitable clinic in a remote village, Mihijam, situated in the border of Bihar in 1918 and soon became a legend. He achieved phenomenal success against all kinds of disease. He could declare with certainty that he would cure both acute and chronic conditions of innumerable common people, who congregated at his village clinic seeking relief from all variety of illnesses. Treating his patients gratis, he naturally had to deal with a vast number of patients every day. If he had followed the classical homeopathic approach to case assessment, he would have been able to examine at most a dozen patients a day. He found that about 80% of his patients suffering from common ailments were curable by specific homeopathic remedies, making his clinical dispensation as quick as lightning. For the remaining 20%, he gave the greatest importance to symptoms narrated by the patients themselves. Thus he achieved success through sheer practical experience. He did not always adhere to Hahnemann's dictum of *"Single simple and minimum."* He did not mind prescribing mixtures of remedies or frequent repetitions of the remedies when required.

5.1 The Banerji Protocols: What are they?

Homeopathy as a school of medicine is very young, only 200 years old. Our family has been associated with it for over 150 years. *It can be said that the Banerji Protocols are the fruit of a cumulative experience and careful analysis of observed trends in patient – medicine interaction and the translation of the same into a system of prescribing with a view to standardize and make easy the practice of an extremely complex system of medicine using ultradilute medicines.*

The use of specific medicines in specific potencies, in fixed dosage patterns, eliminates the necessity for any guess work on the part of novice practitioners and is always a tremendous help for even seasoned doctors. Our approach is more diagnostic than individualistic, i.e. more objective than subjective. These protocols are easy to learn and since the focus is on the diagnostic approach the case-taking time is shortened. That is why it is easy to disseminate to medical students and the general public. In a short time more patients can be treated. Consequently, it also makes the treatment affordable to the weaker sections of society, making it "The People's Medicine." For any scientific medical system it is a rule that interventions should be repeated with almost the same result – meaning, a treatment should have replicability - and the Banerji Protocols fulfill this criterion.

5.2 The Banerji Protocols (BP) in the treatment of cancer

In our clinic in Kolkata, India, an average patient turnout of 1000 to 1200 a day gives us a clear perspective as to disease and treatment trends in the population we serve. We treat an average of 10 to 15% of our patient turnout - 120 to 200 cancer cases a day – whose suffering from this dreaded disease has helped us to formulate set protocols for their treatment. At present, patients from more than seventy countries follow the Banerji Protocols for treatment of their cancer through the website www.pbhrfindia.org, seeking online medical advice and treatment. In our clinics we are privileged to have the opportunity to treat every type of cancer and every stage of the disease. The majority of our patients opt to take only our treatment without any conventional treatments and we also have patients who use our medicines as adjunct therapy along with or after conventional treatments fail. We often also have patients who come to us to seek relief from the various side-effects of conventional chemotherapy and radiation. Our protocols for the different types of cancer are mostly customized according to the location and tissue type, and the specific medicines, in their specific dilutions and dosage patterns, have been standardized by us.

5.3 The Banerji cancer treatment protocols

The main objective we follow while taking on the treatment of our cancer cases is to provide them with a better quality of life and, if possible, to provide a permanent cure. The Banerji Protocols are designed taking into account the diagnosis as well as the various complaints being suffered by the patients. We give a basic set of medicines to treat each cancer type and have 1st line, 2nd line and in most scenarios 3rd line medicines already thought out and designated. This is complemented by preset medicines to give palliative relief to the suffering of the patients brought on by accompanying symptoms. This is the basis of the Banerji Protocols, where quality of life is given paramount importance. The medicines that we use for different types of cancer are listed in detail in Table 1, but require an insight into cancer care for the practitioner in terms of pathology and the cause and effect of the morbid situation affecting the individual.

Type of Cancer	First line	Second line	Third line	Related Symptoms	Symptomatic treatment
Brain	Ruta graveolens 6C, 2xday Calcarea phos 3X, 2xday			Seizures, headache	Arnica montana 3C + Cuprum metallicum 6C
				Confusion	Helleborus 30C liq. 2xday
				Cerebral edema	Lycopodium liq. 30C 2xday
				Hemoptysis	Ferrum phos 3X 5 tablets SOS
				Pleural effusion	Lycopodium 30C liq. 3xday

Type of Cancer	First line	Second line	Third line	Related Symptoms	Symptomatic treatment
Breast cancer	Phytolacca 200C 2xday Carcinosin 30C, on alternate night	Phytolacca 200C 2xday Carcinosin 30C, on alternate night Conium maculatum 3C, 2xday	Stop the above medication and start with a new protocol Thuja occidentalis. 30C, 2xday	In agressive open ulcer with offensive discharge	Psorinum 1000c on alternate morning and Antimonium crudum 200c + Arsenicum album 200c 4xday
Esophageal carcinoma	Condurango 30C liq. 4xday	Nitric Acid 3C liq. 2xday Carbo animalis 200C liq. 2xday	Staphysagria 30C liq. 6xday		
Prostate cancer	Thuja occ. 30C 4xday Carcinosin 30C, on alternate night	Medorrhi-num 200C 2xday Cantharis 200C 2xday	Conium mac. 1000C liq. 1xweek Sabal serrulata Q liq. 2xday Carcinosin 30C,alter-nate nights	Hematuria	Geranium maculatum Q liq. 3xday If this fails then Hamamelis virginica Q liq. 4xday
Prostate (cont'd)				Dysuria	Chimaphila umbellata Q liq. every 1to 2 hours
Pancreas cancer	Carduus mar. Q liq. & Conium mac. 3C liq. every 3 hours alternately Chelidonium majus 6X liq. 3xday	Hydrastis Q liq. & Chelidon-ium 6X liq. every three hours alternately			
Liver cancer	Hydrastis canadensis Q liq. & Chelidon-ium majus 6X liq. every 3 hours alternately Conium maculatum 3C, 2xday	Myrica Q liq. & Hydrastis canadensis Q liq. every 3 hours alternately Carduus marianus Q liq. 2xday			
Rectal cancer	Nitric acid 3C liq. 6xday	Hydrastis 200C & Mercurius solubilis 200C, every 3 hours alternately	Thuja occ. 30C 2xday	Involuntary stool	Veratrum album 200c every 3 hours

Type of Cancer	First line	Second line	Third line	Related Symptoms	Symptomatic treatment
Stomach cancer **Stomach (cont'd)**	Arsenicum alb. 3C liq. 15 minutes before food. plus Hydrastis Q liq. 2xday	Conium maculatum 3C, 2xday Hydrastis Q 2xday			
Uterus, Cervix,Ovary and Appendages cancer	Carbo animalis 200C, 3xday Arnica montana 3C, 3xday	Kreosotum 200C, 4xday	Kreosotum 200C, 4xday Conium maculatum 3C, 2xday		
Osteosarcoma	Symphy-tum offic. 200C, & Calcarea phos 3X, every 3 hours alternately Carcinosin 30C, on alternate nights	Ruta graveolens 200C, & Calcarea phosphorica 3X, every 3 hours alternately			
Colon cancer	Hydrastis Q liq. & Nitric acid 3C liq. every 3 hours alternately	Conium maculatum 3C & Hydrastis 200C every 3 hours alternately	Carbo animalis 200C, 4xday Ferrum phos 3X + Calcarea Fluorica 3X , 2xday	Bleeding per rectum	Hamamelis Virginica Q liq. SOS after every bleeding
				Palpable lump in abdomen	Conium maculatum 3C liq. 1xweek
Throat cancer – pyriform fossa and allied parts	Nitric acid 3C liq, 4xday	Hepar sulphur 200C 4xday Also Hydrastis Canadensis 200c 2xday	Thuja occ. 30C 2xday Kali muriaticum 3X, 4xday	Acute painful deglutition	Mercurius cyanatus 200C, 3xday
Tongue and Cheek cancer	Nitric acid 3C liq, 4xday	Nitric acid 3C liq, 4xday Cistus canadensis. 200C liq.	Mercurius cyanatus 200C liq. 1xday Kali muriaticum 3X, 4xday		

Table 1. Banerji Protocols for treatment of selected cancers. One dose is 2 pills, tablets or drops unless otherwise specified. In Europe, C is equivalent to CH or CK; X is equivalent to D or DH.

5.4 The data collection project of the PBHRF – A unique platform for the research community

In our research foundation the main research activity consists of recording in our electronic data base the treatment and response of all cases of various types of cancer and other life-threatening diseases treated at our clinics. To this end, we maintain a recently upgraded, state-of-the-art computer network with a high-end server and five nodes. Our system also has two stand-alones for internet access and image processing and storage. At present our patient database running on customized software on Oracle and MS Visual Basic has more than 20,000 cases inputted with more than half a million visits recorded. The data consists of approximately 60 cancer types by site, including two cases of cancer of the heart. This data is the epicenter of the PBHRF and makes us attractive to researchers from premiere institutions throughout the world. Clinicians and researchers from many of these institutions have visited our clinics for an insight into our way of treatment. This is an ongoing research initiative that has been active since 2002, though due to our access to cases prior to this date, we have been able to get a wider perspective from even earlier in our experience.

At present, we are in the process of collaborating with researchers from the National Cancer Institute of the United States with the desire to mine the data and use the information to understand better the sphere of efficacy, as well as to fine tune our protocols.

5.5 Cancer treatment outcomes at PBHRF with the Banerji Protocols

In the six months prior to preparation of this manuscript, we saw a total of 1856 cancer cases at PBHRF. Table 2 shows the types of cancer treated during this period.

TYPE OF CANCER	% total cases	# of cases
BRAIN	21%	385
LUNG	14%	260
BREAST	7%	129
GALL BLADDER	5%	98
STOMACH	5%	92
CERVIX	4%	71
ESOPHAGUS	4%	66
RECTUM	3%	55
TONGUE	3%	56
PANCREAS	2%	36
LIVER	2%	36
CHEEK	2%	35
PROSTATE	2%	31
OVARIAN	2%	31
NON HODGKIN'S LYMPHOMA	2%	31
OSTEOSARCOMA	1%	10
OTHER	21%	434
TOTAL	100%	1856

Table 2. Types of cancer cases treated at PBHRF in 6-month period, 2010-2011

Our overall aggregate retrospective data collected on over 20,000 patients with all varieties of cancer treated over an 18-year period (Figure 1) reveals that 21% of the cancers completely regressed, and 23% were improved or stable.

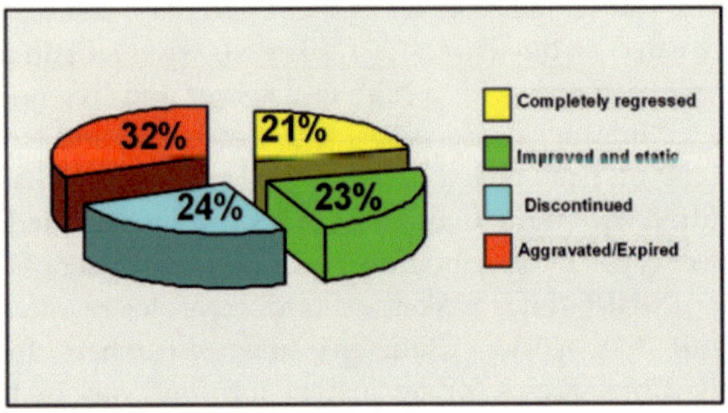

Fig. 1. Results of Treatment of 30,288 Malignant Tumor Cases (1990 - 2008)

Retrospective data collected over a one-year period on patients treated for lung, brain and esophageal cancer showed that complete regressions ranged from 22 to 32% (Figure 2).

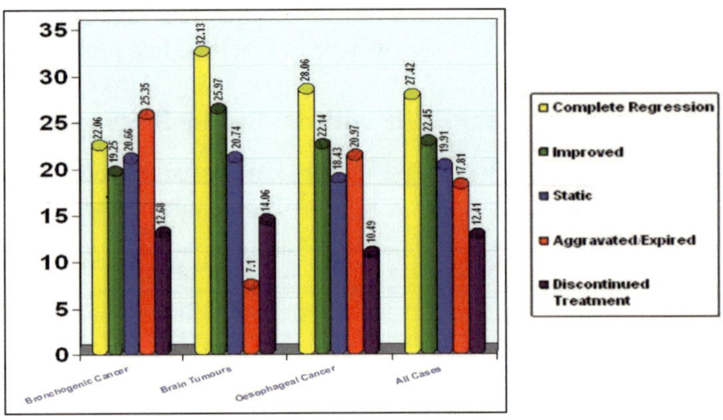

Fig. 2. Results of treatment of 1132 cases of lung, brain and esophageal cancers, August 2006-August 2007

6. Some case studies

We present below three cases, two of which, the lung cancer and the esophageal cancer case, were submitted to the National Cancer Institute of the United States for validation of the results, where they passed strict scrutiny and were presented before the Cancer Advisory Panel.

6.1 Case 1 – Lung cancer

Male, 47 years old, came to the clinic on 30th November 1994. He was suffering from chest pain with severe cough along with loss of weight for the last three months. On examination restricted respiratory movement on the left side with few localized crepitations were present in the upper part of the left chest. Chest X-ray dated the 18th of November 1994 showed "…a well-defined large soft tissue density mediastinal mass in the left upper mediastinum…the lung fields are well expanded. Area of consolidation is seen in the left upper lobe." (Figure 3)

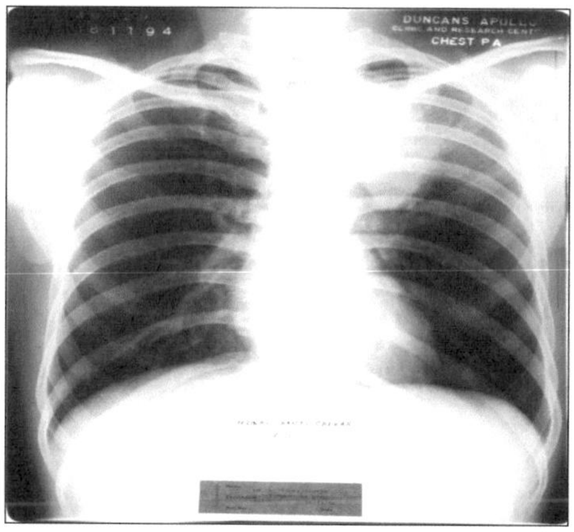

Fig. 3. Case 1, Chest X-ray 18.11.1994

C.T. Scan of chest dated 19th November 1994 shows "an 8.0 cm x 6.4 cm well defined soft tissue mass...in upper mediastinum in left side…with air space consolidation of adjacent left upper lobe." (Figure 4)

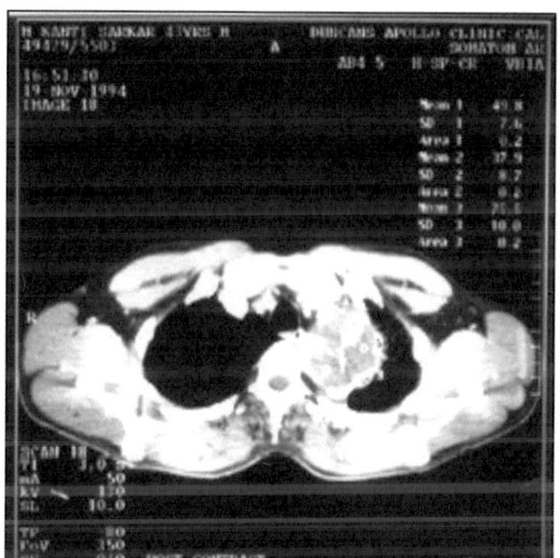

Fig. 4. Case 1, C.T. of chest 19.11.1994

C.T. Guided FNAC of mediastinal mass dated 24th of November 1994 showed "…malignant tumor." (Figure 5)

After undergoing treatment from us with the medicines Kali Carbonicum 200c two drops thrice a week and Ferrum Phosphoricum 3x two tablets twice daily, patient became asymptomatic. X-ray dated 31st of January 1995 showed "...considerable shrinkage in the mediastinal mass..." (Figure 6).

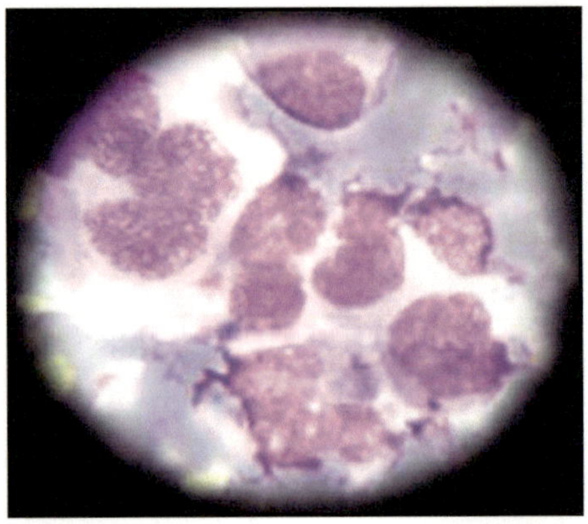

Fig. 5. Case 1, Histopathology 24.12.1994

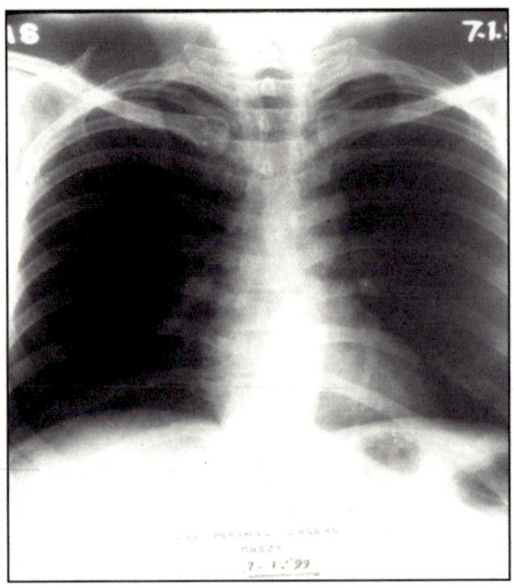

Fig. 6. Case1, Chest X-ray 31.1.1995

X-ray dated 5th of July 1995 showed "....Gradual and excellent regression of the mediastinal mass since original X-ray of 18 November 1994." X-ray dated 9th January 1996 described only a "...small residual opacity still present."

At the National Cancer Institute it was described as a diagnosed case of Malignant Neoplasm. According to TNM classification of the tumor in this case, the growth was T2, N1, M0 - Stage II; if it was a case of metastasis from an unknown primary, then it would be staged at Stage IV. Additional chest X-rays were done on several occasions. The last was on 7th of January 1999, which showed complete resolution of the mediastinal tumor (Figure 7). There were no complications during treatment. We are still reviewing the case off and on but there has been no recurrence.

6.2 Case 2 – Esophageal cancer

Male, aged 75 years, was suffering for two months with difficulty in swallowing food, heartburn and belching, when he came to us for his treatment on 16th of December 1996.

Clinically the patient presented with dysphagia, heartburn and belching. His initial barium swallow showed almost complete obstruction of the esophagus, as shown in Figure 8.

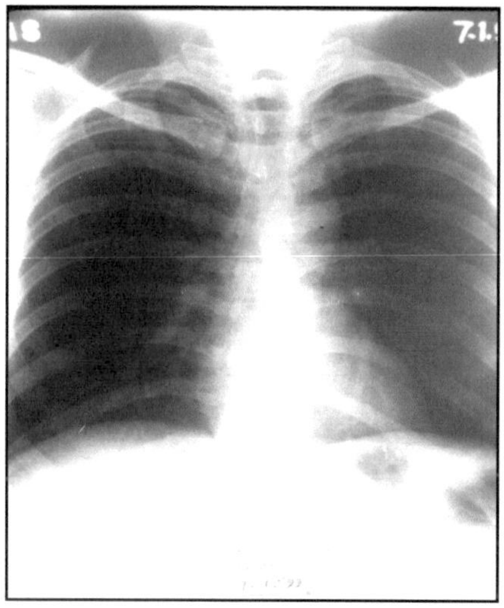

Fig. 7. Case 1, Chest X-ray 7.1.1999

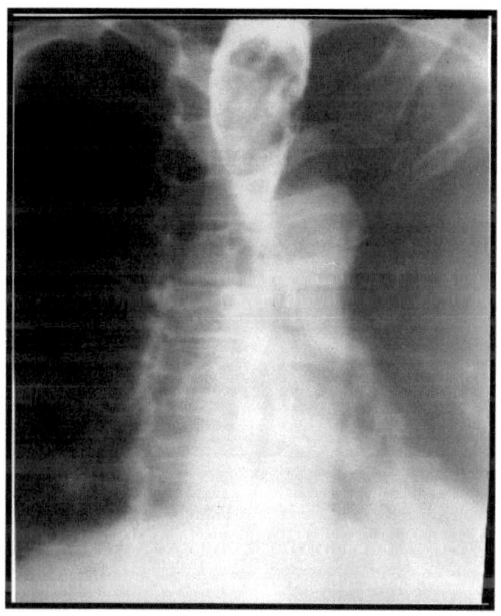

Fig. 8. Case 2, Barium swallow 17.10.1996

Endoscopy done on 29th November 1996 showed "...GE junction at 40cm. At 18 cm. is a growth extending up to 22cm. causing luminal narrowing." A biopsy dated 6th December 1996 showed "...moderately differentiated Squamous Cell Carcinoma" (Figure 9).

After undergoing treatment from us with the medicine Condurango 30c two drops twice daily, the patient's symptoms were resolved within two months. Now the patient is in good health and does not complain of dysphagia. Post treatment barium swallow X-ray of esophagus dated 12th July 1997 showed "...considerable improvement in the patency of the esophagus" (Figure 10). There were no complications during treatment.

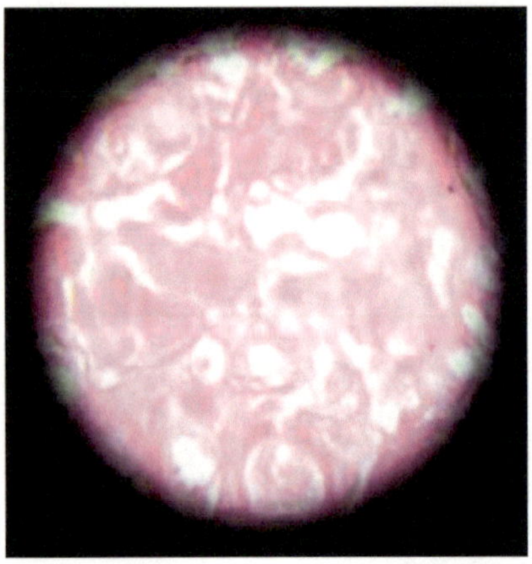

Fig. 9. Case 2, biopsy 29.11.1996

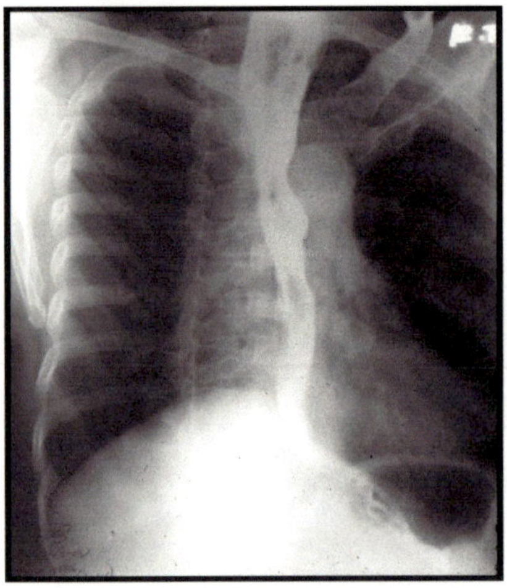

Fig. 10. Case 2, Post-treatment barium swallow 12.7.1997

6.3 Case 3 – Osteosarcoma

Male, aged 8 years, was suffering for 5 to 6 months with swelling in left knee and difficulty in flexing the knee, when he came to us for his treatment on 18th July 2003. On examination the patient presented with a non tender, firm to hard swelling over the left knee joint. X-ray of left knee joint dated 5th June 2003 showed "…a well defined eccentric lesion in metaphyses with sclerosis at edges - ? fibrous cortical defect/aneurismal bone cyst/lymphoma…" (Figure 11).

The child underwent histopathological examination of the swelling and the report dated 12th June 2003 showed "…Section shows histology of a high grade sarcomatous lesion showing many mitotic figures…Poorly differentiated sarcomatous lesion…" (Figure 12). At that time the parents of the child were advised at the Chittaranjan National Cancer Institute, Kolkata, to allow immediate "…above the lesion amputation…" of the affected leg.

After undergoing treatment from us with the medicines Symphytum 200c two doses a day, Calcarea Phosphorica 3X two doses a day and Carcinosin 30c one dose every alternate day, the swelling gradually subsided and now the architecture of the knee has completely returned to normal. X-ray dated 16th December 2003 revealed "…gross healing at osteolytic area..." (Figure 13).

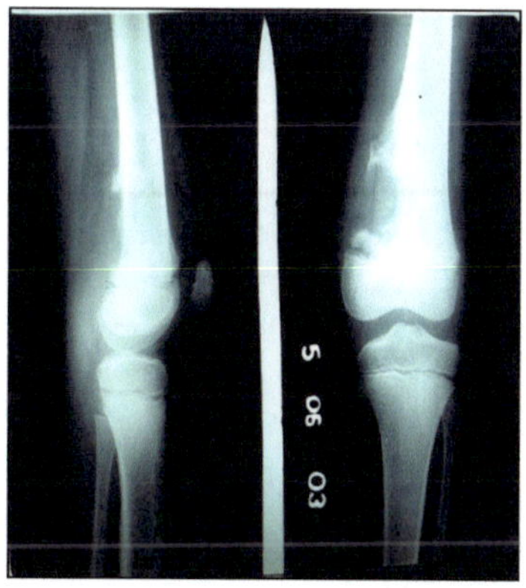

Fig. 11. Case 3, X-ray 5.6.2003

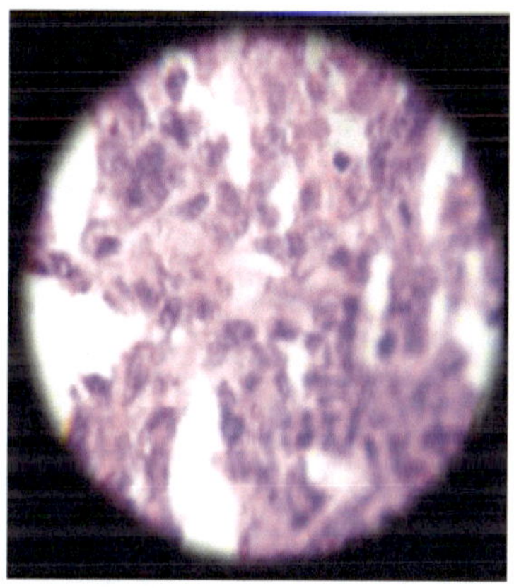

Fig. 12. Case 3, Histopathology 12.6.2003

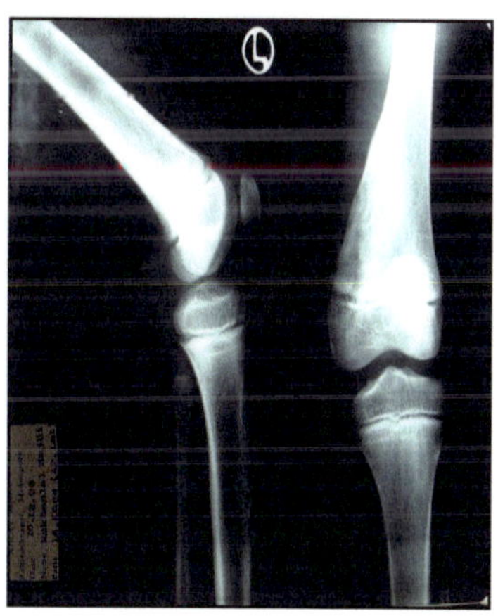

Fig. 13. Case 3, X-ray 16.12.2003

Repeat X-ray dated 14th August 2004 showed "…remineralization seen at the lower third of left femur..." (Figure 14). He then reduced the doses and discontinued our medication after four months.

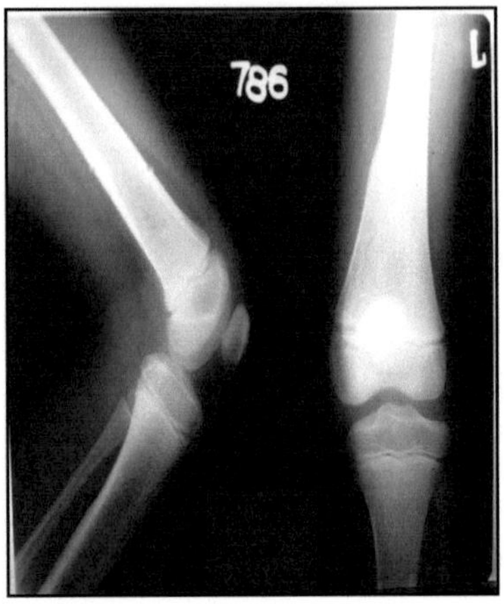

Fig. 14. Case 3, X-ray 14.8.2004

7. Worldwide interest in the Banerji Protocols

However, since 1997, there have been winds of change. It was this year when the National Institutes of Health (NIH) of the United States asked us to produce records of our successes as part of their Best Case Series programme for evaluating clinical data from alternative healthcare practitioners. We submitted complete records of cured cases in 1997, and our presentation of cases was accepted after detailed scrutiny by the National Cancer Institute (NCI) in 1999. Subsequently, we provided a six-hour presentation before a 17-member Cancer Advisory Panel. This panel included cancer specialists from all the leading American Comprehensive Cancer Centers, including the Washington Cancer Institute, The University of Texas M. D. Anderson Cancer Center, The Memorial Sloan Kettering Cancer Center, and The Johns Hopkins Medical Center. The panel accepted our presentation unanimously, and this was indeed a great victory for homeopathy (Banerji, 2008).

Since then we have had many visitors from the United States including: Dr. Jeffrey White, MD, Director, Office of Cancer Complementary and Alternative Medicine, National Cancer Institute; Dr. Moshe Frenkel, Associate Professor of Integrative Medicine and Medical Director of the Integrative Medicine Program, Division of Cancer Medicine Department of Palliative Care and Rehabilitation Medicine at the University of Texas M D Anderson Cancer Center; Dr. Elena Ladas, MS, RD, Director, and Dr. Kara M. Kelly, MD, Medical Director of the Integrative Therapies Program for Children with Cancer, Division of Pediatric Oncology, and others from Columbia University; and Dr. Barbara Sarter, now at the University of San Diego, who spent five months in Kolkata to study the Banerji Protocols and work with us when she held a faculty position in the Department of Family Medicine at the University of Southern California; she has a long background in conventional medicine, and also a degree in classical homeopathy.

An important aspect of the PBHRF's activities is research, and under its banner, Drs. Banerji have been involved in recent years in collaborative research projects with American institutes of international renown which include the University of Texas M. D. Anderson Cancer Center, Columbia University, and the University of Kansas Medical Center. Since 1977, Drs. Banerji have been invited to a large number of prestigious international conferences, symposia, seminars and meetings to deliver lectures, present papers, or discuss important aspects of their work. Patients from more than 70 countries at present follow the Banerji Protocols through the website www.pbhrfindia.org, seeking online medical advice and treatment.

Spain has assumed great importance for our work in recent years. In 2008, a three-member cancer support team from Spain undertook a week-long visit to PBHRF to acquire firsthand knowledge about the Banerji Protocols; two hold senior positions at the University of Barcelona, while the third runs a Valencia-based web portal for cancer support, which is visited by nearly 1000 persons daily, not only in Spain, but also in Spanish-speaking countries elsewhere in the world - with many enquiries on the Banerji Protocols.

The response of Spanish homeopaths, pharmacists and patients to the Banerji Protocols has been extremely enthusiastic. In 2008, Drs. Banerji made a presentation at a conference exclusively for classical homeopaths who enthusiastically welcomed the Banerji Protocols. A documentary film on Dr. Prasanta Banerji is now being made by two Spanish documentary film makers who have undertaken visits to Kolkata and Mihijam.

In 2009, Drs. Banerji visited Japan twice, and there are excellent prospects for the popularization of treatment in this country using the Banerji Protocols. They are scheduled to visit again by invitation from the Royal Academy of Homeopathy, for more seminars in October 2011.

8. Conclusion: Winds of change

Compared to conventional medicine, homeopathy has always suffered from a lack of credibility and recognition the world over, having been acceptable only to those who cannot afford the high costs of conventional medical treatment. However, since 1977, there have been winds of change. There has, on the one hand, been a perceptible lack of success of conventional medicine to cure various ailments and diseases - notably cancer - and, on the other, the serious - and growing - concern of researchers to identify options for medical treatment offered by various streams of alternative medicine, including homeopathy. It is here that the Banerji Protocols of treatment, based on the use of homeopathic medicines, have had an important role to play. Dr. Prasanta Banerji and Dr. Pratip Banerji, along with their assistants, together attend 1000 to 1200 patients every day, including 300 to 400 patients at their free clinic, in Kolkata. By so doing, they keep up the tradition of their revered forefathers, help make the Banerji Protocols a mode of medical treatment for the masses - the second important objective of the PBHRF — and ensure the collection, documentation and use in meaningful research in the years to come. The operations of the PBHRF and the development of the Banerji Protocols have been giving homeopathy a scientific basis and making it eligible for scientific research.

8.1 Looking at the future

To meaningfully serve medical science and humanity, homeopathy required a rebirth. Perhaps nothing can provide this better than the Banerji Protocols and the work of the PBHRF, both aimed at making homeopathy with the use of the Banerji Protocols scientifically acceptable.

Opposition to the Banerji Protocols and the work of the PBHRF from the scientific community and followers of classical homeopathy notwithstanding, everything augurs well for the rebirth of homeopathy. Much is required to make the Banerji Protocols and the role of the PBHRF known everywhere in the world.

9. Acknowledgements

The authors acknowledge the contributions of the following: Dr. Barbara Sarter, PhD, RN, FNP-C, DIHom, Associate Professor, Advanced Practice Programs, Hahn School of Nursing and Health Science, University of San Diego, for her help in writing the manuscript as well as editing the same and making it presentable for publication. This could not have been done without her help. Dr. Aminul Islam, PhD, Department of Zoology, K. C. College, Hetampur, Birbhum, West Bengal, India, for help in collecting information on cancer and alternative medicines. Dr. Apurba Dey, MD(Hom), of the PBHRF, for his diligent editing of the case studies. The assistant doctors of our clinics, who help us to optimize the care rendered to the suffering masses of patients who visit us, lightening our burden sufficiently so that we could apply our minds to this chapter. The patients, the ultimate teachers, who due to the privilege they have accorded us by allowing us to treat them, have taught us the way to fine tune treatments and arrive at the Banerji Protocols for every possible disease.

10. References

Banerjee, A., Pathak, S., Biswas, S. J., Roy-Karmakar, S., Boujedaini, N., Belon, P. (2010). Chelidonium majus 30C and 200C in induced hepato-toxicity in rats. [Research Support, Non-U.S. Gov't]. *Homeopathy: the Journal of the Faculty of Homeopathy, 99*(3), 167-176

Banerji, P., Campbell, D. R., Banerji, P., Campbell, D. R., & Banerji, P. (2008). Cancer patients treated with the Banerji protocols utilising homoeopathic medicine: a Best Case Series Program of the National Cancer Institute USA. *Oncology Reports, 20*(1), 69-74

Becker-Witt, C., Lüdtke, R., Weißhuhn, T., & Willich, S. (2004). Diagnoses and Treatment in Homeopathic Medica Practice. *Forsch Komplementärmed Klass Naturheilkd, 11*, 98-103

Chang, K. H., Brodie, R., Choong, M. A., & Sweeney, K. J. (2011). Complementary and alternative medicine use in oncology: A questionnaire survey of patients and health care professionals. *Biomed Central Cancer, 11*, 196

Ernst, E. (2000). The role of Complementary and Alternative Medicine in Cancer. *Lancet Oncology, 1*, 176 – 180

Ernst, E. (2005). Why Alternative medicines are used. *Pharmaceutical Journals, 275*, 55

Frenkel, M. Homeopathy in cancer care. *Altern Ther Health Med, 16*, 12 – 16

Frenkel, M., Mishra, B. M., Sen, S., Yang, P., Pawlus, A., Vence, L., et al. (2010). Cytotoxic effects of ultra-diluted remedies on breast cancer cells. *International Journal of Oncology, 36*(2), 395-403

Ghosh, A. K. (2010). A short history of the development of homeopathy in India. *Homeopathy, 99*(2), 130-136

Hahnemann, S. (1982). *Organon of Medicine* (J. Kunzli, Trans.). Los Angeles: J. P. Tarcher

Hobhouse, R. (2002). *Life of Christian Samuel Hahnemann*. New Delhi: B. Jain

Honigberger, J. M. (1852). *Thirty-five years in the East: Adventures, discoveries, etc., relating to the Punjab and Cashmere; in connection with medicine, botany, pharmacy, &c*. Vol. 1-2. Boston: Harvard University.

Kassab S, et. al. (2009). Homeopathic medicines for adverse effects of cancer treatments. Cochrane Database Systematic Reviews. 2:CD004845

Kumar, K. B., Sunila, E. S., Kuttan, G., Preethi, K. C., Venugopal, C. N., Kuttan, R., et al. (2007). Inhibition of chemically induced carcinogenesis by drugs used in homeopathic medicine. *Asian Pacific Journal of Cancer Prevention: Apjcp, 8*(1), 98-102

MacLaughlin, B. W., Gutsmuths, B., Pretner, E., Jonas, W. B., Ives, J., Kulawardane, D. V., et al. (2006). Effects of homeopathic preparations on human prostate cancer growth in cellular and animal models. *Integrative Cancer Therapies, 5*(4), 362-372

Marino, R. (2008). Homeopathy and Collective Health: The Case of Dengue Epidemics. *International Journal of High Dilution Research, 7*(25)

Milazzo, S., Russell, N., & Ernst, E. (2006). Efficacy of homeopathic therapy in cancer treatment. *Eur J Cancer, 42*, 282 – 289

Pathak, S., Kumar Das, J., Jyoti Biswas, S., Khuda-Bukhsh, A. R., Pathak, S., Kumar Das, J., et al. (2006). Protective potentials of a potentized homeopathic drug, Lycopodium-30, in ameliorating azo dye induced hepatocarcinogenesis in mice. *Molecular & Cellular Biochemistry, 285*(1-2), 121-131

Pathak, S., Multani, A. S., Banerji, P., Pathak, S., Multani, A. S., Banerji, P., et al. (2003). Ruta 6 selectively induces cell death in brain cancer cells but proliferation in normal peripheral blood lymphocytes: A novel treatment for human brain cancer. *International Journal of Oncology, 23*(4), 975-982

Rostock, M., Naumann, J., Guethlin, C., Guenther, L., Bartsch, H., & Walach, H. (2011). Classical homeopathy in the treatment of cancer patients - a prospective observational study of two independent cohorts. *BMC Cancer, 11*(1), 19

Singh, P., Yadav, R. J., & Pandey, A. (2005). Utilization of indigenous systems of medicine & homoeopathy in India. *Indian Journal of Medical Research, 122*(2), 137-142

Thangapazham, R. L., Rajeshkumar, N. V., Sharma, A., Warren, J., Singh, A. K., Ives, J. A., et al. (2006). Effect of homeopathic treatment on gene expression in Copenhagen rat tumor tissues. *Integrative Cancer Therapies, 5*(4), 350-355

Träger-Maury, S., C, C. T., Maindrault-Goebel, F., Afchain, P., Gramont, A. d., Garcia-Larnicol, M. L., et al. (2007).Use of complementary medicine by cancer patients in a French oncology department. *Bulletin of Cancer, 94*(11), 1017-1025

World Health Organization. (2006). India: Country Cooperation Strategy Brief. http://www.who.int/countries/ind/

Part 3

Feldenkrais Method

6

The *Feldenkrais Method*® of Somatic Education

Patricia A. Buchanan
Des Moines University,
USA

1. Introduction

The *Feldenkrais Method*® of somatic education is an integrative approach to learning and improving function among people of varying abilities across the lifespan. With an emphasis on increasing self-awareness through lessons that stimulate sensing, moving, feeling, and thinking, certified practitioners or teachers of the method propose to take advantage of the human capacity to self-organize behavior (Buchanan & Ulrich, 2001; Ginsburg, 2010).

People have used the *Feldenkrais Method* to enhance their function in many aspects of life, including performance at work, in sports, or in the performing arts. However, estimates are that many more have used it to recover from injury, manage pain, reduce stress, or improve other health-related conditions, either as complementary or alternative approaches to traditional Western medicine. Because of this usage, some groups, such as the United States National Institutes of Health's National Center for Complementary and Alternative Medicine (National Center for Complementary and Alternative Medicine [NCCAM], 2004), view the *Feldenkrais Method* as a form of complementary and alternative medicine, despite the broader self identification as a learning method.

Method founder Moshe Feldenkrais, DSc, (1904-1984) was cautious about the constraints he perceived would be associated with establishing his method within a medical model and the broadly held allopathic emphasis on disease of his time (Feldenkrais, 2010). Despite medicine's growing biopsychosocial perspective, identification with it remains controversial today among practitioners. Some recognize the improved access that may be afforded by that association, while others express apprehension, as did Feldenkrais, about the limitations on this learning method that may follow.

Despite these concerns, Feldenkrais and practitioners of his method would likely agree with the broader definition of health espoused by the World Health Organization. Feldenkrais viewed health as the ability to be flexible and adaptable in life, to recover, and not simply be free from illness or injury (Feldenkrais, 1981, 2010). Similarly, the World Health Organization defined health in the preamble to its constitution as "a state of complete physical, mental and social well-being and not merely the absence of disease or infirmity" (World Health Organization, 1946). Thus, in this context, the *Feldenkrais Method* is an approach to promoting health.

In this chapter, I address four purposes. First, I provide an overview of the *Feldenkrais Method* including background on its originator, descriptions of the two main approaches to delivering lessons (*Functional Integration®* and *Awareness Through Movement®*), and a theoretical foundation grounded in dynamic systems theory. Second, I describe what is known about *Feldenkrais* practitioners (teachers) including the certification process, standards of practice, and the practice profiles of United States practitioners. Third, I place the *Feldenkrais Method* in context with other complementary and alternative medicine approaches. Finally, I review the English language peer-reviewed research regarding the *Feldenkrais Method* and summarize the available evidence regarding its efficacy and safety.

2. The *Feldenkrais Method*

Feldenkrais had a broad view of health and the role that learning plays in being healthy. He argued, "It is certainly not enough to say that not asking for medical or psychiatric help is proof of health" (Feldenkrais, 2010, p. 54). In recognition of the immense number of parts that comprise the human nervous system, he stated: "The health of such a system can be measured by the shock it can take without compromising the continuation of its process. In short, health is measured by the shock a person can take without his usual way of life being compromised" (Feldenkrais, 2010, p. 55). Feldenkrais was among early proponents of the critical role of life experiences in the differentiation of the nervous system and the refinement of our abilities to perceive, feel, act and think. The quality and content of these experiences foster organic learning capable of continuing across the lifespan. From this perspective, health may continue into old age, as is exemplified by artists, writers, musicians and scientists who excel as elders. "The outstanding difference between such healthy people and the others is that they have found by intuition, genius, or had the luck to learn from a healthy teacher, that learning is the gift of life. A special kind of learning: that of knowing oneself. They learn to know 'how' they are acting and thus are able to do 'what' they want—the intense living of their unavowed, and sometimes declared, dreams" (Feldenkrais, 2010, p. 54). This process of learning is what Feldenkrais wanted to promote with his method. The biographical sketch that follows offers insights into how he came to develop his method.

2.1 Founder, Moshe Feldenkrais

Moshe Feldenkrais was born in 1904 in what is now Slavuta, Ukraine and moved at age 5 to Baranovichi, Belarus (Feldenkrais, 1981, 2010; Kaetz, 2007). These towns were literally along the front lines of World War I. They were also Jewish communities that were instrumental in the rise of Hasidic culture that highly valued education grounded in questioning, critical inquiry, self-awareness, and learning for self-improvement. While his family managed to survive, nearly all Jews in these towns were killed in the pogroms (Kaetz, 2007). After the 1917 Balfour Declaration, Feldenkrais left for Palestine in 1918. He used his mathematics and surveyor skills, and his physical labor to help build Tel Aviv (Kaetz, 2007). He also developed skills in self-defense and shared those survival techniques with his peers.

In 1930, Feldenkrais moved to Paris, France to study engineering (Feldenkrais, 1981, 2010). During that time, he met Kano, the originator of Judo, and became one of the first Europeans to earn a black belt. He continued his studies at the Sorbonne and worked in the laboratories of the Joliot-Curies. When the Nazis came to Paris in 1940, Feldenkrais escaped to Great Britain and worked on anti-submarine defense through the remainder of World War II (Feldenkrais, 1981, 1996). During this time, Feldenkrais was functionally impaired by his knees that were first injured during a football (soccer) match in Palestine, and further damaged by escaping France and moving about submarines. Medical options for relief were limited and not very promising. Instead, Feldenkrais began a process of self-exploration that helped him restore his function and developed into his method. He delved into the literature of many disciplines, from mechanics to psychology. Feldenkrais compiled a series of lectures that were well-received by the scientists with him in Scotland (Feldenkrais, 1981, 2010). After Feldenkrais moved to London at the end of the war, he published those lectures as his first book about his method, *Body and Mature Behavior* (Feldenkrais, 1996).

Feldenkrais returned to Israel in 1951; he was soon fully occupied with teaching his method. As the popularity of his work grew, he developed hundreds of lessons that could be delivered verbally to groups of students. Late in life, he taught others to teach his method, beginning in Israel and ending in the United States. He died in 1984 (Feldenkrais, 2010).

It is remarkable, while also understandable given his background, that Feldenkrais "would choose learning as the most useful path for serving the wholeness of both individual and society" (Kaetz, 2007, p. 87). Thus, the *Feldenkrais Method* is first and foremost a learning method, albeit one with reported therapeutic effects. It is an embodied process of self-inquiry that typically occurs in two formats: individual lessons called *Functional Integration*, and group lessons known as *Awareness Through Movement*.

2.2 Individual lessons: *Functional Integration*

Functional Integration lessons (see Fig. 1) use manual contact between teacher and student to guide the student to better understand current patterns of behavior and inform the student in a manner that facilitates self-organization of alternative, improved behavior (Feldenkrais, 1972, 1981, 2010). Students are comfortably clothed during lessons that usually last 30-60 minutes. Teachers use supportive, non-invasive touch that can be informative to both students and teachers. Teachers individualize lessons to target functional goals expressed by students, while using principles and techniques common to the *Feldenkrais Method*. Some of these include: creating a sense of safety with respectful touch and support of body parts; moving limbs through pathways of minimal resistance to suggest more optimal movement trajectories; clarifying existing habitual patterns of positioning and organization to facilitate reorganization; compressing, lengthening, or guiding other movements with emphasis on contact that is as if it were skeleton-to-skeleton; and positioning parts so as to shorten muscles, facilitate decreased contractile activity, and allow more lengthening without stretching (Feldenkrais, 1972, 1981, 2010; Ginsburg, 2010).

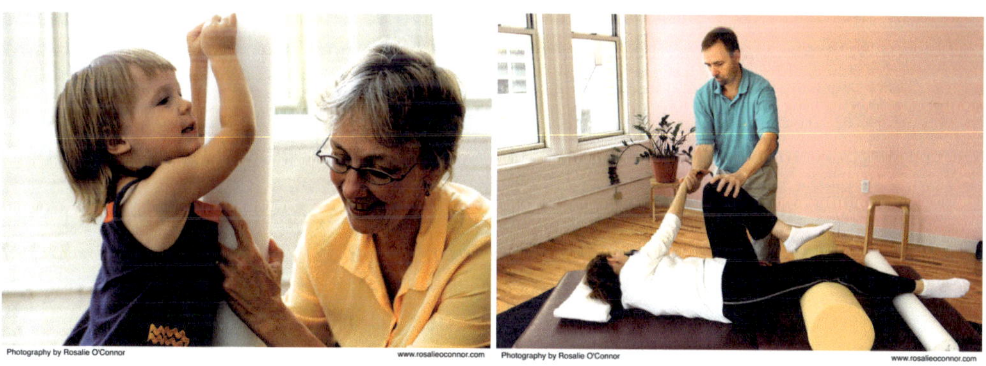

Fig. 1. Examples of *Functional Integration* lessons.

2.3 Group lessons: Awareness Through Movement

Awareness Through Movement lessons (see Fig. 2) are verbally guided explorations that are about 30-60 minutes long. They can be taught to groups of students or to individuals. As with *Functional Integration* lessons, but absent the manual contact, *Awareness Through Movement* lessons use principles to help students notice what they currently do, improve their ability to make finer perceptual distinctions, and guide them to explore modes of action that result in self-improvement (Feldenkrais, 1972, 1981, 2010; Ginsburg, 2010). Students are comfortably clothed, encouraged to move in pain-free ranges, and instructed to reduce effort and move slowly enough to be attentive to what they are doing, sensing, feeling, and thinking. Teachers rarely model movements, but may occasionally highlight alternative approaches students are using to express the verbal instructions. Lessons have one, if not several functional applications, but the overall movement pattern is usually not stated in advance to facilitate individually appropriate learning. Lessons often involve gentle, slow movements, but range from lessons that mainly involve the imagination to more challenging, athletic lessons (Feldenkrais, 1972, 1981, 2010; Ginsburg, 2010).

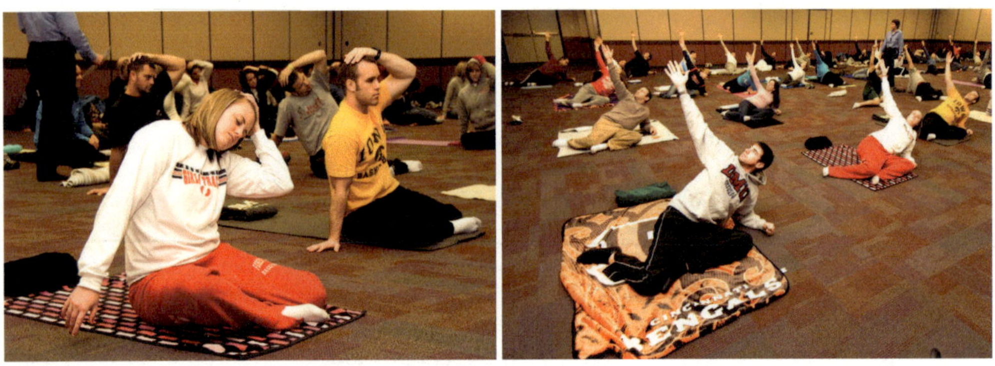

Photographs courtesy of Des Moines University

Fig. 2. Examples of *Awareness Through Movement* lessons.

2.4 *Feldenkrais Method* as an application of dynamic systems theory

As a scientist in the mid-twentieth century, Feldenkrais interacted with numerous leading researchers and scholars of the day. He was privy to and participated in advancing new approaches to understanding the behavior of living and non-living systems (Buchanan & Ulrich, 2001; Feldenkrais, 1981; Ginsburg, 2010). Concurrently, he made significant advances in his concrete application of the relatively abstract and nascent fields of cybernetics, systems theory, complexity, and dynamic systems theory (Ginsburg, 2010). Applications of these new theories to human behavior and development came to prominence during the 1980s and 1990s (Buchanan & Ulrich, 2001; Ginsburg, 2010). When Thelen and Smith published *A Dynamic Systems Approach to the Development of Cognition and Action* in 1994, several *Feldenkrais* teachers quickly saw that they were describing a highly plausible theoretical foundation for the *Feldenkrais Method* (Buchanan & Ulrich, 2001; Ginsburg, 2010; Spencer et al., 2006). This section identifies several of the parallels between the *Feldenkrais Method* and dynamic systems theory.

Feldenkrais explicitly valued life as a process situated in time that is reflective of evolution, culture, and individual history. All of these factors influence human behavior (Feldenkrais, 2010; Ginsburg, 2010). Dynamic systems theory holds that behavior emerges in the moment, while recognizing that change happens on differing time scales and that preceding events influence subsequent events (Spencer et al., 2006; Thelen & Smith, 1994). For example, an infant (or adult) lying on her back and holding her feet may turn the head and begin to roll to the side. Another roll of the head can bring her to her back again. As she goes back and forth, she may look up at someone entering the room and be surprised to find she rolls to sit.

Feldenkrais recognized the limitations of linear and cause-effect scientific approaches. Behavior is dependent on many interacting elements and change, for the better or for the worse, can occur suddenly or gradually (Feldenkrais, 2010; Ginsburg, 2010). Dynamic systems theory proposes that multiple subsystems interact in ways that are often nonlinear to softly assemble behavior. Increasing speed leads me to change from walking to running. A short series of *Awareness Through Movement* lessons can relieve my chronic low back pain.

Feldenkrais argued for the unity of mind and body: "I believe that the unity of mind and body is an objective reality. They are not just parts somehow related to each other, but an inseparable whole while functioning" (Feldenkrais, 2010, p. 28). In another paper, he wrote: "The mental and physical components of any action are two different aspects of the same function. The physical and mental components are not two series of phenomena, which are somehow linked together; but, rather, they are two aspects of the same thing, like two faces of the same coin" (Feldenkrais, 2010, pp. 19-20). Dynamic systems theory similarly argues for an integrated, embodied life of humans who have brains situated in bodies that exist in environments and interact with others such that perception, action and cognition are co-dependent and co-develop. While emotions or feeling are not ignored in dynamic systems, Feldenkrais gave early recognition to this component through his description of learning and development that emerge through sensing, moving, thinking, and feeling (Feldenkrais, 2010). The implications are: there are multiple approaches to facilitating change, and changing one aspect or subsystem can alter the organization of the whole.

Feldenkrais was among the earliest to argue for use-dependant changes in the brain. Early on he wrote that for the most part, "behaviour is acquired and has nothing permanent about it but our belief that it is so" (Feldenkrais, 1996, p. 6). With this perspective, he emphasized the importance of flexible and adaptable behavior, and warned of habits so strong that they "can be likened to a groove into which the person sinks never to leave unless some special force makes him do so. With time, the groove deepens, and stronger forces are necessary to remove him from it" (Feldenkrais, 1996, p. 118). In dynamic systems theory, these grooves are attractors. Strong attractors have little variability in their activity and require large perturbations to provoke change to another state; weak attractors are unreliable and highly variable. More useful are attractors that are sufficiently stable with enough variability to allow for change as needed (Spencer et al., 2006; Thelen & Smith, 1994). With sufficient motivation and clear intention, change—improvement—is available throughout life.

Feldenkrais clearly recognized the influence of one's experience and circumstances in development. Here, his multicultural experiences are evident in his recognition of the influence of sitting styles (e.g., in chairs or on the ground) on the function of the hips and back, and of language on the usage and structure of the vocal apparatus (Feldenkrais, 1981,

1996, 2010). While knowledgeable of human structure and function, he was not prescriptive with his method. Instead, his approach was to help individuals clarify their self-images in order to self-organize individually relevant and appropriate options for acting (Feldenkrais, 2010; Ginsburg, 2010). Dynamic systems theory has similar regard for individual pathways to species-typical behaviors, such as reaching or walking (Spencer et al., 2006; Thelen & Smith, 1994). Learning can be viewed as "carving out individual solutions to the real-world problem" (Spencer et al., 2006, p. 1534). Through exploration, people form stable patterns and ideally conserve their ability for "improvisation on a theme" (Spencer et al., 2006, p. 1534). People can access more than one solution to a problem as conditions change: to walk on pavement or on cobblestones, to sit in a chair or on the floor, to live in the midst of peace or the midst of war.

In this section, I presented an overview of the *Feldenkrais Method* of somatic education and its two components, *Functional Integration* and *Awareness Through Movement*. I shared historical background on its originator, Moshe Feldenkrais—engineer, physicist, martial artist, and survivor of two World Wars. Finally, I presented parallels suggesting that dynamic systems theory offers a foundation for understanding the *Feldenkrais Method*. The next section provides information about *Feldenkrais* practitioners and their training. I present an estimate of their numbers and locations, and offer a profile of United States practitioners.

3. Practitioners/teachers of the *Feldenkrais Method*

People who wish to teach the *Feldenkrais Method* must successfully complete professional education programs that are taught by highly experienced Certified *Feldenkrais* Trainers and Assistant Trainers. All programs follow similar standards established by recognized training accreditation boards (*Feldenkrais Guild®* of North America, 2011; International Feldenkrais Federation). Minimally, students complete 740-800 hours of a structured curriculum over a 3 to 4 year period (*Feldenkrais Guild* of North America, 2011; International Feldenkrais Federation). Consistent with the philosophy of the method, students spend considerable time experiencing lessons, as well as developing teaching skills and learning information from disciplines that are complementary to the method. Usually midway through training programs, students have a practicum in teaching *Awareness Through Movement* lessons. Once they pass, students are authorized to teach *Awareness Through Movment* lessons to the public. They cannot offer *Functional Integration* lessons until they obtain full certification. Graduates can promote themselves as teachers or practitioners of the *Feldenkrais Method*. Actual terminology varies among countries or accreditation boards. For example, Australians use Certified Feldenkrais Practitioner (CFP) (Australian Feldenkrais Guild Inc), while the *Feldenkrais Guild* of North America uses either *Guild Certified Feldenkrais Teacher®* (GCFT) or *Guild Certified Feldenkrais Practitioner*CM (GCFP) (*Feldenkrais Guild* of North America, 2011).

The International Feldenkrais Federation is the association of 17 *Feldenkrais Method* membership organizations. Its representative body adopted a model Standards of Practice in 1994 that describes the *Feldenkrais Method* and its practice (International Feldenkrais Federation). It clearly states "The Method is not a medical, massage, bodywork, or therapeutic technique. The Method is a learning process". The *Feldenkrais Guild* of North America added that "The Method may function as a complement to medical care" (*Feldenkrais Guild* of North America, 2011). The Standards of Practice describe in more detail what a practitioner does and knows than I have presented here. As is typical of professional organizations, member associations have codes of professional conduct and procedures for ethical grievances (*Feldenkrais Guild* of North America, 2011).

3.1 Distribution and numbers of practitioners

Through a review of the International Feldenkrais Federation member organizations' websites and personal communications, I estimated there are at least 6000 *Feldenkrais* teachers in approximately 32 countries in 2011. This estimate is likely quite conservative, as not all certified teachers belong to their country's professional association; therefore, many of those teachers were not counted. Teachers are primarily in Europe and North America. Table 1 lists the ten countries with the most *Feldenkrais* teachers.

Country	Estimated number of *Feldenkrais* teachers
Germany	1700
United States of America	1287
Switzerland	421
Italy	305
Israel	260
Austria	243
Australia	236
Canada	122
United Kingdom	101
France	98

Table 1. Ten countries with the highest estimated number of *Feldenkrais* teachers.

3.2 Practice profile for United States practitioners

Studies of the practice profiles of *Feldenkrais* practitioners are very limited. In a preliminary survey of United States practitioners, most responders did not have additional credentials as traditional health care providers or in other complementary and alternative medicine approaches (Buchanan, 2010). Among responders who did have traditional licenses, most (22.7%) were physical therapists. Of responders with complementary and alternative medicine credentials, massage therapists were most common (10.4%). Information about client visits suggested that most practitioners had part-time practices. On average during a week, they saw 7.6 ± 8.1 students for individual lessons, and 8.4 ± 11.5 students for group lessons. More detailed study of United States teachers is underway. Practice patterns are likely to vary considerably in different countries, but this premise needs to be investigated.

Regardless of country, *Feldenkrais* teachers meet similar certification requirements and follow comparable standards of practice. Most practitioners live in Europe and North America. Much more needs to be investigated about practice profiles, but early studies with United States teachers suggest most have part-time practices, and physical therapy and massage therapy are the most frequent additional credentials. The next section situates the *Feldenkrais Method* among other complementary and alternative medicine approaches.

4. The *Feldenkrais Method* in context

The *Feldenkrais Method* self-identifies as a learning approach for self-improvement. Given its therapeutic applications, it has been identified by others within the broad collection of complementary and alternative medicine approaches.

4.1 Classifications of the *Feldenkrais Method*

Classifications of the *Feldenkrais Method* vary and include these eight categories: manipulative and body-based practices (Barnes et al., 2008, Mamtani & Cimino, 2002; NCCAM, 2004), movement therapy (Kiser & Dagnelie, 2008; Lee, 2004; NCCAM, 2011a), mind and body interventions (Mehling et al., 2005; NCCAM, 2011b), somatic education (Cheever, 2000; Jain et al., 2004), biomechanical-noninvasive/manipulation (Jones, 2005), body work-nonconventional manual manipulation (Nayak et al., 2003), energetic therapy (Witt et al., 2008), and manual healing (Weber, 1998). Classifications of the *Feldenkrais Method* as a mind and body intervention or somatic education seem most fitting, given the integrated approach to self-organized learning through sensing, feeling, moving and thinking espoused by its teachers.

4.2 Comparisons with other approaches

Within these categories, authors grouped the *Feldenkrais Method* with up to 19 of 41 other approaches. The most frequently related approaches were Alexander Technique (12), Trager Approach (11), spinal/peripheral joint manipulation (all forms, 9), Rolfing Structural Integration (8), massage (all forms, 5), Pilates (5), and reflexology (5). The parallels between these approaches and the *Feldenkrais Method* vary considerably. I do not discuss massage since the *Feldenkrais Method* does not use massage techniques and students are fully clothed (*Feldenkrais Guild* of North America, 2011).

The *Feldenkrais Method* has the most in common with the Alexander Technique. Indeed, Feldenkrais studied the Alexander Technique while living in London after World War II and before returning to Israel in 1951 (Feldenkrais, 2010). Both approaches emphasize the organization in upright postures to optimize the carriage of the head, the integration of the spine and pelvis, and the action of the diaphragm in functions that include, but are not limited to, breathing, speaking and singing (Gilman & Yaruss, 2000; Ginsburg, 2010). Both approaches describe themselves as learning methods and use manual and verbal cues to guide awareness and suggest alternatives to existing habits (Jain et al., 2004; Schlinger, 2006). The key distinction may be that the Alexander Technique is more directive in what constitutes improved organization, whereas the *Feldenkrais Method* guides students to discover individually appropriate options for acting (Jain et al., 2004).

The Trager Approach and the *Feldenkrais Method* share perspectives on the need to reduce effort, avoid pain, and perceive differences as part of the process of reorganizing habitual patterns. The Trager Approach utilizes distinctive rhythmical, wavelike movements to release tension and create ease, and offers instruction in self-care movements (United States Trager Association, 2010). The *Feldenkrais Method* includes oscillatory movements in its repertoire, but they are not a hallmark of the method as they are in the Trager Approach. *Feldenkrais* lessons can range from simple, quiet movements to complex, vigorous actions.

Moshe Feldenkrais and Ida Rolf were contemporaries interested in optimizing human function in an environment that is greatly influenced by gravity. Both recognized the relationship of structure and alignment with function, including its emotional and psychological aspects (Gilman & Yaruss, 2000). Rolf developed an approach that emphasizes reorganization of the connective tissue through specific soft tissue mobilization techniques (Rolf Institute of Structural Integration, 2011). Rolfing Structural Integration typically begins with a classic series of ten sessions. Rolf later in life developed a series of movement lessons to increase understanding of more efficient movement patterns. Thus, Rolfing has established protocols for working with individuals and has a major component directed toward physically altering the connective tissues, including fascia. These features are distinct from the *Feldenkrais Method*, which is much more individualized in the application of lessons and does not promote manual techniques to directly alter connective tissue.

Spinal and peripheral joint manipulations are common to chiropractic and osteopathic medicine, as well as rehabilitation approaches such as physical therapy. The effectiveness of the specific application of controlled forces to joints, whether oscillatory or thrusting at end range, may derive from mechanical changes in neighboring tissues and/or be more centrally mediated in response to sensory input (Maitland et al., 2005). The *Feldenkrais Method* does not use thrust manipulation. Students have experienced sensations ("pops" or "cracks") that are consistent with self-mobilization/manipulation within the context of lessons as reorganization occurs. There are techniques within the *Feldenkrais Method* that have some similarities to oscillatory joint mobilizations that are intended to be informative, provide support, increase awareness, and thus facilitate self-reorganization.

Joseph Pilates developed a series of exercises for total body conditioning that emphasizes strength, length, use of the breath, and awareness. The difficulty that many people had with his exercises led him to develop a variety of devices that often incorporated springs (e.g., Reformer, Cadillac trapeze table, chair, etc.) to assist their development (Friedman & Eisen, 1981, Balanced Body). This mindful mode of exercise is attentive to form and is often quite specific in the use of the breath. The *Feldenkrais Method* has numerous lessons that focus on breathing, yet emphasizes the many options for using the breath that varies with context and intention. The use of equipment in the *Feldenkrais Method* typically includes a firm, wide table; rollers of various diameters and densities; and an assortment of pads, towels and other supportive props. Movement activities are framed and intended as lessons that afford self-exploration of habitual patterns and less familiar options that promote individually appropriate self-organization of improved function.

The basis of reflexology, known earlier as zone therapy, is that specific regions of the feet and hands correspond reflexively to organs, glands, and other body areas (International Institute of Reflexology). Techniques that stimulate these reflexes may positively influence the function of the corresponding tissues. The premise and application of reflexology are distinct from the *Feldenkrais Method*. Embodied self-awareness techniques such as the *Feldenkrais Method* can influence the functioning of various organs through the interactions among perceiving, acting, and feeling (Fogel, 2009). Placing muscles in shortened positions can facilitate decreased activation; eye movements can help organize the action of the neck, and breathing explorations can impact the autonomic nervous system to either calm or excite the individual (Fogel, 2009; Ginsburg, 2010). These and many other *Feldenkrais* techniques are used within a learning context to guide self-organized improvement.

The *Feldenkrais Method* self-identifies as an approach to learning that can have therapeutic effects. With the growth in complementary and alternative medicine, it has been categorized, more or less appropriately, with other approaches. A variety of stakeholders are interested in the effectiveness and safety of these approaches, regardless of the claims made by proponents. The next section reviews the literature to address those interests.

5. Systematic review of *Feldenkrais Method* research

Given the relative newness of the *Feldenkrais Method* and limited number of practitioners, research into its effectiveness and safety is still in its early period of development. While some users of the method and a portion of practitioners are quite satisfied with anecdotal accounts and direct experience, others prefer to have access to results from more Western traditional scientific study. This evidence can guide decision making by the public and health care providers, and also suggest future research directions. As this review will document, a growth spurt in *Feldenkrais* research occurred in the past decade. Thus, this review provides a current perspective on the developmental status of *Feldenkrais* research.

The objective of this review was very open, reflecting the small number of peer-reviewed studies available with any one population. Thus, the purpose was to examine the effectiveness and safety of the *Feldenkrais Method* for persons of any age and condition without limitations on comparator groups, outcomes, or study design.

5.1 Methods

Best practices from several sources guided my search and review of the literature (Centre for Evidence Based Medicine; Cochrane Collaboration, 2010; Liberati et al., 2009). I adapted these procedures to extract information from the selected studies, including indicators of possible risk of bias (e.g., description of randomization process, blinding procedures, documentation of attrition, etc.). I did not attempt to contact authors for further information about their studies, but relied solely on the publication contents.

5.1.1 Eligibility criteria

This review included studies of human participants of any age and with any condition who received a *Feldenkrais Method* intervention. Reports of such studies needed to be available in English and published in peer-reviewed journals without limitation on year of publication.

5.1.2 Information sources and search

Between 10 June 2011 to 4 July 2011, I searched several electronic databases for relevant studies. The single search term "Feldenkrais" was sufficient for use in all databases, as the number of records was no greater than 121 in any single search. When available, I added limiters for English language and peer-reviewed journal articles. I queried PubMed and utilized EBSOhost to individually search Academic Search Elite, CINAHL, MEDLINE, PsycINFO, and Rehabilitation & Sports Medicine Source.

In addition to this latest search, I included the results of prior literature searches that I had conducted from September 2001 through April 2009. I incorporated the *Feldenkrais Guild* of North America research bibliography (*Feldenkrais Guild* of North America, 2011). Finally, I added two references obtained through screening of article references.

5.1.3 Study selection

To facilitate screening for duplicates, I entered all search citations into a Microsoft Excel worksheet, sorted entries, and removed duplicates. I identified records for exclusion through review of titles, abstracts, and types of records. Excluded during this screening were materials that clearly were not full research reports published in peer-reviewed journals (e.g., book chapters, dissertations, conference abstracts, other unpublished works).

Another round of screening included electronic searching of full-text documents for the term "Feldenkrais". This process led me to eliminate articles that had minimal relevance to this review. Several records did not study *Feldenkrais* interventions (e.g., referred to the method or to Dr. Feldenkrais, provided background information, or reported on research published elsewhere). This closer screening also identified a few previously unrecognized records that should have been removed earlier.

Through more thorough review of the full-text articles of the remaining records, I pared the list of studies for full review to those that were the original reports of *Feldenkrais Method* interventions. This excluded review articles, tutorials, and studies about knowledge of the *Feldenkrais Method*. Figure 3 summarizes the study selection process.

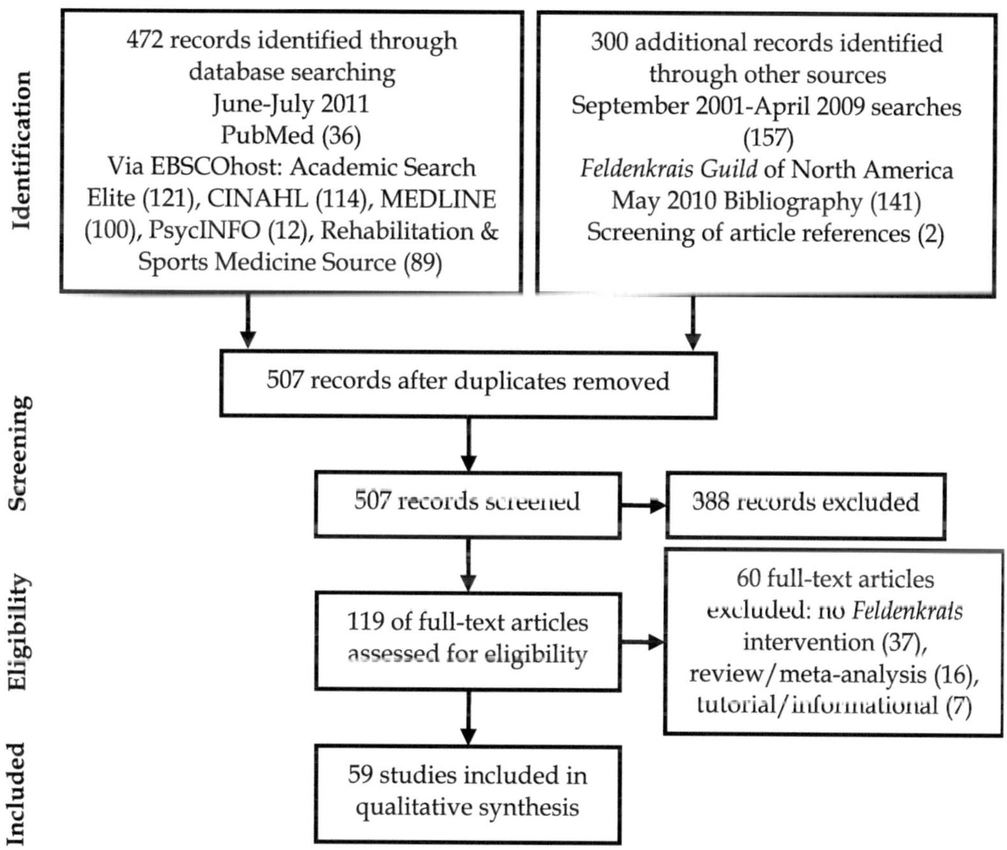

Fig. 3. Flow diagram of study selection.

5.2 Results

Table 2 categorizes 59 studies by level of evidence (1 highest, 4 lowest; level 5 studies were excluded from review) and summarizes their designs, conditions, and participant numbers, genders and ages. Nearly all studies reported some positive effects from interventions that exclusively or partly involved the *Feldenkrais Method*. Three studies found no differences between participants who received *Awareness Through Movement* interventions and those in other interventions or control groups (Brown & Kegerreis, 1991; James et al., 1998; Kolt & McConville, 2000). Only three studies reported any adverse effects. One participant with Alzheimer's disease refused further lessons after three sessions and said the practitioner had hurt him, contrary to staff reports of his improvement (Ann, 2006). One patient in a small study of people with acute myocardial infarcts felt worse after the first *Functional Integration* lesson, but continued the study (Löwe et al., 2002). Lastly, one participant mentioned "giddiness" during a tandem walking activity that was part of an *Awareness Through Movement* series focused on improving balance in the elderly (Vrantsidis et al., 2009).

Lead author	Year	Study design[a]	Condition	Number, Gender[b]	Age in years
Level of evidence: 1					
Smith	2001	RCT	chronic low back pain	16 F 10 M	26-78
Vrantsidis	2009	RCT	elderly with some functional impairments	42 F 13 M	56-94
Level of evidence: 2					
Apel	2006	analytic x-sec survey	Multiple Sclerosis	187 F 67 M	44 +/- 11.6
Bearman	1999	CBA	chronic pain	7 E, 365 C, slightly more F	unclear, wide range
Brown	1991	Q-RCT	healthy adults	9 F 12 M	19-39
Chinn	1994	Q-RCT	neck-shoulder pain	21 F 1 M	18-59
Connors	2011	CBA	various	63, unclear	~75
Gutman	1977	CBA	elderly residents	51 F 16 M	~70s
Hopper	1999	Q-RCT	healthy adults	1: 46 F 29 M 2: 23 F 16 M	17-33
James	1998	Q-RCT	healthy adults	28 F 20 M	~22
Junker	2004	descriptive x-sec survey	dystonia	127 F 53 M	7-79

Lead author	Year	Study design[a]	Condition	Number, Gender[b]	Age in years
Kemp	2005	descriptive x-sec survey	pain	197 F 38 M	65-99
Kirkby	1994	CBA	serious prementrual syndrome	48 F	18-47
Laumer	1997	CBA	disordered eating	27 F 3 M	18-51
Löwe	2002	CBA	acute myocardial infarction	12 F 48 M	60s
Lundblad	1999	Q-RCT	factory workers with neck-shoulder complaints	97 F	~30s
Malmgren-Olsson	2001	CBA	chronic pain	64 F 14 M	~40s
Malmgren-Olsson	2002	CBA	chronic pain	64 F 14 M	~40s
Malmgren-Olsson	2003	CBA	chronic pain	64 F 14 M	~40s
Netz	2003	CBA	healthy adults	147 F	middle aged
Ruth	1992	Q-RCT	healthy adults	18 F 12 M	11-36
Schön-Ohlsson	2006	CBA	chronic low back pain	14 F 10 M	~40s
Schön-Ohlsson	2005	CBA	chronic low back pain	24 unclear	25-65
Stephens	2001	Q-RCT	Multiple Sclerosis	8 F 4 M	~40s-50s
Stephens	2006	Q-RCT	healthy adults	20 F 13 M	21-36
Stephens	2005	CBA	well elderly	19 F 12 M	68-89
Ullmann	2010	CBA	well elderly	33 F 14 M	65+, ~70s
Level of evidence: 3					
DellaGrotte	2008	CBA	chronic pain	11 F 17 M	13-55
Dunn	2000	unimagined side as control	healthy adults	8 F 4 M	18-28

Lead author	Year	Study design[a]	Condition	Number, Gender[b]	Age in years
Johnson	1999	cross-over	Multiple Sclerosis	15 F 5 M	33-54
Kendall	2001	CES no C	fibromyalgia	39 unclear	15-55
Kerr	2002	CES no C	healthy adults	Single: 8 F 5 M Series: 30 F 15 M	adults
Kiser	2008	descriptive x-sec survey	retinitis pigmentosa	50 F 46 M	all ages
Kolt	2000	Q-RCT	healthy adults	35 F 19 M	17-38
Mehling	2011	qualitative	various	Practitioners: 4 F 4 M Clients: 7 F 1 M	adults
Öhman	2011	qualitative	chronic neck-shoulder pain	14 F	32-57
Peper	2004	Q-RCT	adult computer users	23 F 5 M	~30s-40s
Seegert	1999	CBA	healthy adults	25 F	18-25
Level of evidence: 4					
Ann	2006	case series	Alzheimer's disease	4 F 2 M	76-96
Batson	2005	BA no C	post stroke	4 unclear	48-61
Fry	1988	case series	overuse syndrome	175 mix	~12-54
Ginsburg	1986	case series	spinal cord injury, traumatic brain injury	9 F 24 M	adults
Ginsburg	1999	case series	varied	2 F 1 M	adults
Goebel	2006	case series	tinnitus	79 F 165 M	39-77
Halperin	2009	case study	mental illness/disorder	1 F	18-65
Honig	2007	case study	sciatica with piriformis syndrome	1 F	43

Lead author	Year	Study design[a]	Condition	Number, Gender[b]	Age in years
Kepner	2002	case study	chronic low back pain	1 M	45
Lake	1985	case series	back pain	4 F 2 M	26-60
Lyttle	1997	case study	chronic low back pain	1 F	35
Nair	2005	case study	post stroke	1 M	65
Nelson	1989	case study	violinist with neck pain	1 F	20s
Nelson	2005	case series	singers, one post motor vehicle accident	1 F 1 M	19, ?
O'Connor	2002	case series	various	5 unclear	not reported
Schenkman	1989	case series	Parkinson Disease	2 M	67, 68
Stephens	1999	case series	Multiple Sclerosis	4 F	30-46
Stephens	2000	case series	musculoskeletal problems	117 F 63 M	15-86
Wennemer	2006	BA no C	fibromyalgia	20 not reported	not reported
Wilson	2001	case study	disseminated encephalo-myelopathy	1 F	26
Zunin	2009	BA no C	chronic pain	21 F 14 M	25-76

[a]RCT: randomized controlled trial, Q-RCT: quasi-randomized controlled trial, CBA: controlled before and after study; x-xec: cross sectional; BA no C: before and after study, no control; CES no C: comparative effectiveness study, no true control.
[b]F: female participants, M: male participants, E: experimental group, C: controls

Table 2. Summary of reviewed studies' designs and participants' conditions, numbers, genders, and ages; grouped by level of evidence.

Researchers in the United States conducted most of these studies (27), with one study by a *Feldenkrais* teacher who lives and works part time in the United States and Germany. Australian researchers published 12 studies, Swedish investigators reported eight studies, and Germans conducted five studies. Investigators in Canada (2), Israel (2), England (1) and Italy (1) produced the remaining studies.

The most frequent design was controlled before and after (16), followed by case series (11), quasi-randomized controlled trial (10), case studies (7), comparative study without true control (6), cross-sectional survey (3 descriptive, 1 analytic), randomized control trial and qualitative (2 each), and cross-over (1). As suggested by the distribution of study designs, very few studies were of the highest quality. I only assigned the level of evidence 1 to two studies (Smith et al., 2001; Vrantsidis et al., 2009). I rated several studies that reported being randomized controlled trials as level 2 due to the risk of bias in the allocation process (Brown & Kegerreis, 1992; Chinn et al., 1994; Hopper et al., 1999; James et al., 1998; Kolt & McConville, 2000; Lundblad et al., 1999; Peper et al., 2004; Ruth & Kegerreis, 1992; Stephens et al., 2001; Stephens et al., 2006). The most common assessment was level 2 (25), followed by level 4 (21), and level 3 (11). The average level of evidence was 2.8 (SD ± .95). Overall, I assigned a (low) B grade of recommendation to the current body of peer-reviewed literature.

5.2.1 Growth over 35 years

Clearly, the number of studies of the effectiveness and safety of the *Feldenkrais Method* is limited. Readers should remember the relative youth of the discipline and small numbers of practitioners/teachers while evaluating the extant literature. For another perspective (see Table 3), I totaled the numbers of studies across the decades that include the years since Gutman et al. published the first study in 1977. Notable increases in research occurred during the 1990s and 2000s. It remains to be seen if that growth continues in the 2010s.

Set of studies	1970s	1980s	1990s	2000s	2010s
119 screened	1	6	20	79	13
59 eligible	1	5	14	37	3

Table 3. Growth in *Feldenkrais* research, 1977 to mid-2011.

5.2.2 Breadth of studies

Feldenkrais teachers and students have applied this method to numerous situations in which people desire to learn to improve their function. This breadth of utilization is reflected in the range of conditions among the reviewed studies (refer to Table 2). Most studies (11) examined the effects of *Feldenkrais* lessons on healthy persons, primarily adults. Another four studies focused on elderly participants who were generally healthy community dwellers. Many studies focused on people with non-specific pain (7), and with back pain (7). Four studies included people with Multiple Sclerosis, and another four had participants with varied and/or unspecified complaints. Musicians were the focus of three reports. Another three studies involved people with neck, shoulder or other upper quarter conditions. Researchers conducted two studies of people with fibromyalgia and two investigations of persons post stroke. Single projects evaluated the effectiveness of the *Feldenkrais Method* for people with acute myocardial infarct, Alzheimer's disease, disordered eating, disseminated encephalomyelopathy, dystonia, mental illness/disorder, musculoskeletal problems, Parkinson Disease, retinitis pigmentosa, spinal cord injury or traumatic brain injury, serious premenstrual syndrome, and tinnitus.

5.2.3 Discussion

The present body of *Feldenkrais Method* research collectively supports its effectiveness and safety. This assessment must be couched in the recognition that the number of studies remains small and dispersed, findings are often constrained by design limitations, and more rigorous investigations with appropriate methodologies are needed. When I first reviewed the *Feldenkrais* research in 2001 (Buchanan & Ulrich, 2001), I referenced nine articles that evaluated the effects of *Feldenkrais* interventions on nine different populations (Bearman & Shafarman, 1999; Brown & Kegerreis, 1991; Chinn et al., 1994; Gutman et al., 1977; Johnson et al., 1999; Lundblad et al., 1999; Ruth & Kegerreis, 1992; Seegert & Shapiro, 1999; Stephens et al., 1999). This review adds 50 more studies to the mix. Multiple studies targeted healthy adults, persons with non-specific pain and chronic low back pain, and elderly adults. While investigations have increased considerably in the past decade, there is substantial room for improvement and development.

Ives (Ives & Shelley, 1998; Ives, 2003) has been a notable critic of *Feldenkrais* research based on the limited quality and quantity of studies. He pointed out design concerns and I concur there is need for more studies with quality designs. Ives concluded, "From a clinical standpoint, it seems difficult to recommend the *Feldenkrais Method* above other techniques" (Ives, 2003, p. 118). His point is valid in that there are only a handful of studies demonstrating superior results from *Feldenkrais* interventions vs. traditional physical therapy treatment (Lundblad et al., 1999; Malmgren-Olsson et al., 2001; Malmgren-Olsson & Branholm, 2002; Malmgren-Olsson & Armelius, 2003; Schön-Ohlsson et al., 2005).

Ives also argued, "any effects noted appear to be psychological and not physiological" (Ives, 2003, p. 118). I would counter this criticism on two fronts. First, there are now additional studies documenting "physiological" changes; for example, performance on the Posturo-Locomotion-Manual test (Schön-Ohlsson et al., 2005), Timed Up and Go test (Ullmann et al., 2010), Active Knee Extension test (Stephens et al., 2006), Berg Balance Scale (Batson & Deutsch, 2005), and changes in brain activation patterns based on fMRI analyses (Nair et al., 2005). Second, Ives posited a mind-body dualistic perspective as a rationale for disputing the effects of the *Feldenkrais Method*. This is a common criticism levelled against many mind-body approaches. Researchers and practitioners who hold an integrated perspective that can be grounded in dynamic systems theory would argue, as did Feldenkrais (Feldenkrais, 2010), for the unity of mind and body. Self-organization of behavior occurs through the coupling of perception-action-cognition of an organism (human) within an environment (Buchanan & Ulrich, 2001; Ginsburg, 2010; Spencer et al., 2006, Thelen & Smith, 1994). In turn, these theoretical stances impact the methodology choices of researchers and the interpretations that scientists, practitioners and consumers place on studies.

Efforts to apply broadly held scientific methodology and research standards common to the evidenced-based practice of medicine to complementary and alternative approaches has been problematic. In its 2011-2015 Strategic Plan, the National Center for Complementary and Alternative Medicine noted the challenges of developing rigorous studies of mind and body approaches. Four common characteristics pose methodological concerns: 1) blinding of participants and/or practitioners is difficult, 2) benefits are often subjective in nature, 3) interventions are often individualized and can be complex, creating difficulties for standardizing protocols and assessing outcomes, and 4) objective measures may not exist to adequately measure biological processes that are not yet well understood (NCCAM, 2011a).

Mehling (2005) examined the challenges of reducing the risk of bias in quantitative studies with various forms of mind-body therapies, including the *Feldenkrais Method*. After reviewing existing higher quality studies, he offered several suggestions associated with the lack of blinding. First, researchers should include more objective outcome measures and blind assessors to allocation. Second, investigators can ask participants at the end whether they thought they were in intervention or control groups, and make similar inquiries of assessors. Third, researchers may track participants' expectations for their group's activity in order to evaluate for effectiveness expectations. Fourth, researchers need to recognize and monitor the expectations associated with different kinds of control groups. Lastly, the use of pre-consent randomization may minimize expectations by limiting knowledge to the allocated group activity and restricting information about alternative activities. For challenges with control, Mehling suggested that researchers: control the amount of time, settings, and provider characteristics; control the amount and quality of attention given to participants without mimicking the specifics of the target intervention; include a no-treatment control along with a placebo; and consider a multimodal control intervention parallel to the multimodal approach that includes the targeted method. To better manage volunteer bias and attrition, Mehling proposed that investigators: offer meaningful control interventions; recruit from settings with patients open to research but without existing preference for complementary and alternative approaches; in particular, recruit through physician referral; and consider partial randomization in which participants can declare their preferences for allocation and those without strong preferences are randomly assigned.

Traditionally trained researchers may reasonably evaluate the *Feldenkrais* literature and conclude that it is too heavy in case studies situated near the bottom of the level of evidence ratings, and is in need of more level 1-2, third person objective, analytical studies of the quality of Lundblad (1999), Schön-Ohlsson (2005), Smith (2001), and Vrantsidis (2009). Others would argue that more phenomenological and qualitative, first person subjective studies similar to Ginsburg (1999), Mehling (2011), and Öhman (2011) would advance knowledge of this method. Ginsburg (1999, p. 82) is among those who have argued the value of both research perspectives, stating: "the phenomenology of the Feldenkrais method allows one to connect changes in the domain of inner experience with changes in the organization of outer behaviour. It thus provides a way to observe the correlations between the domain of phenomenology and the domain of external observation." Whether within individual investigations or across the body of literature, there is value in a mixed methods approach to deepening knowledge of the effectiveness and safety of the *Feldenkrais Method* and enhancing understanding of its underlying mechanisms.

In sum, research into the effectiveness and safety of the *Feldenkrais Method* has developed considerably since 1977. The number of studies has increased, with multiple reports of interventions with healthy adults, adults with chronic pain, and well elderly groups. Still, the available support for the effectiveness and safety of the *Feldenkrais Method* should be viewed cautiously. Much more research needs to be done utilizing a range of methodologies with appropriate rigor befitting a learning method that is grounded in the self-organization of human behavior that emerges in relation to intention, others, and the environment.

6. Conclusion

Feldenkrais encapsulated his method in this statement: "Organic learning is essential. It can also be therapeutic in essence. It is healthier to learn than to be a patient or even be cured. Life is a process not a thing. And, processes go well if there are many ways to influence them. We need more ways to do what we want than the one we know—even if it is a good one in itself" (Feldenkrais, 1981, p. 29).

In this chapter, I have expanded on Feldenkrais' statement and made these key points:

- The *Feldenkrais Method* of somatic education self-identifies as a learning method that may have therapeutic effects. It presents itself as an approach to health promotion, when health is viewed broadly and not just as the absence of disease or injury.
- Through individual *Functional Integration* lessons and group *Awareness Through Movement* lessons, *Feldenkrais* teachers guide students to sense, move, think and feel in ways intended to facilitate self-improvement and create more individually appropriate options for functioning.
- The *Feldenkrais Method* shares many principles with dynamic systems theory, including: emergence of self-organized behavior via subsystem interactions; perception-action-cognition coupling; and an ideal of reliable, yet flexible and adaptable, behavior.
- Practitioners around the world complete similarly structured curricula typically spanning four years to earn certification, and follow comparable standards of practice.
- Others have categorized the *Feldenkrais Method* with a range of complementary and alternative medicine approaches, most appropriately with the Alexander Technique.
- *Feldenkrais Method* effectiveness and safety research has increased considerably in the past decade. Results are mostly favorable, but remain sparse and subject to design limitations. Much more research is needed that rigorously combines appropriate quantitative and qualitative methodologies to further evaluate the *Feldenkrais Method.*

I encourage readers unfamiliar with the method to gain direct experience with a few of the widely available *Awareness Through Movement* lessons or via *Functional Integration* lessons from area practitioners. In particular, I invite researchers and practitioners to collaborate on quality investigations of the *Feldenkrais Method* for the benefit of all stakeholders.

7. Acknowledgment

I thank Des Moines University for the support that allowed me to produce this chapter. I thank Sam Kegerreis for introducing me to the *Feldenkrais Method* some 25 years ago. I am grateful to many unnamed but known *Feldenkrais* colleagues and research colleagues around the world, particularly members of Esther Thelen's "family." Credit to all; errors are mine.

8. References

Ann, J. (2006). Individuals with dementia learn new habits and are empowered through the Feldenkrais method. *Alzheimer's Care Quarterly*, Vol. 7, No. 4, pp. 278-86.

Apel, A., Greim, B., König, N., & Zettl, U. (2006). Frequency of current utilisation of complementary and alternative medicine by patients with multiple sclerosis. *Journal Of Neurology*, Vol. 253, No. 10, pp. 1331-6.

Australian Feldenkrais Guild Inc. (2010). 07.08.2011, Available from http://www.feldenkrais.org.au/.

Balanced Body. (n.d.). 07.08.2011, Available from http://www.pilates.com/BBAPP/V/index.html.

Barnes, P. M., Bloom, B., & Nahin, R. L. (2008). Complementary and alternative medicine use among adults and children: United States, 2007. *National Health Statistics Reports; No. 12.*

Batson, G., & Deutsch, J. (2005). Effects of Feldenkrais awareness through movement on balance in adults with chronic neurological deficits following stroke: a preliminary study. *Complementary Health Practice Review,* Vol. 10, No. 3, pp. 203-10.

Bearman, D., & Shafarman, S. (1999). The Feldenkrais Method in the treatment of chronic pain: a study of efficacy and cost effectiveness. *American Journal of Pain Management,* Vol. 9, No. 1, pp. 22-7.

Brown, E., & Kegerreis, S. (1991). Electromyographic activity of trunk musculature during a Feldenkrais Awareness through Movement lesson. *Isokinetics and Exercise Science,* Vol. 1, No. 4, pp. 216-21.

Buchanan, P. (2010). A preliminary survey of the practice patterns of United States Guild Certified Feldenkrais Practitioners^CM. *BMC Complementary and Alternative Medicine,* Vol. 10, No. 12 (Electronic).

Buchanan, P., & Ulrich, B. (2001). The Feldenkrais Method: a dynamic approach to changing motor behavior. *Research Quarterly for Exercise and Sport,* Vol. 72, No. 4, pp. 315-323.

Centre for Evidence Based Medicine. (n.d.). 07.06.2011, Available from http://www.cebm.net.

Cheever, O. (2000). Connected knowing and `somatic empathy' among somatic educators and students of somatic education. *ReVision,* Vol. 22, No. 4, pp. 15-23.

Chinn, J., Trujillo, D., Kegerreis, S., & Worrell, T. (1994). Effect of a Feldenkrais intervention on symptomatic subjects performing a functional reach. *Isokinetics and Exercise Science,* Vol. 4, No. 4, pp. 131-136.

Cochrane Collaboration. (2010). 07.06.2011, Available from http://www.cochrane.org/cochrane-reviews.

Connors, K., Galea, M., & Said, C. (2011). Feldenkrais Method balance classes improve balance in older adults: a controlled trial. *Evidence-Based Complementary and Alternative Medicine.,* Vol. 2011, No. 873672 (Electronic).

DellaGrotte, J., Ridi, R., Landi, M., & Stephens, J. (2008). Postural improvement using core integration to lengthen myofascia. *Jornal of Bodywork and Movement Therapies,* Vol. 12, pp. 231-45.

Dunn, P., & Rogers, D. (2000). Feldenkrais sensory imagery and forward reach. *Perceptual And Motor Skills,* Vol. 91, No. 3 Pt 1, pp. 755-7.

Feldenkrais Guild of North America. (2011). 07.06.2011, Available from http://www.feldenkrais.com/.

Feldenkrais, M. (1972). *Awareness Through Movement: Health Exercises for Personal Growth.* Harper and Row, ISBN 0-06-250322-7, New York.

Feldenkrais, M. (1981). *The Elusive Obvious.* Meta Publications, ISBN 0-916990-09-5, Cupertino, CA.

Feldenkrais, M. (1996). *Body and Mature Behavior: A Study of Anxiety, Sex, Gravitation and Learning.* International Universities Press, ISBN 0-8236-8009-6, Madison, CT. (Originally published 1949.)

Feldenkrais, M. (2010). *Embodied Wisdom: The Collected Papers of Moshe Feldenkrais.* Somatic Resources, ISBN 978-1-55643-906-3, San Diego, CA.

Fogel, A. (2009). *The Psychophysiology of Self-Awareness: Rediscovering the Lost Art of Body Sense.* W. W. Norton, ISBN 978-0-393-70544-7, New York.

Friedman, P., & Eisen, G. (1981). *The Pilates Method of Physical and Mental Conditioning.* Warner Books, Inc, ISBN 0-446-97859-0, New York.

Fry, H. (1988). The treatment of overuse syndrome in musicians. Results in 175 patients. *Journal Of The Royal Society Of Medicine,* Vol. 81, No. 10, pp. 572-5.

Gilman, M., & Yaruss, J. (2000). Stuttering and relaxation: applications for somatic education in stuttering treatment. *Journal of Fluency Disorders,* Vol. 25, No. 1, pp. 59-76.

Ginsburg, C. (1986). The shake-a-leg body awareness training program: dealing with spinal injury and recovery in a new setting. *Somatics,* Vol. 5, No. 4, pp. 31-42.

Ginsburg, C. (1999). Body-image, movement and consciousness: examples from a somatic practice in the Feldenkrais Method. *Journal of Consciousness Studies,* Vol. 6, No. 2-3, pp. 79-91.

Ginsburg, C. (2010). *The Intelligence of Moving Bodies: A Somatic View of Life and Its Consequences.* AWAREing Press, ISBN 978-0-9824235-0-9, Santa Fe, NM.

Goebel, G., Kahl, M., Arnold, W., & Fichter, M. (2006). 15-year prospective follow-up study of behavioral therapy in a large sample of inpatients with chronic tinnitus. *Acta Oto-Laryngologica,* Vol. 126 (Supplement), pp. 70-9.

Gutman, G., Herbert, C., & Brown, S. (1977). Feldenkrais versus conventional exercises for the elderly. *Journal Of Gerontology,* Vol. 32, No. 5, pp. 562-72.

Halperin, G., & Boz-Mizrahi, T. (2009). The Amitim program: an innovative program for the social rehabilitation of people with mental illness in the community. *The Israel Journal Of Psychiatry And Related Sciences,* Vol. 46, No. 2, pp. 149-56.

Honig, P. (2007). A case report of the treatment of piriformis syndrome: applying modalities of therapeutic bodywork. *Massage Today,* Vol. 7, No. 1, pp. 10 1.

Hopper, C., Kolt, G., & McConville, J. (1999). The effects of Feldenkrais awareness through movement on hamstring length, flexibility, and perceived exertion. *Journal of Bodywork & Movement Therapies,* Vol. 3, No. 4, pp. 238-47.

International Feldenkrais Federation. (n.d.). 01.07.2011, Available from http://feldenkrais-method.org/en/node/295.

International Institute of Reflexology. (n.d.). 01.08.2011, Available from http://reflexology-usa.net/.

Ives, J. (2003). Comments on "the Feldenkrais Method: a dynamic approach to changing motor behavior." *Research Quarterly For Exercise And Sport,* Vol. 74, No. 2, pp. 116-23.

Ives, J., & Shelley, G. (1998). The Feldenkrais Method® in rehabilitation: a review. *Work,* Vol. 11, No. 1, pp. 75-90.

Jain, S., Janssen, K., & DeCelle, S. (2004). Alexander technique and Feldenkrais method: a critical overview. *Physical Medicine & Rehabilitation Clinics of North America,* Vol. 15, No. 4, pp. 811-25.

James, M., Kolt, G., McConville, J., & Bate, P. (1998). The effects of a Feldenkrais program and relaxation procedures on hamstring length. *Australian Journal of Physiotherapy,* Vol. 44, No. 1, pp. 49-54.

Johnson S. K., Frederick J., Kaufman M., & Mountjoy B. (1999). A controlled investigation of bodywork in multiple sclerosis. *Journal of Alternative and Complementary Medicine,* Vol. 5, No. 3, pp. 237-43.

Jones, C. (2005). The spectrum of therapeutic influences and integrative health care: classifying health care practices by mode of therapeutic action. *Journal Of Alternative And Complementary Medicine,* Vol. 11, No. 5, pp. 937-44.

Junker, J., Oberwittler, C., Jackson, D., & Berger, K. (2004). Utilization and perceived effectiveness of complementary and alternative medicine in patients with dystonia. *Movement Disorders,* Vol. 19, No. 2, pp. 158-61.

Kaetz, D. (2007). *Making Connections: Hasidic Roots and Resonance in the Teachings of Moshe Feldenkrais.* River Centre Publishing, ISBN 978-0-9784014-0-5, Metchosin, British Columbia, Canada.

Kemp, C., Ersek, M., & Turner, J. (2005). A descriptive study of older adults with persistent pain: use and perceived effectiveness of pain management strategies. *BMC Geriatrics,* Vol. 5, No. 12 (Electronic).

Kendall, S. A., Ekselius, L., Gerdle, B., Sörén, B., & Bengtsson, A. (2001). Feldenkrais intervention in fibromyalgia patients: a pilot study. *Journal of Musculoskeletal Pain,* Vol. 9, No. 4, pp. 25-35.

Kepner, J., Strohmeyer, V., & Elgelid, S. (2002). Wide dimensions to yoga therapy; comparative approaches from Viniyoga, Phoenix Rising Yoga Therapy, and the Feldenkrais Method®. *International Journal of Yoga Therapy,* No. 12, pp. 25-38.

Kerr, G., Kotynia, F., & Kolt, G. (2002). Feldenkrais® awareness through movement and state anxiety. *Journal of Bodywork & Movement Therapies,* Vol. 6, No. 2, pp. 102-7.

Kirkby, R. (1994). Changes in premenstrual symptoms and irrational thinking following cognitive-behavioral coping skills training. *Journal of Consulting and Clinical Psychology,* Vol. 62, No. 5, pp. 1026-1032.

Kiser, A., & Dagnelie, G. (2008). Reported effects of non-traditional treatments and complementary and alternative medicine by retinitis pigmentosa patients. *Clinical & Experimental Optometry,* Vol. 91, No. 2, pp. 166-76.

Kolt, G., & McConville, J. (2000). The effects of a Feldenkrais® Awareness Through Movement program on state anxiety. *Journal of Bodywork & Movement Therapies,* Vol. 4, No. 3, pp. 216-20.

Lake, B. (1985). Acute back pain. Treatment by the application of Feldenkrais principles. *Australian Family Physician,* Vol. 14, No. 11, pp. 1175-8.

Laumer, U., Bauer M., Fichter M., & Milz, H. (2004). Therapeutic effects of the Feldenkrais Method (Awareness Through Movement) in eating disorders. *Feldenkrais Research Journal,* Vol. 1. (English Translation of German Article Originally Published 1997). 15.06.2011, Available from http://iffresearchjournal.org/volume/1/laumer.

Lee, C. O. (2004). Clinical trials in cancer part I: Biomedical, complementary, and alternative medicine: finding active trials and results of closed trials. *Clinical Journal of Oncology Nursing,* Vol. 8, No. 5, pp. 531-535.

Liberati, A., Altman, D. G., Tetzlaff, J., Mulrow, C., Gotzsche, P. C., Ioannidis, J. P. et al. (2009). The PRISMA statement for reporting systematic reviews and meta-analyses of studies that evaluate health care interventions: explanation and elaboration. *PLoS Medicine,* Vol. 6, No. 7 (Electronic).

Löwe, B., Breining, K., Wilke, S., Wellmann, R., Zipfel, S., & Eich, W. (2002). Quantitative and qualitative effects of Feldenkrais, progressive muscle relaxation, and standard medical treatment in patients after acute myocardial infarction. *Psychotherapy Research,* Vol. 12, No. 2, pp. 179-191.

Lundblad, I., Elert, J., & Gerdle, B. (1999). Randomized controlled trial of physiotherapy and Feldenkrais interventions in female workers with neck-shoulder complaints. *Journal of Occupational Rehabilitation,* Vol. 9, No. 3, pp. 179-94.

Lyttle, T. (1997). The Feldenkrais Method: application, practice and principles. *Journal of Bodywork & Movement Therapies,* Vol. 1, No. 5, pp. 262-9.

Maitland, G. D., Hengeveld, E., Banks, K., & English, K. (2005). *Maitland's Vertebral Manipulation.* Elsevier, ISBN 0-7506-8806-8, Edinburgh.

Malmgren-Olsson, E., & Armelius, B. (2003). Non-specific musculoskeletal disorders in patients in primary care: subgroups with different outcome patterns. *Physiotherapy Theory & Practice,* Vol. 19, No. 3, pp. 161-73.

Malmgren-Olsson, E., Armelius, B., & Armelius, K. (2001). A comparative outcome study of body awareness therapy, Feldenkrais, and conventional physiotherapy for patients with nonspecific musculoskeletal disorders: changes in psychological symptoms, pain, and self-image. *Physiotherapy Theory & Practice,* Vol. 17, No. 2, pp. 77-95.

Malmgren-Olsson, E., & Bränholm, I. (2002). A comparison between three physiotherapy approaches with regard to health-related factors in patients with non-specific musculoskeletal disorders. *Disability And Rehabilitation,* Vol. 24, No. 6, pp. 308-17.

Mamtani, R., & Cimino, A. (2002). A primer of complementary and alternative medicine and its relevance in the treatment of mental health problems. *The Psychiatric Quarterly,* Vol. 73, No. 4, pp. 367-81.

Mehling, W., Wrubel, J., Daubenmier, J., Price, C., Kerr, C., Silow, T. et al. (2011). Body awareness: a phenomenological inquiry into the common ground of mind-body therapies. *Philosophy, Ethics, And Humanities In Medicine,* Vol. 6, No. 6 (Electronic).

Mehling, W. E., DiBlasi, Z., & Hecht, F. (2005). Bias control in trials of bodywork: a review of methodological issues. *The Journal of Alternative and Complementary Medicine,* Vol. 11, No. 2, pp. 333-342.

Nair, D., Fuchs, A., Burkart, S., Steinberg, F., & Kelso, J. (2005). Assessing recovery in middle cerebral artery stroke using functional MRI. *Brain Injury,* Vol. 19, No. 13, pp. 1165-76.

National Center for Complementary and Alternative Medicine. (2004). Expanding Horizons of Health Care: Strategic Plan 2005-2009. *NIH Publication 04-5568 d251.*

National Center for Complementary and Alternative Medicine. (2011a). Third Strategic Plan 2011-2015: Exploring the Science of Complementary and Alternative Medicine. *NIH Publication No. 11-7643 D458.*

National Center for Complementary and Alternative Medicine. (2011b). 05.06.2011, Available from http://nccam.nih.gov/health/whatiscam/.

Nayak, S., Matheis, R. J., Schoenberger, N. E., & Shiflett, S. C. (2003). Use of unconventional therapies by individuals with multiple sclerosis. *Clinical Rehabilitation,* Vol. 17, No. 2, pp. 181-191.

Nelson, S. (1989). Playing with the entire self: the Feldenkrais method and musicians. *Seminars In Neurology,* Vol. 9, No. 2, pp. 97-104.

Nelson, S., & Blades, E. (2005). Singing with your whole self: the Feldenkrais Method and voice. *Journal of Singing,* Vol. 62, No. 2, pp. 145-157.

Netz, Y., & Lidor, R. (2003). Mood alterations in mindful versus aerobic exercise modes. *Journal Of Psychology,* Vol. 137, No. 5, pp. 405-19.

O'Connor, M., & Webb, R. (2002). Learning to rest when in pain. *European Journal of Palliative Care,* Vol. 9, No. 2, pp. 68-71.

Öhman, A., Åström, L., & Malmgren-Olsson, E. (2011). Feldenkrais therapy as group treatment for chronic pain--a qualitative evaluation. *Journal Of Bodywork And Movement Therapies,* Vol. 15, No. 2, pp. 153-61.

Peper, E., Gibney, K., & Wilson, V. (2004). Group training with healthy computing practices to prevent repetitive strain injury (RSI): a preliminary study. *Applied Psychophysiology And Biofeedback,* Vol. 29, No. 4, pp. 279-87.

Rolf Institute of Structural Integration. (2011). 01.08.2011, Available from http://rolf.org/.

Ruth, S., & Kegerreis, S. (1992). Facilitating cervical flexion using a Feldenkrais method: Awareness through movement. *Journal of Orthopaedic & Sports Physical Therapy,* Vol. 16, No. 1, pp. 25-9.

Schenkman, M., Donovan, J., Tsubota, J., Kluss, M., Stebbins, P., & Butler, R. B. (1989). Management of individuals with Parkinson's Disease: rationale and case studies. *Physical Therapy,* Vol. 69, 11, pp. 64-75.

Schlinger, M. (2006). Feldenkrais Method, Alexander Technique, and yoga -- body awareness therapy in the performing arts. *Physical Medicine & Rehabilitation Clinics of North America,* Vol. 17, No. 4, pp. 865-75.

Schön-Ohlsson, C., Willén, J., & Johnels, B. (2005). Sensory motor learning in patients with chronic low back pain: a prospective pilot study using optoelectronic movement analysis. *Spine,* Vol. 30, No. 17, pp. E509-16.

Schön-Ohlsson, C. U., Willén, J. A., & Johnels, B. E. (2006). Optoelectronic movement analysis to measure motor performance in patients with chronic low back pain: test of reliability. *Journal of Rehabilitation Medicine,* Vol. 38, No. 6, pp. 360-367.

Seegert, E., & Shapiro, R. (1999). Effects of alternative exercise on posture. *Clinical Kinesiology: Journal of the American Kinesiotherapy Association,* Vol. 53, No. 2, pp. 41-7.

Smith, A., Kolt, G., & McConville, J. (2001). The effect of the Feldenkrais method on pain and anxiety in people experiencing chronic low back pain. *New Zealand Journal of Physiotherapy,* Vol. 29, No. 1, pp. 6-14.

Spencer, J., Clearfield, M., Corbetta, D., Ulrich, B., Buchanan, P., & Schöner, G. (2006). Moving toward a grand theory of development: in memory of Esther Thelen. *Child Development,* Vol. 77, No. 6, pp. 1521-38.

Stephens, J. (2000). Feldenkrais method: background, research, and orthopaedic case studies. *Orthopaedic Physical Therapy Clinics of North America,* Vol. 9, No. 3, pp. 375-94.

Stephens, J., Call, S., Evans, K., Glass, M., Gould, C., & Lowe, J. (1999). Responses to ten Feldenkrais awareness through movement lessons by four women with multiple sclerosis: improved quality of life. *Physical Therapy Case Reports,* Vol. 2, No. 2, pp. 58-69.

Stephens, J., Davidson, J., DeRosa, J., Kriz, M., & Saltzman, N. (2006). Lengthening the hamstring muscles without stretching using "awareness through movement.". *Physical Therapy,* Vol. 86, No. 12, pp. 1641-50.

Stephens, J., C. Pendergast, B.A. Roller, & R.S. Weiskittel. (2005). Learning to improve mobility and quality of life in a well elderly population: The benefits of Awareness Through Movement. *Feldenkrais Research Journal,* Vol. 2. 15.06.2011, Available from http://iffresearchjournal.org/volume/2/stephens.

Stephens, J., DuShuttle, D., Hatcher, C., Shmunes, J., & Slaninka, C. (2001). Use of Awareness Through Movement improves balance and balance confidence in people with Multiple Sclerosis: a randomized controlled study. *Neurology Report,* Vol. 25, No. 2, pp. 39-49.

Thelen, E., & Smith, L. B. (1994). *A Dynamic Systems Approach to the Development of Cognition and Action.* MIT Press, ISBN 0-262-20095-3, Cambridge, MA.

Ullmann, G., Williams, H., Hussey, J., Durstine, J., & McClenaghan, B. (2010). Effects of Feldenkrais exercises on balance, mobility, balance confidence, and gait performance in community-dwelling adults age 65 and older. *Journal of Alternative & Complementary Medicine,* Vol. 16, No. 1, pp. 97-105.

United States Trager Association. (2010). 01.08.2011, Available from http://tragerus.org/.

Vrantsidis, F., Hill, K., Moore, K., Webb, R., Hunt, S., & Dowson, L. (2009). Getting Grounded Gracefully©: effectiveness and acceptability of Feldenkrais in improving balance. *Journal of Aging & Physical Activity,* Vol. 17, No. 1, pp. 57-76.

Weber, D. (1998). Complementary and alternative medicine: considering the alternatives. *Physician Executive,* Vol. 24, No. 6, pp. 6-14.

Wennemer, H., Borg-Stein, J., Gomba, L., Delaney, B., Rothmund, A., Barlow, D. et al. (2006). Functionally oriented rehabilitation program for patients with fibromyalgia: preliminary results. *American Journal of Physical Medicine & Rehabilitation,* Vol. 85, No. 8, pp. 659-66.

Wilson, B., Gracey, F., & Bainbridge, K. (2001). Cognitive recovery from "persistent vegetative state": psychological and personal perspectives. *Brain Injury,* Vol. 15, No. 12, pp. 1083-92.

Witt, C., Ludtke, R., Mengler, N., & Willich, S. (2008). How healthy are chronically ill patients after eight years of homeopathic treatment?--Results from a long term observational study. *BMC Public Health,* Vol. 8, No. 413 (Electronic).

World Health Organization. (1946). *Constitution of the World Health Organization.* New York, 1946. 01.03.2011, Available from http://whqlibdoc.who.int/hist/official_records/constitution.pdf.

Zunin, I., Orenstein, S., Chang, M., & Cho, S. (2009). Comprehensive pain program outcomes evaluation: a preliminary study in Hawai'i. *Hawaii Medical Journal,* Vol. 68, No. 7, pp. 158-61.

Part 4

Tai Chi

7

The Use of *Qigong* and *Tai Chi* as Complementary and Alternative Medicine (CAM) Among Chronically Ill Patients in Hong Kong

Judy Yuen-man Siu
David C. Lam Institute for East-West Studies,
Hong Kong Baptist University,
Hong Kong

1. Introduction

Practicing *qigong* and *tai chi* in public parks is a common activity in mornings of Hong Kong. Many people have the impression that *qigong* and *tai chi* practice is mainly an exercise for the elderly. However, many young people are also practicing *qigong* and *tai chi* in Hong Kong. There were more than 300,000 people participating in the morning *tai chi* classes in 2001 (Hong Kong Tai Chi Association 2001: 194), and the number keeps increasing. As some followers practice *qigong* in other classes, presumably there should be more than 300,000 *qigong* and *tai chi* followers in Hong Kong.

Qigong and *tai chi* are common complementary and alternative medicine (CAM) in Chinese communities. Not only do *qigong* and *tai chi* practitioners aim at the balance of *qi*, the maintenance of health, and the prolongation life, but both practices also become a popular therapeutic remedy among patients who receive biomedical treatment. Some patients' resource centres and self-help groups in hospitals provide *qigong* and *tai chi* classes for their patients.

When societies have multiple medical systems, biomedicine usually occupies a dominant position. As is the situation in other countries, Hong Kong is a medically pluralistic society. Global and cosmopolitan medical system (such as biomedicine) coexists with regional medical systems (such as traditional Chinese medicine), and other local medical systems including folk remedies. In this context of medical pluralism, this chapter will discuss how and why people are motivated to practice *qigong* and *tai chi*, though biomedicine is the mainstream medical system in Hong Kong. The increasing number of followers who use *qigong* and *tai chi* in an attempt to maintain health status shows that *qigong* is one of the popular forms of CAM in Hong Kong.

Practicing *qigong* and *tai chi*, as shown by the participants, is a coping strategy for them to respond to, explain, and control their illness experiences. More on psychological and spiritual perspective during the therapeutic process is not the only reason that drives patients to seek CAM. The subjective feeling of patients about how they can be treated, which depends largely on their cultural background and knowledge and the fact that alternative remedies often fit with their cultural ideas on health, also takes account. As CAM is most often deeply rooted in the cultural ideas, they serve the cultural needs which cannot be fulfilled by the mainstream biomedical system. This explains why every society has its own CAM therapy.

The motivations for seeking CAM therapies are many. Taking the *qigong* and *tai chi* practice in Hong Kong as an example, the personal experiences of patients of the inefficacy of biomedicine in treating their diseases are a strong motivating force. This relates to the understanding of the cultural perceptions of disease and medicine (ie. Biomedicine and traditional Chinese medicine in this chapter) of people. Other motivations including the seeking of social network and support as well as emotional well-being also motivates these patients to engage in the practice.

1.1 Brief introduction of *qigong*

Limited literature provides a clear definition of *qigong*. As Dong (1990) stated, "[*q*]*igong* is an ancient Chinese system of 'breathing' or 'vital energy' mind control exercises" (Dong, 1990: 1). However, the definition of *qigong* is never static and rigid. In general, *qigong* can be described as a form of "breathing exercise".

Two categories of *qigong* are noted in literature, namely hard *qigong* and soft *qigong*. Hard *qigong* is considered as a kind of martial arts, which involves the breaking of steel rods, splitting bricks by hand, and resisting attacks by assailants with weapons. Soft *qigong* concerns with enabling one to maintain health (Dong, 1990). As this chapter examines how people use *qigong* as a form of CAM, therefore, soft *qigong* is the main focus.

Four major traditions are noted within the category of soft *qigong*, namely Taoist, Buddhist, Confucian, and medical. Taoist *qigong* emphasizes the training of body and mind, focusing on the relationship between the individual and cosmic environment. Prolongation of life expectancy is one of its main goals. Buddhist *qigong* emphasizes the cultivation of mind and moral will, aiming at escaping from the "hard life". Confucian tradition places its emphasis on conceptual mind, righteousness, honesty of higher thought, altruism, the obtain of rest, steadiness, and tranquillity. Medical *qigong* aims at preventing and treating diseases as well as to maintain health (Dong, 1990).

Although there are several traditions in soft *qigong* theoretically, the boundary of these traditions is not clear-cut in practice. The existence of *tai chi* leads to further difficulties in definition. However, most literature refers *qigong* and *tai chi* as the same thing (Miura 1989: 348). This chapter will also follow this idea as referring *qigong* and *tai chi* as the same thing.

2. Aims and objectives

This chapter aims to investigate the motivations for practicing *qigong*. The participants had encountered different experiences before they decided to engage in the practice. Their motivation thus is often a hybridization of their experiences.

Cultural perceptions are important in shaping ideas and beliefs on diseases. People have their own interpretations and explanations of diseases that can be different from biomedical explanations. Cultural interpretations influence how people view diseases, which in turn influences their decisions in seeking alternative therapies, such as *qigong*.

Cultural perceptions of medical systems influence how people perceive the strengths and weaknesses of different medical systems, which influence them in choosing a suitable therapy.

Beliefs and expectations also motivate people to practice *qigong*. The health benefits that they either expect or have already experienced serve as a motivation.

Although biomedicine is the mainstream medical system in Hong Kong, there are quite a number of followers practicing *qigong* for health purposes. Their experiences in seeking biomedical remedies also explain their motivations to practice *qigong*.

3. Research methods and participants

A qualitative approach by using an anthropological study approach was adopted to investigate the in-depth experiences and perceptions of the sampled *qigong* and *tai chi* followers in Hong Kong. Participant-observation and semi-structured in-depth interviews were conducted in the data collection procedure.

Participant-observation involves "getting close to people and making them feel comfortable with your presence so that you can observe and record information about their lives" (Bernard, 2002: 322). Participant-observation was conducted in three morning *tai chi* classes which were organized by the Leisure and Cultural Services Department of the Hong Kong government. Each class consisted of 40 followers. The majority of the followers were females, with only 12 male followers among these three classes. Most of the followers in these classes were in the mid-aged from 40s to 50s. Only a few were in their 20s and 60s to 70s. All the followers in these three classes were suffering from chronic conditions and requiring regular follow-ups in biomedical settings. The common chronic conditions that the followers were suffering included cancers in the recovering stage, hypertension, diabetes mellitus, heart diseases, and bone and joint problems.

Semi-structured interviews were conducted with 30 participants who were sampled in these 3 classes by purposive sampling. The interviews were conducted with an interview question guide which covered the main areas of concern. Participant information sheets were distributed to the participants prior to the interviews so to ensure their clear understanding of the research. Twenty participants who had learnt *qigong* and *tai chi* for more than five years and another 10 participants who had just started the learning were purposively sampled. To examine the motivations of the practice in relation to their health conditions, the participants with chronic conditions and were receiving biomedical follow-ups were purposively sampled.

4. Perceived role of biomedicine and TCM in health maintenance and disease treatment

Biomedicine and TCM are the two largest medical systems in Hong Kong. Perceptions and understandings of these two approaches by the participants enable the understanding of the perceived strengths and weaknesses of these medical systems, and so the underlying motivations for practicing *qigong*. For the remedy to appear effective, it is often important that the remedy ideas are compatible with the cultural ideas of patients.

Health maintenance has never been in the concept of biomedicine to the participants. The followings were the most common impressions of the participants on biomedicine:

I have never heard western medicine [biomedicine] has such concept. Perhaps taking vitamins is an approach. However, I would not think it is a good approach to maintain health. To me, vitamins are drugs, and I think taking drugs definitely would not have any positive effect on health. Besides vitamins, I cannot think of any other approaches that can maintain health from the viewpoint of western medicine. [P3]

I think [biomedical] doctors would only ask you to do more exercise and have a balanced diet to maintain your health. However, I think the advice is so vague that it seems they have recommended nothing at all for people to keep up their health. What western medicine recommends is only a common sense that even a primary school kid can tell you the same thing. [P14]

Although more participants perceived that TCM could help to maintain health, many of them believed that its concept of health maintenance is not strong. Participants perceived biomedicine and TCM as forms of therapy, to which they would only turn to when they suffered from health problems. Although many participants believed that TCM has the concept of health maintenance, they would only consult TCM practitioners when they encountered health problems. This comment represents the most typical viewpoint among the participants:

I would just only see [TCM] doctors when I was ill. If I saw a doctor just merely for health maintenance, I would feel very strange, though I think it can still be reasonable to see a Chinese medicine practitioner just for the purpose of health maintenance. It is just the same case with western medicine [biomedicine]. How could I ask him to give me some drugs just for maintaining health? The doctor will think I have gone crazy! [P6]

5. Perceived role of *qigong* in health maintenance and disease treatment

In contrast to their views of biomedicine and TCM, the participants perceived *qigong* as having more role in maintaining health. They perceived *qigong* as a form of exercise, and exercise is one of the approaches to maintaining health. However, the form of exercise represented by *qigong* and the form of exercise that the biomedical doctors mention are, to them, two different things. As this female informant stated:

Tai chi is different from other exercises like running. Western [biomedical] doctors often recommend people to do running or swimming; but these exercises are "hard exercises"; they train your muscles only. Tai chi is different. Though it is also an exercise, it is an exercise that can strengthen you internally; you can feel the "hot qi" flowing from inside to outside. This "hot qi" is very good for you; your health becomes better because of this "hot qi". Having those "hard" exercises cannot produce "hot qi". You feel hot only, but not due to the "hot qi". The exercises with no "hot qi" are not as good as qigong. [P22]

On the other hand, most participants would not perceive *qigong* as a form of standalone therapy that can treat diseases. They would not think one can rely solely on the practice of *qigong* for recovery. Rather, they believed they still had to consult doctors, no matter biomedicine or TCM. *Qigong* could only serve as a form of complementary remedy for them after prior diagnosis and treatment by biomedicine or TCM:

Tai chi of course cannot be used as a major form of therapy for most diseases; it can only serve as a complement. You still need to see doctors and take the medicine. If you only practiced tai chi when you were sick, then the situation may become worse. Tai chi is good for health, but it is mainly used as prevention or complement, when you are sick, you still need doctors to help you. [P11]

However, a minority of participants believed one can use *qigong* only as a therapy for emotional problems, stress, depression, and psychiatric and psychological illnesses, since they perceived biomedicine and TCM were unable to deal with these problems:

Qigong can be used as a major therapy for some diseases, though not all. If you often feel stressed, nervous, or have psychiatric diseases, I think it is enough for you to practice qigong only, since qigong can help you to relax. For these mind problems, qigong is the best and you can practice it alone. Western doctors can only give you some tranquilizers or other drugs, but it is difficult for you to have a full recovery, and I have never heard Chinese medicine can treat these problems, so I think qigong alone is enough already. [P2]

6. Degree of participation of patients

6.1 Biomedicine

The perceived degree of patient participation in biomedicine and TCM as active or passive also provides another aspect to understand the motivations to practice *qigong* as related to the perceptions of patients' role in treatment.

The majority of participants perceived their role in biomedical remedies as passive. "Active" in the therapeutic process, to the participants, means they have the opportunity to ask questions; whereas a "passive" role means that they rarely have the opportunity to ask questions and have little room for making decisions.

Participants always felt difficulty in raising questions in the biomedical encounter due to the short consultation time. However, short consultation time was not the only reason for their inability to ask questions in many cases. Limited knowledge of biomedicine also led to their sense of helplessness, since they did not know how and what to ask. Even if they asked their doctors about their health problems, they would not necessarily get the feedbacks as doctors held absolute control and power to determine what and how they would tell the participants:

I do not know what I should ask the [biomedical] doctors, because I do not have much knowledge in western medicine [biomedicine] and its medication. I can just only ask them whether I need to avoid eating some food. That's all. I had tried asking doctors about my diseases in the past, but they would only tell you about the diagnosis. If you asked them about the drugs, they would just tell you that the nurses would tell you later, and all you need to do is to follow the instructions of the nurses. All I can do is to believe in doctors. [P11]

The biomedical encounter is a setting with clear power relations. Professional knowledge of medicine and treatment is under the absolute control of doctors. The experience for those participants with higher education level was better in communicating with doctors than those with lower education level, since a higher education level often enabled them to ask questions. However, their feelings about the responses of biomedical doctors were similar:

In western medicine [biomedicine], it is impossible for a patient to be active. It is the [biomedical] doctors to take the leading role in the therapeutic process. It is the doctors who give the prescription and help you, though you still need to put the drugs into your mouth by yourself. Sometimes I tried to be more active by asking doctors some questions relating to my diseases, and sometimes I asked the doctors whether there were any other possibilities with my case. However, the doctors would start becoming unhappy and keep silent. Even worse, they would just reply me with one sentence – "if I said yes, then it would be yes". Perhaps they thought that even if they explained to me, I would not understand; or they were unhappy about that I was challenging them. [P9]

Some participants also noted that the "order" of biomedical doctors could make them feel they were expected and required to be obedient during the therapeutic procedure. Such feeling was particularly strong when they were under physical and clinical examination:

The instructions from [biomedical] doctors are orders. You need to obey him when you are in the consultation room. You have to open your mouth if the doctors ask you to; you have to take off your clothes if the doctors ask you to. You can choose not following his instructions afterwards; but when you are in the consultation room, you have to obey all of his instructions, no matter whether his orders are reasonable or not. [P21]

The participants' experiences in biomedical encounters illustrated the hierarchical doctor-patient relationship. This relationship could lead to a sense of helplessness on the participants. The pretence that they were being given a choice of remedies also led to a sense of helplessness among the participants in the context of biomedical treatment:

My doctor had suggested several therapeutic options as well as their advantages and disadvantages to me. Then he asked me to choose which remedy I would pick. However, I really think that I do not have much room to choose. During the discussion, the doctor would reveal his preference and indicate which one is the best option. Will you dare to choose another option? [P19]

The one-way communication from doctors to patients was a major factor contributing to the passive feeling of the participants in the remedy process. This, in turn, served as a motivating force for them to seek other forms of remedy which enabled them to take a more active control on their own health.

6.2 TCM

Participants perceived their role in TCM as more active than biomedicine, though it was still passive to them. Being able to ask more questions enabled them to experience a more active role in the therapy, as both the patients and TCM practitioners shared a common cultural knowledge in TCM. Longer consultation time and their deeper knowledge of TCM contributed to such sense:

Although my role is still passive in Chinese medicine, I think I can be more active than western medicine [biomedicine]. The whole consultation process of Chinese medicine is more like Q and A [questioning and answering]. I know how to ask and what to ask. I know more about Chinese medicine. I can ask whether I am too "hot" or too "cold". I can ask about the prescription of Chinese medicine, because I know the names, nature, and usage of some common herbs. I can have more time and opportunity to ask questions and tell him more about my discomforts. At the same time, he is willing to listen and explain to me without losing patience. I can have more interaction with him as a result. How can I ask the [biomedical] doctors about the drugs? I know nothing about it, and so don't know how to ask. [P15]

Although participants perceived themselves as more active during the therapeutic process in TCM than biomedicine's, still they perceived their role as not active enough. As a result, they are motivated to search for other alternatives, such as *qigong*, which served as a solution for them.

6.3 *Qigong*

The practice of *qigong* enhances and empowers participants with an active role in their health. Compared with biomedicine and TCM, most participants believed that the participation role is most active in the practice of *qigong*:

You need to be active in the practice of tai chi, because you need to keep on practicing by yourself. You practice because you are willing to practice, and because you want to keep up your health. Nobody can force you to practice if you are unwilling to do so. It is different from western medicine [biomedicine] and Chinese medicine. You go to see doctors because you are ill; you need their help, because you cannot treat yourself, so the role is passive when you need treatment. [P4]

I practice qigong besides receiving the western [biomedical] treatment. I think I need to do something for my health. If I just sit here and wait for the doctors to give me treatment, then I would feel I could do nothing for my health. I learn qigong because through the practice, I feel like I can do something for my health. [P10]

The doctor said my disease had been cured after my stomach had been taken out. I did not need to take any biomedical drugs and therapy after the surgery, but I still think that I have not yet fully recovered. I think it is better for me to practice tai chi after the surgery, because western [biomedical] treatment cannot treat you thoroughly. I don't feel very good if I just rely on western medicine [biomedicine]. I do not feel comfortable if I do not do something by myself. Practicing tai chi can make me feel more secure that I am doing something for my health. [P21]

"There is a potential for people to resist the passive patient role" (Lupton, 2000: 115). The search of "feel like they can do something for their health" reveals their unconscious desire to regain an active role in their health, and they were able to regain an active control on their health through the practice of *qigong*.

Alternative therapies ascribe the causes of ill health to more than just the purely biological, and encourage individuals to take responsibility for their own health by rejecting the disempowered role of the submissive patient. The emphasis is upon the perception of health as a value in itself, and upon the individual actively participating in the ongoing maintenance of good health… Unlike biomedical medicine, alternative therapies can provide satisfactory explanations for the questions 'Why me?' and 'Why now?'… (Lupton, 2000: 125 – 126).

7. Motivations of the *qigong* practice

Both biomedicine and TCM were inadequate to fulfil participants' cultural perceptions and needs of health and diseases. As they perceived biomedicine and TCM as a form of therapy, they turned to *qigong* for health maintenance and body strengthening after the therapeutic process. To the participants, only *qigong* could provide them with such a concept. The passive role of patients in biomedicine and TCM, in addition, explains why the participants were driven to practice *qigong* as an alternative for remedies and health maintenance. As the followings demonstrate, the practice of *qigong* is often due to a hybridization of concerns, including health, social and emotional concerns.

The concept of remedy, if it is to appear effective, needs to be compatible with the cultural ideology and needs of patients. As biomedicine and TCM are inadequate to provide satisfactory explanations and fulfil the needs in treatment, the participants were attracted to the practice of *qigong*, which is more compatible with their cultural understandings on health and illnesses.

7.1 Health motivations of *qigong* practice

Health concerns and illness experiences were the chief motivations in the practice of *qigong* among the participants. The particularly high sense of health consciousness was apparent among the participants, who were mostly middle-aged persons and having been suffering from chronic diseases.

7.1.1 Concept of "legitimacy" of health maintenance

Definition of "legitimacy" among the participants on perceiving a suitable health maintenance method was greatly influenced by their cultural perceptions. Health maintenance shopping is common among the participants. Although they also tried exercising, still they perceived *qigong* as the most "legitimate" form of health maintenance approach:

Before I came here to learn tai chi, I had tried having many kinds of exercises. I had tried jogging and dancing in the past. However, I really think that if you want to maintain your health, you should find a more "legitimate" practice. Simply moving your hands and legs is definitely not enough. I think tai chi is more "legitimate" because you have to follow the procedures in the practice. [P6]

The concept of "legitimacy" was often closely tied to the concept of "healing" and "tradition":

What I mean by "legitimate" is…hmm…is…[pause for 5 seconds]. Qigong has a very long history; it is our tradition, and a traditional way to maintain health. The Chinese in the past also practiced qigong, so it should be good. Only good things can survive for a long time, so it [qigong] should be "legitimate". Also, you cannot find another method that can help you to maintain health and treat your disease in a single practice. Running, swimming, or having ballgames can only train your physical fitness, but it cannot treat you [disease], so qigong seems more "legitimate". [P18]

7.1.2 Deteriorating of health status

The participants were mainly aged 30s to 50s, and one of the major motivations was their deteriorating health status associated with their age. All the participants reaching such middle age indicated that they have experienced some extent of deteriorating health status. They caught diseases much easier than when they were young, though these diseases were not necessarily serious and life threatening:

When I was young, I rarely got sick. I rarely caught cold and flu. However, when I entered 40s, I started catching more and more minor diseases, such as cold and cough. In the past, even if I caught a cold and flu, I could drink some "box tea" [an over-the-counter Chinese medicine which treats cold and flu] and then recovered quickly. However, now I need to see doctors when I got a cold and flu; otherwise, it could be very difficult for me to get recovered. [P7]

Because of their experiences of deteriorating health status, they felt the strong need of keeping up their health through exercising. In view of their decreasing health status and physical fitness, they perceived exercises with soft and slow motion - such as *qigong* and *tai chi* - as the most suitable option. They perceived vigorous exercises as damaging, and even life threatening, for them:

Vigorous exercise is not suitable for everybody. I am old, so I am not capable of doing such vigorous exercises like running. Running can lead to injury of legs and knees. Also, I don't know whether my heart is still capable of coping with such vigorous exercise. You know, newspapers often report middle-aged people died suddenly when they were playing ballgames, even though they appear to be normal and healthy. Therefore, I choose tai chi, since it is mild and slow, and I can cope with it. [P27]

The suffering of menopause was a significant reason that motivated middle-aged women to practice *qigong*. The classes had a gender imbalance with a high proportion of female followers. The participants suffered from different degrees of discomfort associated with menopause, and the prevention of such discomforts was a key concern for these middle-aged female followers. Quite a number of middle-aged female followers were attracted to practice *qigong* because of the frequent reports about its efficacy in preventing osteoporosis:

My doctor said he could prescribe some hormones for me to alleviate my discomforts. However, I am reluctant to take these drugs, because it is said that taking such medicine for a long time can increase the probability of getting cancers. Also, medicine is medicine, and it is unnatural, so it can have a lot of side effects. The newspaper reports said tai chi can help to prevent osteoporosis, and said tai chi is good to bones and health for old people, so I come to try. [P25]

7.1.3 Suffering from diseases

Disease suffering was a major motivation for the participants. Two main categories of diseases were identified from the participants: 1) the life threatening diseases such as cancers, and 2) chronic illnesses. Although all participants had already completed the major therapeutic procedure, many of them felt uncertainty, which was a strong motivation for them to practice *qigong*:

Although I have finished the surgery and chemotherapy in the hospital, I still need to go to the hospital regularly for check-ups. Superficially, it seems that I have recovered, and the regular check-up is just for safety concern. But I understand that there is still a possibility for the cancer to relapse. It may not be in the same place [organ], but can transfer to other places [organs]. If I really have recovered, then why should I have to go to the hospital regularly? Is it really for safety purpose? Perhaps it is, because it is often safer to check whether the cancer will relapse. Qigong may not help preventing the cancer from relapsing, but at least I have tried something. I have tried my best to do as much as possible, and to practice qigong as frequently as possible. If the cancer really relapses, then that's my fate that I have to accept. However, I think my health will become better if I practice qigong; even if it [cancer] relapses, my body will be stronger to accept and able to cope with the therapy procedures. [P16]

Some participants were second-time learners of *qigong*. They had the experience of practicing *qigong* many years ago but stopped practicing after some time. The suffering of diseases motivated them to re-engage in the practice:

I had learnt tai chi many years ago because I felt I was not healthy. However, I did not have time to practice it because of work. Also, I did not have much patience and physical ability at that time. I had to work until late at night, so how could I wake up early to attend the lectures? Therefore, I gave up the practice. Only when I caught cancer that I suddenly recognized that health is really very important. I regret that I did not keep on practicing it at that time. If I had kept on practicing at that time, perhaps I would not need to suffer from this disease. As I have the chance [to get the recovery] now, so I would not miss this chance again. Suffering from cancer is a warning signal for me. It reminds me that health is very important, and I should do everything that can help to maintain health. Hence, I pick up the practice again. [P1]

Some participants were "forced" to practice *qigong* because of their diseases. Although they thought *qigong* is boring, still they practiced it because they believed *qigong* could help with their diseases:

Honestly speaking, I really have no interest in learning tai chi. It is very boring. If I were not sick, I would not have come to learn tai chi. [P11]

Some young participants were reluctant to practice *qigong* because they believed such practice was not appropriate for their generation. However, they were "forced" to practice *qigong* because of their health problem:

If I were healthy, of course I would not have come here to learn tai chi. You know, tai chi is an activity for the elderly. I am still young, so I should choose other kinds of sports instead of tai chi. I had been struggling for a long time whether I should come, because I am afraid that my friends would tease me. However, I have no choice. My bones have problems; if I play sports, I would further injure myself. As I heard that tai chi can help with the bones, so I come and try. [P8]

Suffering from chronic diseases was another common motivation, since biomedicine and TCM failed to ensure total recovery for them:

I often feel pain in my knees, especially when walking upstairs and downstairs. I could not take buses, because sitting for a long time could make my knees and legs feel numb. If you look at my knees, you can see they are swollen and larger than the normal size. I had seen a western [biomedical] doctor before, but he told me there is no remedy for it. He just told me that I could only have more swimming. However, swimming is not a remedy; it is just an exercise! Then I realize there should be no good remedy for me. But I cannot wait until I could not walk, and I should try my best to heal myself, so I come to learn tai chi to see if it can help. [P26]

7.1.4 Seeking a faster recovery

Qigong was expected to provide faster recovery to many participants. They believed the recovery process would be shortened if they practiced *qigong* in addition to the biomedical treatment.

"Recovery" was a subjective perception to participants, as they often had their own definition of "recovery". This subjective perception motivated them to practice *qigong* for attaining full recovery:

I really think that I still have not recovered yet. If I was recovered, then I would not need to take drugs and pay regular visits to the hospital. You know, I need to take the drugs for the rest of my life. The doctor told me that I can be considered as having recovered, but I don't think so, because I still need to take drugs and pay regular visits to the hospital. I think it is impossible for me to gain full recovery, because I have to take drugs on a long-term basis. I cannot rely on doctors, but rather I should rely on myself, so I learn tai chi. [P28]

The subjective understanding of "recovery" was thus different from the clinical definition. This revealed the conflicting explanatory models between biomedical doctors and patients. The conflict in the explanatory models, I argue, is due to the different concerns on "disease" and "illness". Unlike biomedical doctors who concerned about "disease", participants concerned about their "illness" experience. Indeed, past literature shows that the distinction between "disease" and "illness" is often vague for chronically ill patients:

In chronic disorders…it may be difficult to distinguish the disease from the illness. In such disorders, illness may exist when the disease is in remission, and recurrence of the disease itself may be due to the illness… illness can occur in the absence of disease, for example, in…chronic "functional" complaints… In that sense, illness is a reaction to an imagined, perceived, or even desired disease… (Kleinman, 1980: 74).

Patients recovering from cancers often require long-term care and regular medical check-ups. Such experiences made these recovering participants felt that they were still "sick", because they were under the influence of their illness experience.

The idea of the "five-year recovery period" as mentioned by biomedical doctors also motivated participants to keep on practicing *qigong*:

I also want to consider myself as recovered. However, it is difficult to tell whether you can really recover, especially if you are a cancer patient like me. I asked the [biomedical] doctor whether I could be considered as recovered, but the doctor just said if I did not suffer from a relapse [of cancer] in the coming five years, then I can be considered as recovered in their sense. However, how about having it again more than 5 years later? It still has this possibility. I just know that I need to continue practicing tai chi, at least I want to pass these five years. [P30]

7.1.5 Alleviating chronic pain

Alleviation of chronic and long-term pain was another motivating factor for their *qigong* practice. This motivation was particularly apparent among those participants who were suffering from rheumatic and bone pain. Although biomedicine could relieve their pain quickly, the efficacy was short unless they took painkillers on a long-term basis. As they had a negative impression on biomedical drugs, they searched for a more natural approach to alleviate their pain. This led them to *qigong* practice:

I want to get rid of my rheumatic pain through learning tai chi. Western [biomedical] doctors cannot deal with this. They can do nothing besides prescribing painkillers and injection to me. I think both are useless in my pain, because they fail to give me a complete cure. The pain will come back again after several hours. However, tai chi is different. If you have patience, then it can cure your pain. Even if you still suffer from the pain, the frequency and level [of pain] is reduced. I have not used any painkillers since I started practicing tai chi. [P24]

The desire for long-term alleviation of chronic pain was often spurred by their desire to avoid physiotherapy. Some participants perceived physiotherapy as a painful experience, both physically and emotionally. *Qigong* could thus serve as an escape for them:

I have suffered from sciatica [low back pain] for many years. I used to seek western medical [biomedical] remedies for my pain. When I need western medical attention, my pain is so serious that I need to be hospitalized. The doctors would prescribe me a heavy dosage of painkillers or even a morphine injection. However, the pain returned after several hours. I also needed to receive physiotherapy. It is really very painful for me. I needed to go into the hospital for treatment every few months. It is really an endless therapy and a nightmare for me. The most discouraging thing is my situation did not get any better. I just felt like I was wasting time on doing useless and painful things. I therefore learned tai chi. I do not feel pain anymore since I started practicing it. Therefore, I will keep on practicing it with the hope that I will not need western medical treatment again. [P13]

The concept of "Chinese" physiotherapy was mentioned by the participants. They perceived *tai chi* as a Chinese form of physiotherapy. However, unlike biomedical physiotherapy, this "Chinese physiotherapy" was much better in the perception of the participants:

I think tai chi is just like physiotherapy, since you need to move your body, hands, and legs during the practice. It is very similar to western [biomedical] physiotherapy. However, tai chi is a lot less painful than [biomedical] physiotherapy. If you could not do some certain motion in tai chi, then you could choose not doing that motion, or just only do part of that motion. You will feel comfortable with the practice, and will be willing to continue with it. But you cannot choose what to do or not to do in physiotherapy. You have to follow all the instructions of the nurse [physiotherapist]. You cannot say I don't want to do it because I feel pain. The nurse [physiotherapist] will ask you to do it even harder if you feel pain! If the outcome of both is similar, then of course I will choose the painless tai chi. [P5]

7.1.6 Restoring of health after surgical treatment

The desire to restore health after surgery was another most common motivation for those participants who received surgical treatment. Surgery was perceived as harmful to their body and could lead to "depletion" as a result. As "depletion" is a Chinese concept, they believed only a "Chinese" approach could help. *Qigong* was the first approach that they could think of.

I learn tai chi because I had a major surgery ten years ago. After the surgery, I felt "depleted". I often felt dizzy and tired, and my friends told me that I looked really pale. My relatives had prepared some Chinese medicine tonics for me after the surgery. I felt a little bit better, but I still felt it was not enough – I still could not return to the health status I had before surgery. Some of my friends who had surgery before also practiced tai chi at that time and they told me that it could help. Hence, I went to learn tai chi. [P3]

7.1.7 Experiencing the side effects of biomedical treatment

The side effects induced by biomedical treatment were a common motivation. In many cases, they experienced side effects of long-term medication due to their chronic disease suffering. They believed practicing *qigong* was the first step to rebuild their health.

The idea of side effects was also a subjective feeling of the participants. In some cases, they did not really experience any side effects, but they perceived they did because the popular belief on biomedicine led them to link biomedical drugs with the side effects together:

I need to take western [biomedical] drugs for a long time. I want to stop the drug treatment, because I think it is not good to the body if I take these drugs for a long time. I have asked the doctor whether I can stop taking drugs if I feel better, but he just told me to follow his instructions. I really feel uncomfortable after taking these drugs. How uncomfortable? [paused for 10 seconds]. I do not know how to tell you, but I feel really uncomfortable. This uncomfortable feeling must be due to the side effects of the drugs. I believe tai chi can rebuild my health, and the side effects will no longer appear. [P16]

In other cases, the "side effects" that the participants experienced were the symptoms of their diseases. However, they perceived the uncomfortable feelings as due to the biomedical drugs. The attempt to alleviate the "side effects" of the biomedical drugs could motivate them to practice *qigong*:

Because of hypertension and diabetes, I need to take [biomedical] drugs on a long-term basis. However, I often feel dizzy and have a headache after taking the drugs. I told the doctor but he [biomedical] just told me that the uncomfortable feelings are due to the diseases but not to the drugs. I asked the doctor whether I can stop taking them, but he just told me to take the drugs accordingly. I really think that these feelings are due to the side effects of the drugs. I really think that the drugs have depleted my health. If I cannot stop taking the drugs, then I need to learn tai chi so to strengthen my health in order to get rid of these uncomfortable feelings. [P11]

7.1.8 Escaping from the biomedical treatment

Unpleasant experiences in receiving biomedical treatment served as a motivating force for some participants. The unpleasant experiences were often related to perceived inappropriate biomedical treatment. This drove them to try keeping their exposure to biomedicine to an absolute minimum. They attempted to gain better health and avoid seeking biomedical advice through the continuous practice of *qigong*:

If you were sick, of course you needed to see the doctor; but whether you can get proper treatment is another matter. Sometimes I feel it heavily depends on luck whether you can meet a good and experienced doctor. If you met an unscrupulous doctor, then you could not get proper treatment even though you have seen the doctor. The reason why I learn qigong is partly due to such unscrupulous doctor. When I played squash with my friend, I suddenly felt sick. I found difficulty in breathing. Therefore I rested immediately. I was very afraid at that time, and so I went to see the doctor ...

The doctor just carried out some simple examination roughly. He told me [part of] my lungs was "burst" and so he referred me to a private hospital immediately. At first, I felt doubtful, because I felt difficulty in breathing at that moment only; but as he had been my family doctor since I was a child, so I trust him. When I was in the ward, he suddenly told me that the best way to treat my case was by operation, and he recommended a surgeon to handle this operation. Then I felt strange; why the operation was decided so suddenly without telling me first? So I told him I needed to think about this and I requested to leave. The doctor seemed quite unhappy with this...

I found another doctor who was recommended by a friend; and this doctor gave me another diagnosis that my heart has a problem. I was very disappointed. Why did he [the family doctor] cheat me? I had been seeing him for such a long time. It is hard for me to believe it. Even a familiar doctor can treat you in this way, so how can I trust other doctors? Even if this new doctor does not cheat me that my heart has problem, I still feel doubtful about him. I feel doubtful with the doctors; it is better to see them as few times as possible. If qigong can really help, then I can recover and need not to see them. [P14]

The desire to avoid surgical treatment also motivated some participants to practice *qigong*:

The [biomedical] doctor suggested removing the gallstone by surgery as soon as possible; otherwise, I would have a 3% probability of suffering from cholecystitis. You know, surgery is really horrible. I heard from others that practicing qigong can help to dissolve the gallstone, so I come to learn qigong. If qigong could really help, then I can avoid having surgery. I take Chinese medicine as well, because my friends told me that some Chinese medicine can also dissolve the gallstone. [P20]

7.2 Positive belief on health of *qigong*

Strong belief in *qigong* on health was a remarkable motivator for the *qigong* practice. Participants believed that *qigong* could serve as a long-term health maintenance approach, provided that they have the patience to practice it continuously. They believed that even if *qigong* did not bring health benefits, it would not have harmful effects on them either.

Their belief in the positive effects of *qigong* on their health was often due to their experiences of improved health, which gave them confidence in continuing with the practice. Even those participants who had not experienced obvious health improvement still believed in its efficacy provided they would continue with the practice. They would blame themselves for being lazy and unserious in their practice if they failed to experience these benefits:

Although I still cannot experience the benefits of tai chi, I strongly believe that it will be effective on my case. I am still a beginner in tai chi. I am sure if I have patience in the practice, I will see its benefits. Tai chi has a long tradition in China, hence it is already a clear evidence. I think I still have not devoted myself to the practice, since I do not practice it everyday. Therefore, I will not blame tai chi as useless to me. It is my fault if I cannot enjoy the efficacy of tai chi, since I am not hardworking enough in the practice. [P5]

A strong belief in the efficacy of *qigong* for health was noted. Even though some participants still suffered from their diseases after they have practiced *qigong*, they still maintained their beliefs of *qigong* in their health:

Honestly speaking, I could not feel any better with my "wind wet" pain [rheumatic pain], though I have practiced tai chi for almost one year. However, if I did not practice it, my "wind wet" pain may have become even worse. [P13]

The strong belief in the efficacy of *qigong* did not diminish even when the participants experienced adverse effects from it. Even though they felt worse with their ailment after practice, they believed it as the healing process of *qigong*:

I have had low back pain for many years. After I have taken the Omega oil capsules, my back pain has gone already. However, the pain returns after I practice qigong. I often move vigorously when I am practicing, and my back moves even more vigorously. Perhaps due to the vigorous movement, the back pain returns. However, as the master said, body moves because qigong is treating the diseased area. The vigorous movement of a certain part indicates that part has problem, and qigong can treat your problem by moving that part more. I believe qigong is treating my back pain. [P23]

7.3 Social and emotional motivations of *qigong* practice

Besides their health concerns and their hope for treatment and recovery, the social support, bonding, and network that had been built up during the practice was also a significant motivation for their continuing practice.

7.3.1 Emotional attachment with *qigong* masters and fellow followers

The close relationship between *qigong* masters and fellow followers was particularly apparent in the morning *tai chi* class. Owing to their continuing practice, their relationship has become closer and closer. Such emotional attachment encouraged them to continue with the practice. Besides relationship in class, such close bonding could be recognized from the activities and gatherings other than lectures. It was a common practice for them to go to Chinese restaurants to have breakfast together after class. At the end of each course and during some important Chinese festivals, the followers would invite the master for a "thank master feast". Such emotional attachment among fellow followers and with the master was an important consideration for them in the practice:

We have practiced together for several years. Our relationship is not just only a master-follower relationship, but we have become very good friends as well. After the lecture, we would go to yum cha [Chinese dining with dim sum] together, and we would go shopping together afterwards. We would chat everything, including children, family, health, etc. We would not view the master as a master, and the master would not view us as her followers. I do not want to leave my practice. If I really quit my practice, then it would be more difficult to keep up our relationship. Perhaps we can still be friends if any of us quit the practice, but I think the relationship cannot be kept as good as present. Indeed, the master is really very nice. Although she is stern during lecture, she is serious in her teaching and cares about us. She is very nice after lectures. [P26]

I often visit the master outside lectures. We often have meals and buy things together. I think we are very good friends with each other, because we share all our happiness and unhappiness together. [P10]

I think the relationship between my master and myself is very similar to a father-son relationship. When he scolded me, I did not dare to resist him. Even though he has retired to Zhongshan [in the Mainland China] now, I often phone him and visit him when I have a holiday. [P9]

The family atmosphere was significant in motivating the followers to continue with the practice. The master was viewed as a core of spirit for the followers, whereas the senior followers in the class often served as the "elders" in a family, supervising the practice of other followers. In the first lecture of the course, the master announced:

All the followers here should be treated as family members with one another. As you participate in this class, you are just like a member in our family. Therefore, we should take care of one another, and be devoted to the practice.

7.3.2 Social networking

As most participants have followed the master for a long time in the morning class, learning new things was not their aim. Although some of them practiced in the hope to sharpen their skills, the morning class was also a kind of social gathering for the followers and master in reality.

The participants also sought for a social relationship and a wider social network, which was a motivation for the continuous practice. The search for a social support was apparent as most participants were housewives or having been retired, they would perceive the class practice as a form of social resource for support.

I feel happy to come to practice tai chi here every morning, because I feel like I am back to the family. We will greet and chat each other, and will have gatherings other than lectures. The class is just like another home for me. Before I come to practice, my life was just concentrated with my husband and children. I felt lonely and helpless if any problems emerged in my family. However, after I have joined the tai chi class, I can have support from my fellow classmates. I know where I can get support and advice if any problems emerge. The master and classmates are so warm and we are just like family members who will support each other. [P22]

8. Conclusions

As discussed in this chapter, there are many motivations for the participants' practice of *qigong*. In many cases, these motivations were intertwining together to motivate the practice. These motivations related to their experiences in seeking medical treatment, their illness experiences, their search for a social support network as well as an emotional attachment with fellow followers and masters. Besides, their perceptions on biomedicine and TCM in the role of health maintenance and disease treatment, in addition to their search for a more active control in their health also accounted for their practice.

9. References

Baer, Hans A. 2001. *Biomedicine and Alternative Healing Systems in America: Issues of Class,* Race, Ethnicity, and Gender. Madison, Wisconsin: The University of Wisconsin Press.

Baer, Hans A., Merrill Singer, and Ida Susser. 1997. *Medical Anthropology and the World System: A Critical Perspective*. Westport, CT: Bergin and Garvey.

Bernard, H.R. 2002. *Research methods in anthropology: qualitative and quantitative approaches.* Walnut Creek, CA: AltaMira Press.

Brady, Erika. 2001. *Healing Logics: Culture and Medicine in Modern Health Belief Systems.* Logan, Utah: Utah State University Press.

Chen, Nancy N. 1995. "Urban Spaces and Experiences of Qigong." In Deborah S. Davis et al., *Urban Spaces in Contemporary China: The Potential for Autonomy and Community in Post-Mao China*, pp. 347 - 361. New York: Cambridge University Press.

Cheng, Tin-hung, and Wun-kong Tsui, eds. 1996. *The Record of Tai Chi Martial Arts of Master Cheng Tin-hung*". Hong Kong: Hong Kong Tai Chi Association.

Croizier, Ralph C. 1968. *Traditional Medicine in Modern China: Science, Nationalism, and the Tensions of Cultural Change*. Cambridge, MA: Harvard University Press.

Dong, Paul, and Aristide H. Esser. 1990. *Chi Gong: The Ancient Chinese Way to Health*. New York: Marlowe and Company.

English-Lueck, J. A. 1994. "Taijiquan and Qigong." In Dingbo Wu and Patrick D. Murphy, eds., *Handbook of Chinese Popular Culture*, pp. 137 - 151. Westport, CT: Greenwood Press.

Fabrega, Jr., Horacio. 1999. *Evolution of Sickness and Healing*. Berkeley: University of California Press.

Farquhar, Judith. 1994. *Knowing Practice: The Clinical Encounter of Chinese Medicine*. Boulder, CO: Westview Press.

Frohock, Fred M. 1995. *Healing Powers: Alternative Medicine, Spiritual Communities, and the State*. Chicago: The University of Chicago Press.

Greenhalgh, Susan. 2001. *Under the Medical Gaze: Facts and Fictions of Chronic Pain*. Berkeley: University of California Press.

Good, Bryon J. 2001. *Medicine, Rationality, and Experience: An Anthropological Perspective.* Cambridge: Cambridge University Press.

Hahn, Robert A. 1995. *Sickness and Healing: An Anthropological Perspective*. New Haven: Yale University Press.

Hatty, Suzanne E., and James Hatty. 1999. *The Disordered Body: Epidemic Disease and Cultural Transformation*. NY: State University of New York Press.

Helman, Cecil G. 2001. *Culture, Health, and Illness*. London: Arnold.

Hong Kong Tai Chi Association. 2001. *"The Three Hundred Questions of Tai Chi Quan"*. Hong Kong: Hong Kong Tai Chi Association.

Hsu, Elisabeth. 1999. *The Transmission of Chinese Medicine*. Cambridge: Cambridge University Press.

Kleinman, Arthur. 1980. *Patients and Healers in the Context of Culture: An Exploration of the Borderland between Anthropology, Medicine, and Psychiatry*. Berkeley, CA: University of California Press.

Kleinman, Arthur. 1988. *The Illness Narratives: Suffering, Healing, and the Human Condition*. NY: Basic Books.

Kleinman, Arthur. 1997. *Writing at the Margin: Discourse between Anthropology and Medicine*. Berkeley: University of California Press.

Laderman, Carol, and Marina Roseman, eds. 1996. *The Performance of Healing*. London: Routledge.

Leisure and Cultural Services Department. 2002. *Leisure and Cultural Link*. Hong Kong: Leisure and Cultural Services Department.

Loustaunau, Martha O., and Elisa J. Sobo. 1997. *The Cultural Context of Health, Illness, and Medicine*. Westport, CT: Bergin and Garvey.

Lupton, Deborah. 2000. *Medicine as Culture: Illness, Disease and the Body in Western Societies*. London: Sage Publications Ltd.

Mattingly, Cheryl. 1998. *Healing Dramas and Clinical Plots: The Narrative Structure of Experience*. Cambridge: Cambridge University Press.

Mattingly, Cheryl, and Linda C. Garro, eds. 2000. *Narrative and the Cultural Construction of Illness and Healing*. Berkeley: University of California Press.

McGuire, Francis A., Rosangela K. Boyd, and Raymond E. Tedrick. 1999. *Leisure and Aging: Ulyssean Living in Later Life*. Champaign, IL: Sagamore Publishing.

Miura, Kunio. 1989. "The Revival of Qi: Qigong in Contemporary China." In Livia Kohn and Yoshinobu Sakade, eds., *Taoist Meditation and Longevity Techniques*, pp. 331 – 358 Ann Arbor: Center for Chinese Studies, University of Michigan.

Morris, David B. 1998. *Illness and Culture in the Postmodern Age*. Berkeley: University of California Press.

Palmer, David A. 2003. "Modernity and Millenialism in China: *Qigong* and the Birth of Falun Gong." *Asian Anthropology* 2(3): 79 – 109.

Penny, Benjamin. 1993. "Qigong, Daoism and Science: Some Contexts for the Qigong Boom." In Mabel Lee and A.D. Syrokomla-Stefanowska, eds., *Modernization of the Chinese Past*, pp. 166 – 179. Sydney: Wild Peony.

Romanucci-Ross, Lola, Daniel E. Moerman, and Laurence R. Tancredi, eds. 1997. *The Anthropology of Medicine: From Culture to Method*. Westport, CT: Bergin and Garvey.

Scheid, Volker. 2002. *Chinese Medicine in Contemporary China: Plurality and Synthesis*. Durham, NC: Duke University Press.

Siu, J.Y.M., Sung H.C., & Lee, WL. 2007. Qigong practice among chronically ill patients during the SARS outbreak. *Journal of Clinical Nursing*, 16(4): 769-776.

Strathern, Andrew, and Pamela J. Stewart. 1999. *Curing and Healing: Medical Anthropology in Global Perspective*. Durham, NC: Carolina Academic Press.

Yuen, Chung Lau Natalis, and Natalie Y. K. Yuen. 2001. "Scientific Bases of Qigong." *United Services Recreation Club*, pp.16.

Zhu, Xiaoyang and Benjamin Penny. 1994. "The Qigong Boom." *Chinese Sociology and Anthropology* 27(1): 3 – 94.

Part 5

Herbalism

8

Medical Herbalism and Frequency of Use

Behice Erci
Nursing Department, Malatya Health School, İnönü University, Malatya, Turkey

1. Introduction

Medical herbalism is today a sophisticated system of natural medicine using plant extracts and herbs to help treat physical and mental disorders. Herbalism is a traditional medicinal or folk medicine practice based on the use of plants and plant extracts. Herbalism is also known as botanical medicine, medical herbalism, herbal medicine, herbology, and phytotherapy. The scope of herbal medicine is sometimes extended to include fungal and bee products, as well as minerals, shells and certain animal parts. Medical Herbalism is the modern version of traditional herbal medicine which has been used throughout the world for thousands of years. Herbalists use concentrated whole plant extracts, in the form of tinctures, infusions, salves, creams and pills, as part of a holistic treatment plan to address the underlying causes of your condition (Kennedy et al., 2009; Tapsell et al. 2006; Fabricant, 2001)

Ancient Indians, Chinese and Europeans discovered origins of medicinal herbs. They have been using them for curative purposes successfully. In India itself, there are more than 1100 medicinal plants grown all over the wild forests. Of these, some 60 geniuses are used immensely in medicinal preparations. Despite their demands today, they are not grown in a controlled manner. Rather tribes use them as their livelihood in some belts where they are grown in the wild. Unlike India, in China, the spurt in demand for traditional medicines has made the government to allow growth of these plants for further research and development. About 100 units have nearly 600 plant types, grown for their medicinal value. Herbal medicines are used in Ayurveda, Naturopathy, and Homeopathy, traditional and Native American medicines. About 74 plant types are used in modern medicines. (Vickers & Zollman, 1999; Goldman, 2001; Tapsell et al. 2006; Fabricant, 2001)

Herbal medicine in China has for centuries been a well-organized system of knowledge based on observations, experiments, and clinical trials, and the effectiveness of a significant number of these remedies has been verified by modern science. Elsewhere, the latest effort in plant codification has been undertaken by a consortium of medical researchers, pharmaceutical companies, and herbalists who are investigating the flora of the rain forests in the hope of discovering new plant resources that might yield cures for heart disease, cancer, AIDS, and other deadly disease (Goldman, 2001).

Herbal medicine is the use of plants-their leaves, stems, bark, flowers, fruits, and seeds to prevent or cure disease. Four billion people or about 80% of the world's population uses herbal medicine today as part of health care (Sonal Sekhar et al., 2008). Different cultures use herbs located in their geographical locations for curing common illnesses. They have been successful to a certain extent and over many centuries, some of the herbal cures have proved to be far more useful than allopathic drugs (Sonal Sekhar et al., 2008; Tapsell et al., 2006; Fabricant, 2001). The most frequently used Chine Medicine therapies were Chinese herbal medication (93.6%) (Lin et al., 2010).

Many of today's synthetic drugs originated from the plant kingdom, and only about 200 years ago our pharmacopoeia was dominated by herbal medicines. Medical herbalism (i.e. the medicinal use of preparations that contain exclusively plant material) went into rapid decline when pharmacology established itself as a leading branch of therapeutics. In much of the English speaking world, herbalism virtually vanished from the therapeutic map about a century ago. In contrast, many developing countries never abandoned medical herbalism (e.g. Ayurvedic medicine in India, Kampo medicinein Japan, and Chinese herbalism in China) and in othercountries, e.g. Germany and France, medical herbalism continued to co-exist with modern pharmacology, albeitat an increasingly lower level (Ernst, 2000). In recent years, this situation has started to change again. The usage of herbal medicines by the general US population, for instance, increased by 380% (from a1-year prevalence of 2.5–12.1%) between 1990 and1997 (Eisenberg et al., 1998). A more recent US survey suggested that 16.4% of all patients attending an internal medicine clinic were current users of herbal medicines (Rhee et al., 2004).

Herbal medicine has become a popular form of healthcare. Even though several differences exist between herbal and conventional pharmacological treatments, herbal medicine can be tested for efficacy using conventional trial methodology. Several specific herbal extracts have been demonstrated to be efficacious for specific conditions. Even though the public is often misled to believe that all natural treatments are inherently safe, herbal medicines do carry risks. It is need to know which herbal remedies do more harm than good for which condition (Ernst, 2000).

The aim of this chapter is to provide a general introduction to using herbal medicine, type of herbal medicine, characteristics of herbal medicine user, adverse-effects of herbal medicine, method of application of herbal medicine, and cost of herbalism.

2. Methods

Search's stages involved: Searching literature, result examination, result synthesis. All database searches ran from 1997 to 2011 inclusive. Although only English papers were extracted, no geographical or methodological limitations were placed on the literature. The majority of articles were found in the health care databases, Medline, Cinahl, Social Science, Web of Science, Science Direct and Wiley-Blackwell. Google scholar however proved a useful adjunct to the traditional databases. Articles searched were considered for review. Abstracts and full-text of articles were reviewed. Total 84 articles were reviewed and 36 of these articles were used for the chapter.

The chapter's subheadings and keywords used for literature searching. Search keywords were herbal medicine, using frequency, botanical medicine, phytotherapy, adverse-effects, application of herbs and cost of herbalism.

3. Results

3.1 Frequency of herbal medicine use

The prevalence of herbal use among diverse racially/ethnically varies from culture to culture and population to population. The most common types of complementary alternative medicine used were herbal therapies (34%) (Huillet et al., 2011). Overall, 36% of one study sample reported ever using herbs. The proportions of herbal users varied across racial/ethnic groups, with use being reported by 50% of Hispanics, 50% of Asians, 41% of Whites, and 22% of African-Americans. Herbal use by other family members was reported to be 41% (57% among Hispanics, 45% among Asians, 37% among Whites, and 30% among African-Americans). About 40% of all of the survey respondents, but especially Asians (55%) and Whites (47%), believed that taking prescription medications and herbal medicines together was more effective than taking either alone. About 41% of Hispanic respondents believed that herbal medicines were superior to prescription medications, as compared to 12% of Whites. One hundred sixty-two of the 485 respondents answered affirmatively to using herbal medication (34%). Broken down by gender, 116 of 331 female respondents (35%) and 46 of 153 male respondents (30%) use herbal medication. The ingestion of herbal medicines was similar in the Asian and Caucasian respondents (38%, 35% respectively). Frequency of herbal medicine use was as follows: daily by 63 patients (39% of herbal medicine users), week by 16 patients (10%), once a month by 20 patients (12%) and less than once a month by 48 patients (30%). Other group patients were taking 65 different preparations containing at least 45 distinct ingredients. The most frequent herbal medicine consumed was echinacea, glucosamine, garlic, ginkobiloba, St.John's wort and "chinese mix" alsocommon. Thirty-five patients (22%) did not know the once a name of the medication they were taking. The largest numbers of consumers of herbal medicines (31.5% of users) were in the 31–45-yr-oldrange, which was also our largest group of patients. The46–60-yr-old group accounted for 25% of overall use and the over-60 group in our institution accounted for 17% (Lennox & Henderson, 2003). Research studied in surgery patients showed thirty-eight percent of the study population had consumed herbal medicine in the 2 years before surgery and 16% continued the use of herbal medicine in the month of surgery (Adusumilli et al., 2004). A survey conducted with 1200 pregnant Nigerian women demonstrated that 12% used native herbs (Gharoro & Igbafe, 2000). Herbal medicine product use was more prevalent amongst nulliparous women (42%). A study conducted in South Africa showed that out of 229 pregnant women, 55% had used herbal medicine products during pregnancy (Mabina et al., 1997). Herbal medicine product use was more prevalent amongst nulliparous women (42%). A study conducted in South Africa showed that out of 229 pregnant women, 55% had used herbal medicine products during pregnancy (Mabinaet al., 1997). In other study, one hundred and nine out of 392 women (27.8%) reported to have been taking one or more herbal products during pregnancy, in the 36.7% of cases throughout all pregnancy (Ayaz &Yaman Efe, 2010). Results of studies confirmed that herbal medicine has been frequently used by variety patient groups, pregnant and healthy people

3.2 Type of herbal medicine used

More than 100 different types of herbal remedies were cited. The most frequently reported ones were lime, mint, rosehip, lemon, clary, parsley, garlic, nettle, thyme and camomile. The most commonly used herbs were lime, mint, rosehip and lemon (Nur, 2010). Traditional herbal medicines constitute major parts of the consumption of therapeutic remedies, often the combination with allopathic medicines. Different cultures use herbs located in their geographical locations in different forms for curing common illnesses. Aromatherapy is the use of oils from herbs and other aromatic plants to achieve relaxation or relief from a disorder. Ayurveda and Chinese herbal medicines are ancient healing systems from India and China stresses the mind and body relationship in the maintenance of good health (Sonal Sekhar et al., 2008). Adusumilli et al. determined that patients taking herbal medicine often consumed more than one type of product. Patients also consumed cod liver oil (15.2%), primrose oil (11.2%), herbal tea (53.3%), herbal vitamins (15%), and other herbal supplements (11.3%) (Adusumilli et al., 2004).

Sixty three percent (63%) of Asian women used most common was a vegetarian diet, followed by use of dietary and herbal supplements and alternative medical systems. Females reported a significantly higher use a vegetarian diet, and use of dietary and herbal (ˇSari´c-Kundali´c et al., 2010). Herbal practitioners will consider a woman's symptoms and health before creating a treatment plan. There are many herbs that may be used such as black cohosh, ginseng, dong quai and agnuscastus, dependent on the symptoms (Gollschewski et al., 2004).

The most commonly used herbal medicine products during pregnancy were garlic, aloe, chamomile, peppermint, ginger, echinacea, pumpkin seeds, and ginseng (Gharoro & Igbafe, 2000). A survey of 200 pregnant US women demonstrated that 15% used 'home remedies' (most commonly ginger, vitamin B6, chamomile, and cola) in an attempt to relieve morning sickness (Gibson & Powrie, 2001). The most frequently herbs taken by interviewees were chamomile, licorice, fennel, aloe, valerian, echinacea, almond oil, propolis, and cranberry (Ayaz &Yaman Efe, 2010).

The most frequently prepared formulation was an infusion (used in 42.68% of the individually mentioned applications). Other applied preparations mentioned with decreasing frequency were decocts (17.24%), ointments (10.40%), direct application of plants without prior preparation (5.88%), fluid unctions (5.47%), syrups (4.10%) and tinctures or a collars (3.69%), freshly pressed juices(3.42%), powders (2.33%) and finally macerations (1.09%) (ˇSari´c-Kundali´c et al., 2010).

3.3 Characteristics of herbal medicine user

A research showed that majority of user was male, immigrants, college graduates, and had access to care. Older age, female gender, unmarried, and higher income was associated with use of dietary and herbal supplements; Asian women who reported being vegetarian were more likely to be female, unmarried, spiritual, and self-reported their physical health to be fair or poor (ˇSari´c-Kundali´c et al., 2010). Another study was found herbal users were mostly female, were more highly educated and were more likely to live in smaller house holds of one to four people (Nur, 2010). The same study was determined herbal remedies are likely to be used by the young people, females, those with higher education, those with good or excellent perceived health status and those with chronic illness, and it seems essential to offer informational programmes for them (Nur, 2010).

In a study found that there was significant association of herb use with/without drugs with age and employment status. Prevalence of herb use alone was lowest in people aged 65 years and older and highest in 35–44 and 45–54 year-olds whilst concomitant herb–drug use was highest in people aged 65 years and older and lowest in 18–24 year-olds (Picking et al., 2011). Another study stated approximately 18.9% of adults used herbs in the preceding year, but use varied significantly by socio-demographic category and socioeconomic status. Women, for example, were more likely to use herbs than men. Use rates were highest in middle age (21.9% of adults aged 45 to 64 years) and lowest in older adults (10.4% of adults aged:-75 years). Hispanics (17.4%) were slightly less likely to use herbs than non-Hispanics (19.1%). Persons of multiple race (32.2%), Asians (24.6%), and American Indian or Alaskan natives (21.9%) had relatively high use rates, whereas blacks were less likely to use herbs (14.3%). Residents of the western United States were relatively heavy users of herbal medicines (24.9%) compared with those in the South (16.3%). Herb use was positively correlated with socioeconomic status. College graduates were more likely to report medicinal herb use (25.3%) than adults who did not graduate from high school (10.4%). Adults with annual family incomes less than US $20,000 were less likely to use herbs (15.8%) than those who earned more (20.1%). Those with public insurance reported the lowest use rates (13.8 %), where as those with private insurance only reported the highest use rates (21.2%), and18.1% of uninsured adults used herbs in the preceding 12 months. Herb use was also associated with good health and positive health behaviours. Adults who described their health as excellent (19.3%) or very good (19.6%) were more likely to use herbs than those who described their health as fair (17.4%) or poor (14.3%) who had quit smoking were more likely to use herbs (21.7%) than those who had never smoked (18.2%) or current smokers (18.3%). Adults who exercised >3 times per week used herbs more often (26.3%) than those who did not (16.5%). The relationship between herb use and conventional medical care access and utilization was complex. Many or most adults appeared to use herbal treatments as a complement to conventional medical treatment. Herb use was relatively common among adults who used prescription medicines (20.6%) or over-the-counter medicines (20.6%), and use of herbs increased as total health expenditures increased, with the highest rates among adults from families that spent US $5000 or more annually on medical care (24.5%).However, there is also some evidence that herbs are being used as an alternative to conventional medical treatment. Adults who delayed (27.7%) or avoided (27.2%) needed medical care due to cost were more likely to use herbs than those who did not. Adults who could not afford to purchase a prescribed drug (26.9%) were more likely to use herbs medicinally than those who could afford their prescriptions or were not prescribed any medications (18.3%). Most users considered herbs and other natural products somewhat important (29.7%) or very important (27.8%) in maintaining their health or wellbeing. Two common acute conditions, head or chest cold (29.7%) and stomach or intestinal illness (10.6%), were the most frequently cited illnesses treated with herbs, but respondents also reported using herbs to treat a variety of chronic conditions (eg, arthritis, anxiety/depression, recurring pain) (Kennedy, 2005). Results of studies given showed that herbal medicine user have been women, person with high education, people with middle and older, individual who have chronic illness, and person those with good or excellent perceived health status.

3.4 Use reasons of herbal medicine

Species of the genera Achillea, Hypericum, Mentha, Teucrium,Thymus, and Urtica were particularly highly recommended by the majority of the informants. The most frequently mentioned indications were urogenital tract disorders, respiratory system disorders, gastrointestinal tract disorders, skin ailments, blood system disorders, nervoussystem disorders, cardiovascular system disorders, and rheumatism (ˇSari´c-Kundali´c et al., 2010). Ivy leaf contains spooning which are considered to have mucolytic, spasmolytic, bronchodilatory and antibacterial effects (Sieben et al., 2009; Gepdiremen et al., 2005). Despite widespread use of ivy leaf extracts, the effectiveness for the treatment of acute cough is not well established (Holzinger & Chenot, 2011). Other study found most frequently used herbal medicine were species from the genera Urtica (4.13%), Olea (4.13%), Salvia (3.83%), Arctium (3.39%), Hypericum (3.10%), Rubus (2.80%), Centaurium (2.65%), Allium (2.65%), Matricaria (2.51%), Malva (2.21%), Aesculus (2.21%), Betula (2.06%), Achillea (2.06%), Plantago (1.92%), Lavandula (1.92%), Juniperus (1.92%), Mentha (1.77%), Equisetum (1.77%), Fragaria (1.62%), Tilia (1.47%), Thymus (1.47%), Symphytum (1.47%), Artemisia (1.47%) and Arnica (1.47%). The most frequent indications were urogenital tract disorders (16.05% of the mentioned applications), respiratory system disorders (16.05%), gastrointestinal tract disorders (14.40%), skin ailments (11.52%), blood system disorders (8.78%), nervous system disorders (7.13%), cardiovascular system disorders (6.58%) and rheumatism (5.90%). Less frequent indications were metabolism disorders (strengthening of the organism; 3.84%), senses disorders (eyes, ears; 2.06%), influenzal infections (2.06%), lever and gall disorders (1.92%), parasitic induced ailments (1.65%), inflammations (0.96%), musculoskeletal system disorders (0.82%) and endocrinological disorders (0.27%) (ˇSari´c-Kundali´c et al., 2010). A study determined the reasons for using herbal remedies included that they are natural products (79.8%), for health enhancement (58.9%) and to overcome health problems (32.2%). Nearly three in five people in this study reported using an herbal remedy to overcome health problems or for health enhancement. The major purposes for using the herbal remedies were health enhancement or to prevent possible health problems (58.9%), to treat specific conditions (47.2%), or to cure gastrointestinal (35.8%) or urinary problems (19.2%) (Nur, 2010). Cui et al. found that the most common reason for using Chinese herbal medicine among breast cancer patients was cancer treatment (81.5%), followed by immune system enhancement (12%), metastasis prevention or side effect management (7.9%), and the reduction of menopausal symptoms (4.7%) (Cui et al., 2004). According to these and other survey data, medical herbalism was most commonly employed for allergies, insomnia, respiratory problems, and digestive problems (Ernst, 2005). Alternative herbal based therapies are prevalent and popular in urologic disease in general and prostatic disorders in particular. Typical herbal therapies recommended for benign prostatic hypertrophy (BPH) with some clinical evidence of efficacy includes saw palmetto (Serenoarepens), stinging nettle (Urticadioica) and Pygeumafricanum (Hirsch, 2000). Bee pollen extract (cernilton) has also been used with less evidence of efficacy for BPH. Lower urinary tract symptoms (LUTS) provide a complex but common connection between BPH and chronic prostatitis. Therefore, alternative agents, whether use alone or in combination for treatment of BPH, are also recommended for men with prostatitis (Shoskes & Manickam, 2003). Alternative and complementary therapies are also popular in men with prostate cancer. Since these agents either target prostate cancer cells or the side effects of therapy, they are seldom used in men with prostatitis. Another well-known supplement is zinc. It was one of the earliest factors identified in seminal plasma with an antimicrobial effect. The initial discovery that many men with chronic bacterial prostatitis have low levels of zincin the semen has led to the longstanding recommendation for zinc supplements in men with all forms of prostatitis (Shoskes & Manickam, 2003). The most commonly used therapy of hypertensive patient was herbal therapy, usually taken as a tea or infusion (Gohar et al., 2008). Some herbalists still recommend white willow to treat headaches, arthritis, and other painful conditions, contending that it is less likely to produce stomach upset and other adverse effects of aspirin (Goldman, 2001). The reasons for taking herbal medicines were diverse, including constitutional symptoms, respiratory complaints, arthritis, gastrointestinal disorders, hormonal and bladder symptoms (Lennox & Henderson, 2003). Kelly et al. stated the reason for taking any product containing herbal and other natural supplements was examined for subjects interviewed in 2002; the 2 most common reasons reported by both sexes were vitamin and supplement diet, at 21% and 12%, respectively. Other common reasons among men were energy (7.0%) and prevention. Women reported health (7.2%) and physician recommended (4.7%) at similar proportions as among males. Energy, menopausal symptoms, and immune booster each accounted for approximately 4% of the use of herbal and other natural supplements among women (Kelly et al., 2005). In general, herbs are effective for treating minor ailments such as digestive problems, flu, cough, headache, and rash. Herbal practitioners will consider a woman's symptoms and health before creating a treatment plan. There are many herbs that may be used such as black cohosh, ginseng, dong quai and agnuscastus, dependent on the symptoms (Gollschewski et al., 2004). Herbal medicine has been used for remedy of so many diseases and decreasing of symptoms and health promotion.

3.5 Recommendations source for herbal medicine use

The decision to use herbal products was mainly based on personal judgement and on the conviction that these natural substances would be safer than traditional medicines (Cuzzolin et al., 2010). The decision to use herbal remedies was mainly based on recommendations from the mass media (45.1%). Only 29.1% of users obtained information from their physicians or health providers, and only 37.9% informed their doctors. The decision to use herbal remedies was mainly based on the recommendations of mass media (45.1%), family members (43.1%), friends (32.0%) and neighbours (26.3%). Herbal remedy users obtained herbs from multiple sources. However, purchasing herbal remedies from herb sellers or folk remedy shops were the most common (67.8%) (Nur, 2010).

The most common sources of herbal information were friends and family (68%) and doctors (44%). Among those who reported using herbals, 53% had discussed their herbals use with a physician and 47% had seen a herbals practitioner (Huillet et al., 2011). About half of the patients learned about CAM from their relatives or friends, with more women than men using the therapies (Gohar et al., 2008). Only a small proportion of users (5.2%) consulted a complementary and alternative medicine provider about herbs or other natural products, and only a third (33.4%) told a physician or other conventional medical provider about their herb use (Kennedy, 2005). As expected, factors associated with herbal use included race/ethnicity, having an immigrant family history, and herbal use by other family members. In addition, it was found interactions between having an immigrant family history and herbal use by other family members (Kuo et al., 2004). Seventy-four patients (46%) had informed their family physician that they were on herbal medicines, while 72 patients (44%) stated that their family physician was unaware that they were taking these medications. Of the 162 patients using herbal medicines, 54 were taking them on the advice of their doctor (33%) and 88 were self-prescribing (54%) (Lennox & Henderson, 2003). Women reported physician recommended (4.7%) at similar proportions as among males (Kelly et al., 2005). Of the patients who took herbal medicines, 36% of the patients learned about herbal medicines from friends,27% from family members, 11% from magazines, 8% from audiovisual media, 6% from newspapers, and 12% of the patients from the Internet and health food shops (Adusumilli et al., 2004). Patients who reported using herbs indicated that they received information about those herbs mainly from family members and relatives. Nevertheless, most patients reported that they preferred receiving herbal information (e.g., on effectiveness, side-effects, and drug interactions) through hand outs or brochures from there. Physicians or pharmacists, followed by having access to a consultation service or a Web site (Kuo et al., 2004).

3.6 Method of herbal medicine application or use

Infusions were the most frequently prepared formulation. Other applied preparations mentioned with decreasing frequency were decocts, ointments, direct application of plants without prior preparation, fluid unction, sirups and tinctures or collars, freshly pressed juices, powders, and finally macerations. Balms known as "mehlems" were special to Bosnia and were prepared from freshly chopped or freshly pressed herbal parts of various plants. Warmed resins from Abies or Picea species, bees wax, raw cow or pig lard, olive oil and honey were used as additives in the mehlem formulations. Representatives of the genera Arctium, Carlina, Euphrasia, Hypericum, Plantago, Teucrium, and Urtica were most frequently used in these balms (ˇSari´c-Kundali´c et al., 2010).

For medical purpose, dried herbs are usually recommended because their increased concentration makes them more potent than the fresh plants. Leaves and flowers are dried in an airy, shady place; sun bakes out their oils and may also damage other medicinal ingredients. Roots and heavy stems are cleaned, chopped, dried, and then stored in glass jars or other non-metallic containers in a cool, dry place until they are used. Medicinal herbs are most often steeped in boiling water and consumed as a tea. These teas, which can be unpleasantly bitter or strong-tasting, should not be confused with the pleasant, commercially available herbal teas, which contain only a small fraction of the herbs used in a medicinal brew (Sonal Sekhar et al., 2008). It is seem that herbals are used variety shape. This condition increases frequency use.

3.7 Adverse effect of herbal medicine

Herbal therapies may produce adverse effects, cause toxicity, or interact with conventional medicines. Moreover, in the majority of countries (with the notable exceptions of Germany, France, and Sweden) herbal products are marketed without proof of testing for efficacy or safety. They are sold as food and dietary supplements under regulations for Current Good Manufacturing Practice, which ensures that they are produced under sanitary conditions but provides no guarantee of purity or efficacy (Nicholson, 2006).

One study determine four out of 109 women (3.7%) reported side effects: constipation after a tisane containing a mix of herbs, rash and itching after local application of aloe or almond oil (Cuzzolin et al., 2010). Users were more often affected by morbidities pregnancy-related and their neonates were more frequently small for their gestational age. A higher incidence of threatening miscarriages and preterm labours was observed among regular users of chamomile and licorice (Cuzzolin et al., 2010). Many plants are highly toxic. Herbal medicine probably presents a greater risk of adverse effects and interactions than any other complementary therapy. Serious adverse events after administration of herbal products have been reported, and in most cases, the herbs involved were self-prescribed and bought over the counter or were obtained from a source other than a registered practitioner.

In the most notorious instance, several women developed rapidly progressive interstitial renal fibrosis after taking Chinese herbs prescribed by the staff of a weight loss clinic. Herbal products may be contaminated, adulterated, or misidentified. Adverse effects seem more common with herbs imported from outside Europe and North America. In general, patients taking herbal preparations regularly should receive careful follow-up and have access to appropriate biochemical monitoring (Vickers & Zollman, 1999).

Many herbs are highly toxic, even in small doses. Be cautions of homemade remedies, and if you gather wild herbs, be sure you know what you are picking. The following herbs can be fatal: Aonite, Arnica, Beladonna, Yohimbe, Lobelia etc. Researches confirmed some herbals are toxic. So, herbals should be used with physician's suggest.

3.8 Cost of herbal medicine

In the UK, cough liquids accounted for sales worth 102 million pounds in 2008 (Proprietary Association of Great Britain, 2009). Coca and Nink (2008) "Supplementary statistical overview," in pharmaceutical prescription among these non-antibiotic cough remedies, herbal preparations containing extracts from the leaves of ivy enjoy great popularity in many European countries (Coca & Nink, 2008; Glaeskeet al., 2008; Guo et al., 2006). In 2007, more than 80%of herbal expectorants prescribed in Germany comprised ivy extract and amounted to nearly 2 million prescriptions nationwide and a volume of sales exceeding 13 million Euros (Coca & Nink, 2008).

Most patients reported collecting their own medicinal plants (214/264, or 81%) and a few were supplied with bush medicines by friends or relatives, but little use was made of herbal shops, herbalists, or bush medicine doctors. Bush medicines were used at least every week by 107/264, or 41% of patients surveyed. The frequency of bush medicine use was not clear for 56/264 (21%) of users, possibly because they only took bush medicines when specific illnesses were experienced (Mahabir & Gulliford, 1997).

In most industrialised countries, herbal medicinal products (HMPs) have become increasingly popular and in the Third World they have always been a main source of medical treatment. Survey data show that between 1990 and 1997 the use by US citizens of herbal remedies has increased by approximately 100%. More and more physicians are either referring patients to herbal practitioners or practising phytotherapy themselves (Gepdiremen et al., 2005). US sales figures for herbal remedies have risen almost exponentially and, in 1997, exceeded $US350 million (Sieben et al., 2009). HMPs are used to treat a large variety of conditions as well as for 'maintenance of health', i.e. disease prevention. HMPs come in guises ranging from a commercially marketed product to a self-made tea produced from home-grown plants. The issue is further complicated by the fact that several different 'cultures' exist, e.g. European herbalism (often using single herb remedies) and Chinese or Indian herbalism (typically using mixtures of many herbs). The consumer is often led to believe that 'natural' can be equated with 'harmless', yet HMPs are associated with numerous risks. The high level of usage renders rigorous safety assessment of HMPs an ethical imperative (Gepdiremen et al., 2005). The following article attempts to give a short introduction to this area by providing several examples of HMPs causing concern in recent years (Ernst, 2004). It could be not reached adequate literatures about cost of herbal medicine. It is difficult to say about the cost dimension for overall world.

4. Conclusion

Herbal remedy use was common in world wise, especially among females, the more highly educated and those with health-related problems, particularly. Nearly three of five users reported using herbal remedies for health enhancement or to prevent health problems, while almost half of the users wished to over come specific conditions. Almost a third of users were concurrently taking drugs while four of five were not aware of potential interactions with regular medication. Precautions many plants are poisonous. Make sure that you know exactly what is in an herbal remedy before you take it internally. Before using any herbal remedy for a child's illness, consult a paediatricians or paediatric nurse. Take only the recommended dosage. Herbal products that are safe in small amounts can produce severe side effects when taken in larger doses.

Despite the complexity of herbal products, investigations of their efficacy are feasible and desirable, particularly vis-a-vis their popularity. For some but by no mean sell herbal medicines, efficacy data are now emerging. Some herbal medicines are efficacious for certain indications. All herbal medicines are associated with safety issues which are often complex.

Generally speaking, research into herbal medicines is much less active than research into conventional drugs. Lack of commercial impetus due to lack of paten protection is one obvious reason. Another reason may lie in the legal status of herbal medicines: as dietary supplements they are not under any formal obligation to prove efficacy. Based on the data available today, it is impossible to draw general conclusions about the therapeutic value of herbal medicines. Healthcare professionals have therefore been cautious in recommending herbal medicines.

5. References

Adusumilli, P.S., Ben-Porat, L., Pereira, M., Roesler, D. & Leitman I. M. (2004). The Prevalence and Predictors of Herbal Medicine Use in Surgical Patients. *Journal of the American College of Surgeons*, 198,583–590.

Ayaz, S. & Yaman Efe, S. (2010). Traditional practices used by infertile women in Turkey. *International Nursing Review* 384-387.

Coca, V. & Nink, K., Supplementary statistical overview, in *Pharmaceutical Prescription Report*, U. Schwabe and D. Paffrath, Eds., pp. 963–1071, Springer, Heidelberg, Germany, 2008 (German).

Cui, Y., Shu, X.O., Gao, Y., Wen, W., Ruan, Z.X., & Jin, F. (2004). Use of complementary and alternative medicine by Chinese women with breast cancer. *Zheng Breast Cancer Res Treatment*, 85, 263-270.

Cuzzolin, L., Francini-Pesenti, F, Verlato, G, Joppi, M., Baldelli, P. & Benoni, G. (2010). Use of herbal products among 392 Italian pregnant women: focus on pregnancy outcome. *Pharmaco epidemiology and drug safety,* 19: 1151–1158.

Eisenberg D., David R.B., Ettner S.L., Appel, S., Wilkey, S., Van Rompay, M. & Kessler, R.C. (1998) Trends in alternativemedicine use in the United States; 1990–1997. *JAMA,* 280, 1569–1575.

Ernst E. (2004), Risks of herbal medicinal products. *Pharmacoepidemiology and drug safety;* 13: 767–771.

Ernst, E. (2005). The efficacy of herbal medicine - an overview. *Publishing Fundamental & Clinical Pharmacology,* 19, 405–409.

Ernst, E. (2000). Herbal medicine. A concise overview for professionals, *Butterworth Heinemann,* Oxford.

Fabricant, D.S. (2001). The Value of Plants Used in Traditional Medicine for Drug Discovery. Environmental Health Perspectives. *Reviews in Environmental Health,* 109 (1): 69-75.

Gepdiremen, A., Mshvildadze, V., Süleyman, H. & Elias, R. (2005). Acute anti-inflammatory activity of four saponins isolated from ivy: alpha-hederin, hederasaponin-C, hederacolchiside-E and hederacolchiside-F in carrageenan-induced rat paw edema. *Phytomedicine,* 12(6-7), 440–444.

Gharoro, E.P. & Igbafe, A.A. (2000). Pattern of drug use amongst antenatal patients in Benin City, Nigeria. *Medical Science Monitor,* 6, 84–87.

Gibson, P.S., Powrie, R. & Star, J. (2001). Herbal and alternative medicine use during pregnancy: a cross sectional survey. *Obstetrics Gynecology,* 97: S44–S45.

Glaeske, G., Schicktanz, C. & Janhsen, K. (2008). GEK Pharmaceutical report," GEK Statutory health insurance, German.

Gohar F., Greenfield S.M, Beevers D.G., Lip G.Y.H. Jolly K. (2008). Self-care and adherence to medication: a survey in the hypertension outpatient clinic. *BMC Complementary and Alternative Medicine,* 8,4 doi:10.1186/1472-6882-8-4

Goldman, P. (2001). Herbal Medicines Today and the Roots of Modern Pharmacology. *Annals of Internal Medicine,* 135, 594-600.

Gollschewski, S, Anderson, D, Skerman, H, & Lyons-Wall, P. (2004). The Use of Complementary and Alternative Medications by Menopausal Women in South East Queensland. *Women's Health Issues,* 14, 165–171.

Guo, R., Pittler, M.H. & Ernst, E. (2006). Herbal medicines for the treatment of COPD: a systematic review. *European Respiratory Journal,* 28, 2, 330–338,

Hirsch, I.H. (2000). Integrative urology: a spectrum of complementary and alternative therapy. *Urology* 56:185–189

Holzinger, F, & Chenot, J.O. (2011). Systematic Review of Clinical Trials Assessing the Effectiveness of Ivy Leaf (Hedera Helix) for Acute Upper Respiratory Tract Infections. *Evidence-Based Complementary and Alternative Medicine,* 2011, pagesdoi: 10.1155/2011/382789)

Huillet, A, Erdie-Lalena, C., Norvell, D., Davis B.E., Complementary and Alternative Medicine Used by Children in Military Paediatric Clinics. *The Journal of Alternative and Complementary Medicine,* 17, (6), 2011, pp. 531–537.

Kelly, J.P., Kaufman, D.W., Kelley, K, Rosenberg L, Anderson T. E., Mitchell A.A., (2005). Recent Trends in Use of Herbal and Other Natural Products. *Archives of Internal Medicine,*165, 281-286.

Kennedy, D.A., Hart, J., Seely, D. (2009). Cost effectiveness of natural health products: a systematic review of randomized clinical trials. *Evidence-Based Complementary and Alternative Medicine*, 6, 3, 297–304,

Kennedy, J. (2005). Herb and Supplement Use in the US Adult Population. *Clinical Therapeutics*, 27, 11, 1847-1858.

Kuo, G.M, Hawley, S.T, Weiss, L.T, Balkrishnan, R. & Volk, R. J. (2004). Factors associated with herbal use among urban multiethnic primary care patients: a cross-sectional survey. BMC Complementary and Alternative Medicine, 4,18 doi:10.1186/1472-6882-4-18.

Mahabir, D. & Gulliford, M. C. (1997). Use of medicinal plants for diabetes in Trinidad and Tobago. *Revista Panamericana de Salud Pública,*1(3), 174-179.

Nicholson, T. (2006). Complementary and alternative medicines (including traditional Maori treatments) used by presenters to an emergency department in New Zealand: a survey of prevalence and toxicity. *Journal of the New Zealand Medical Association*, 119, 1233.

Nur, N. (2010). Knowledge and behaviours related to herbal remedies: a cross-sectional epidemiological study in adults in Middle Anatolia, Turkey. *Health and Social Care in the Community*, 18(4), 389–395

Lennox, P.H. & Henderson C.L. (2003). Herbal medicine use is frequent in ambulatory surgery patients in Vancouver Canada. *Canadian Journal of Anesthesia*, 50, 1, 21–25.

Picking, D., Younger, N., Mitchell, S. & Delgoda, R. (2011). The prevalence of herbal medicine home use and concomitant use with pharmaceutical medicines in Jamaica. *Journal of Ethnopharmacol*, doi:10.1016/j.jep.2011.05.025.

Proprietary Association of Great Britain, (2009). *PAGB Annual Review 2009*, PAGB, London, UK.

Rhee, S.M., Garg, V.K., Hershey, C.O. (2004). Use of complementary and alternative medicines by ambulatory patients. *Archives of Internal Medicine*, 164,1004–1009.

Shoskes, D.A. & Manickam, K. (2003). Herbal and complementary medicine in chronic prostatitis. *World Journal of Urology*, 21, 109–113

Sieben, A., Prenner, L., Sorkalla, T., Wolf, A., Jakobs, D., Runkel, F. & Haberlein, H. (2009). *α*-Hederin, but not hederacoside c and hederagenin from Hedera helix, affects the binding behavior, dynamics, and regulation of *β*2- adrenergic receptors. *Biochemistry*, 48, 15, 3477–3482.

Sonal Sekhar, M., Aneesh, T.P.K. Varghese J., Vasudaven, D.T. (2008). KGRevikumar: Herbalism: A Phenomenon of New Age In Medicine. *The Internet Journal of Pharmacology*, 6 (1). Mabina, M.H., Pitsoe, S.B. & Moodley J. (1997). The effect of traditional herbal medicines on pregnancy outcome. South African Medical Journal, 87, 1008–1010.

Tapsell, L.C., Hemphill, I., Cobiac, L., Patch, C.S., Sullivan, D.R., Fenech, M., Roodenrys, S., Keogh, J.B., Clifton, P.M., Williams, P.G., Fazio, V.A., Inge, K.E. (2006). Health benefits of herbs and spices: the past, the present, the future. *The Medical journal of Australia*, 185, 4-24.

Vickers, A. & Zollman, C. (1999). ABC of complementary medicine: Herbal medicine - Clinical review. *British Medical Journal, 319 (7211): 693–696.*

9

Diabetic Nephropathy – Using Herbals in Diabetic Nephropathy Prevention and Treatment – The Role of Ginger (*Zingiber officinale*) and Onion (*Allium cepa*) in Diabetics' Nephropathy

Arash Khaki[1,*] and Fatemeh Fathiazad[2]
[1]*Department of Pathology, Tabriz Branch, Islamic Azad University, Tabriz,*
[2]*Department of Pharmacognosy, Faculty of Pharmacy,*
Tabriz University of Medical Sciences, Tabriz,
Iran

1. Introduction

Diabetic nephropathy is a kidney disease or damage that results as a complication of diabetes. See also: Type 1 diabetes, Type 2 diabetes, Risk factors for diabetes, Chronic kidney disease causes, incidence, and risk factors. The exact cause of diabetic nephropathy is unknown, but it is believed that uncontrolled high blood sugar leads to the development of kidney damage, especially when high blood pressure is also present. In some cases, your genes or family history may also play a role. Not all persons with diabetes develop this condition.Each kidney is made of hundreds of thousands of filtering units called nephrons. Each nephron has a cluster of tiny blood vessels called a glomerulus. Together these structures help remove waste from the body. Too much blood sugar can damage these structures, causing them to thicken and become scarred. Slowly, over time, more and more blood vessels are destroyed. The kidney structures begin to leak and protein (albumin) begins to pass into the urine.Persons with diabetes who have the following risk factors are more likely to develop this condition:

- African American, Hispanic, or American Indian origin
- Family history of kidney disease or high blood pressure
- Poor control of blood pressure
- Poor control of blood sugars
- Type 1 diabetes before age 20
- Smoking

Diabetic nephropathy generally goes along with other diabetes complications including high blood pressure, retinopathy, and blood vessel changes. Early stage diabetic nephropathy has no symptoms. Over time, the kidney's ability to function starts to decline. Symptoms develop late in the disease and may include: Fatigue, Foamy appearance or

* Corresponding Author

excessive frothing of the urine, Frequent hiccups, General ill feeling, Generalized itching, Headache, Nausea and Vomiting, Poor appetite, Swelling of the legs, Swelling usually around the eyes in the mornings; general body swelling may occur with late-stage disease.

1.1 Signs and tests

The main sign of diabetic nephropathy is persistent protein in the urine. (protein may appear in the urine for 5 to 10 years before other symptoms develop.) If your doctor thinks you might have this condition, a microalbuminuria test will be done. A positive test often means you have at least some damage to the kidney from diabetes. Damage at this stage may be reversible. The test results can be high for other reasons, so it needs to be repeated for confirmation.High blood pressure often goes along with diabetic nephropathy. You may have high blood pressure that develops rapidly or is difficult to control.

1.2 Expectations (prognosis)

Nephropathy is a major cause of sickness and death in persons with diabetes. It is the leading cause of long-term kidney failure and end-stage kidney disease in the United States, and often leads to the need for dialysis or kidney transplantation.The condition slowly continues to get worse once large amounts of protein begin to appear in the urine or levels of creatinine in the blood begin to rise.Complications due to chronic kidney failure are more likely to occur earlier, and get worse more rapidly, when it is caused by diabetes than other causes. Even after dialysis or transplantation, persons with diabetes tend to do worse than those without diabetes.Complications,Possible complications include: Anemia, Chronic kidney failure (rapidly gets worse), Dialysis complications, End-stage kidney disease, Hyperkalemia, Severe hypertension, Hypoglycemia, Infections, Kidney transplant complications, Peritonitis (if peritoneal dialysis used).

1.3 Prevention

All persons with diabetes should have a yearly checkup with their doctor to have their blood and urine tested for signs of possible kidney problems.Persons with kidney disease should avoid contrast dyes that contain iodine, if possible. These dyes are removed through the kidneys and can worsen kidney function. Certain imaging tests use these types of dyes. If they must be used, fluids should be given through a vein for several hours before the test. This allows for rapid removal of the dyes from the body.Commonly used nonsteroidal anti-inflammatory drugs (NSAIDs), including ibuprofen, naproxen, and prescription COX-2 inhibitors such as celecoxib (Celebrex), may injure the weakened kidney. You should always talk to your health care provider before using any drugs.

2. Herbalism

Herbalism is a traditional medicinal or folk medicine practice based on the use of plants and plant extracts. Herbalism is also known as botanical medicine, medical herbalism, herbal medicine, herbology, herblore and phytotherapy. The scope of herbal medicine is sometimes extended to include fungal and bee products, as well as minerals, shells and certain animal parts. Traditional use of medicines is recognized as a way to learn about potential future medicines. In 2001, researchers identified 122 compounds used in mainstream medicine which were derived from "ethnomedical" plant sources; 80% of these compounds were used in the same or related manner as the traditional ethnomedical use.

Plants have evolved the ability to synthesize chemical compounds that help them defend against attack from a wide variety of predators such as insects, fungi and herbivorous mammals. By chance, some of these compounds, whilst being toxic to plant predators, turn out to have beneficial effects when used to treat human diseases. Such secondary metabolites are highly varied in structure, many are aromatic substances, most of which are phenols or their oxygen-substituted derivatives. At least 12,000 have been isolated so far; a number estimated to be less than 10% of the total. Chemical compounds in plants mediate their effects on the human body by binding to receptor molecules present in the body; such processes are identical to those already well understood for conventional drugs and as such herbal medicines do not differ greatly from conventional drugs in terms of how they work. This enables herbal medicines to be in principle just as effective as conventional medicines but also gives them the same potential to cause harmful side effects. Many of the herbs and spices used by humans to season food yield useful medicinal compounds.

Similarly to prescription drugs, a number of herbs are thought to be likely to cause adverse effects. Furthermore, "adulteration, inappropriate formulation, or lack of understanding of plant and drug interactions have led to adverse reactions that are sometimes life threatening or lethal.

2.1 Biological background

All plants produce chemical compounds as part of their normal metabolic activities. These are divided into primary metabolites, such as sugars and fats, found in all plants, and secondary metabolites, compounds not essential for basic function found in a smaller range of plants, some useful ones found only in a particular genus or species. Pigments harvest light, protect the organism from radiation and display colors to attract pollinators. Many common weeds, such as nettle, dandelion and chickweed, have medicinal properties.

The functions of secondary metabolites are varied. For example, some secondary metabolites are toxins used to deter predation, and others are pheromonesused to attract insects for pollination. Phytoalexins protect against bacterial and fungal attacks. Allelochemicals inhibit rival plants that are competing for soil and light.

Plants upregulate and downregulate their biochemical paths in response to the local mix of herbivores, pollinators and microorganisms. The chemical profile of a single plant may vary over time as it reacts to changing conditions. It is the secondary metabolites and pigments that can have therapeutic actions in humans and which can be refined to produce drugs.

Plants synthesize a bewildering variety of phytochemicals but most are derivatives of a few biochemical motifs.

- Alkaloids contain a ring with nitrogen. Many alkaloids have dramatic effects on the central nervous system. Caffeine is an alkaloid that provides a mild lift but the alkaloids in datura cause severe intoxication and even death.

- polyphenol, also known as phenolics, contain phenol rings. The anthocyanins that give grapes their purple color, the isoflavones, the phytoestrogens from soy and the tannins that give tea its astringency are phenolics.
- Terpenoids are built up from terpene building blocks. Each terpene consists of two paired isoprenes. The names monoterpenes, sesquiterpenes,diterpenes and triterpenes are based on the number of isoprene units. The fragrance of rose and lavender is due to monoterpenes. The carotenoids as terpenoids produce the reds, yellows and oranges of pumpkin, corn and tomatoes.
- Glycosides consist of a glucose moiety attached to an aglycone. The aglycone is a molecule that is bioactive in its free form but inert until the glycoside bond is broken by water or enzymes. This mechanism allows the plant to defer the availability of the molecule to an appropriate time, similar to a safety lock on a gun. An example is the cyanoglycosides in cherry pits that release toxins only when bitten by a herbivore.

The word drug itself comes from the Dutch word "droog" (via the French word Drogue), which means 'dried plant'. Some examples are inulin from the roots of dahlias, quinine from the cinchona, morphine and codeine from the poppy and digoxin from the foxglove.

The active ingredient in willow bark, once prescribed by Hippocrates, is salicin, which is converted in the body into salicylic acid. The discovery of salicylic acid would eventually lead to the development of the acetylated form acetylsalicylic acid, also known as "aspirin", when it was isolated from a plant known as meadowsweet. The word *aspirin* comes from an abbreviation of meadowsweet's Latin genus *Spiraea*, with an additional "A" at the beginning to acknowledge acetylation, and "in" was added at the end for easier pronunciation. "Aspirin" was originally a brand name, and is still a protected trademark in some countries. This medication was patented by Bayer company.

2.2 Popularity

A survey released in May 2004 by the National Center for Complementary and Alternative Medicine focused on who used complementary and alternative medicines (CAM), what was used, and why it was used. The survey was limited to adults, aged 18 years and over during 2002, living in the United States.

According to this survey, herbal therapy, or use of natural products other than vitamins and minerals, was the most commonly used CAM therapy (18.9%) when all use of prayer was excluded.

Herbal remedies are very common in Europe. In Germany, herbal medications are dispensed by apothecaries (e.g., Apotheke). Prescription drugs are sold alongside essential oils, herbal extracts, or herbal teas. Herbal remedies are seen by some as a treatment to be preferred to pure medical compounds which have been industrially produced.

In the United Kingdom, the training of medical herbalists is done by state funded Universities. For example, Bachelor of Science degrees in herbal medicine are offered at Universities such as University of East London, Middlesex University, University of Central Lancashire, University of Westminster, University of Lincoln and Napier University in Edinburgh at the present. Avid public interest in herbalism in the UK has been recently confirmed by the popularity of the topic in mainstream media, such as the prime-time hit

TV series BBC's Grow Your Own Drugs,which demonstrated how to grow and prepare herbal remedies at home.

In the United States, a Bachelor of Science degree in herbal sciences is offered at Bastyr University, and a Master of Science in herbal medicine is offered at Tai Sophia Institute. There are also many smaller organizations and teachers offering certifications.

A 2004 Cochrane Collaboration review found that herbal therapies are supported by strong evidence but are not widely used in all clinical settings.

2.3 Types of herbal medicine systems

Use of medicinal plants can be as informal as, for example, culinary use or consumption of an herbal tea or supplement, although the sale of some herbs considered dangerous is often restricted to the public. Sometimes such herbs are provided to professional herbalists by specialist companies. Many herbalists, both professional and amateur, often grow or "wildcraft" their own herbs.

Some researchers trained in both western and traditional Chinese medicine have attempted to deconstruct ancient medical texts in the light of modern science. One idea is that the yin-yang balance, at least with regard to herbs, corresponds to the pro-oxidant and anti-oxidant balance. This interpretation is supported by several investigations of the ORAC ratings of various yin and yang herbs.

In America, early settlers relied on plants imported from Europe, and also from local Indian knowledge. One particularly successful practitioner, Samuel Thomson developed a hugely popular system of medicine. This approach was subsequently broadened to include concepts introduced from modern physiology, a discipline called Physiomedicalism. Another group, the Eclectics, were a later offshoot from the orthodox medical profession, who were looking to avoid the current medical treatments of mercury and bleeding, and introduced herbal medicine into their practices. Both groups were eventually overcome by the actions of the American Medical Association, which was formed for this purpose. Cherokee medicine tends to divide herbs into foods, medicines and toxins and to use seven plants in the treatment of disease, which is defined with both spiritual and physiological aspects, according to Cherokee herbalist David Winston.

In India, Ayurvedic medicine has quite complex formulas with 30 or more ingredients, including a sizable number of ingredients that have undergone "alchemical processing", chosen to balance "Vata", "Pitta" or "Kapha."

In Tamil Nadu, Tamils have their own medicinal system now popularly called the Siddha medicinal system. The Siddha system is entirely in the Tamil language. It contains roughly 300,000 verses covering diverse aspects of medicine such as anatomy, sex ("kokokam" is the sexual treatise of par excellence), herbal, mineral and metallic compositions to cure many diseases that are relevant even to-day. Ayurveda is in Sanskrit, but Sanskrit was not generally used as a mother tongue and hence its medines are mostly taken from Siddha and other local traditions.

In addition there are more modern theories of herbal combination like William LeSassier's triune formula which combined Pythagorean imagery with Chinese medicine ideas and resulted in 9 herb formulas which supplemented, drained or neutrally nourished the main organ systems affected and three associated systems. His system has been taught to thousands of influential American herbalists through his own apprenticeship programs during his lifetime, the William LeSassier Archive and the David Winston Center for Herbal Studies. Different chemicals in herbs are more abundant than in a single drug. Some chemicals in herbs may work as growth hormones or antibiotics, nutrients, and toxin neutralizers.

Many traditional African remedies have performed well in initial laboratory tests to ensure they are not toxic and in tests on animals. Gawo, a herb used in traditional treatments, has been tested in rats by researchers from Nigeria's University of Jos and the National Institute for Pharmaceutical Research and Development. According to research in the African Journal of Biotechnology, Gawo passed tests for toxicity and reduced induced fevers, diarrhoea and inflammation.

2.4 Routes of administration

The exact composition of a herbal product is influenced by the method of extraction. A tisane will be rich in polar components because water is a polar solvent. Oil on the other hand is a non-polar solvent and it will absorb non-polar compounds. Alcohol lies somewhere in between. There are many forms in which herbs can be administered, these include:

- Tinctures - Alcoholic extracts of herbs such as Echinacea extract. Usually obtained by combining 100% pure ethanol (or a mixture of 100% ethanol with water) with the herb. A completed tincture has a ethanol percentage of at least 25% (sometimes up to 90%). The term tincture is sometimes applied to preparations using other solvents than ethanol.
- Herbal wine and elixirs - These are alcoholic extract of herbs; usually with an ethanol percentage of 12-38% Herbal wine is a maceration of herbs in wine, while an elixir is a maceration of herbs in spirits (e.g., vodka, grappa, etc.)
- Tisanes - Hot water extracts of herb, such as chamomile.
- Decoctions - Long-term boiled extract of usually roots or bark.
- Macerates - Cold infusion of plants with high mucilage-content as sage, thyme, etc. Plants are chopped and added to cold water. They are then left to stand for 7 to 12 hours (depending on herb used). For most macerates 10 hours is used.
- Vinegars - Prepared at the same way as tinctures, except using a solution of acetic acid as the solvent.
- Whole herb consumption - This can occur in either dried form (herbal powder), or fresh juice, (fresh leaves and other plant parts).
- Syrups - Extracts of herbs made with syrup or honey. Sixty five parts of sugar are mixed with 35 parts of water and herb. The whole is then boiled and macerated for three weeks.
- Extracts - Include liquid extracts, dry extracts and nebulisates. Liquid extracts are liquids with a lower ethanol percentage than tinctures. They can (and are usually) made by vacuum distilling tinctures. Dry extracts are extracts of plant material which are evaporated into a dry mass. They can then be further refined to a capsule or tablet. A nebulisate is a dry extract created by freeze-drying.
- Inhalation as in aromatherapy can be used as a mood changing treatment to fight a sinus infection or cough , or to cleanse the skin on a deeper level (steam rather than direct inhalation here)

Topicals:

- Essential oils - Application of essential oil extracts, usually diluted in a carrier oil (many essential oils can burn the skin or are simply too high dose used straight - diluting in olive oil or another food grade oil such as almond oil can allow these to be used safely as a topical).
- Salves, oils, balms, creams and lotions - Most topical applications are oil extractions of herbs. Taking a food grade oil and soaking herbs in it for anywhere from weeks to months allows certain phytochemicals to be extracted into the oil. This oil can then be made into salves, creams, lotions, or simply used as an oil for topical application. Any massage oils, antibacterial salves and wound healing compounds are made this way.
- Poultices and compresses - One can also make a poultice or compress using whole herb (or the appropriate part of the plant) usually crushed or dried and re-hydrated with a small amount of water and then applied directly in a bandage, cloth or just as is.

2.5 Examples of plants used as medicine

Few herbal remedies have conclusively demonstrated any positive effect on humans, possibly due to inadequate testing. Many of the studies cited refer to animal model investigations or in-vitro assays and therefore cannot provide more than weak supportive evidence.

- Aloe vera has traditionally been used for the healing of burns and wounds. A systematic review (from 1999) states that the efficacy of aloe vera in promoting wound healing is unclear, while a later review (from 2007) concludes that the cumulative evidence supports the use of aloe vera for the healing of first to second degree burns.
- Artichoke (*Cynara cardunculus*) may reduce production cholesterol levels according to *in vitro* studies and a small clinical study.
- Blackberry (*Rubus fruticosus*) leaf has drawn the attention of the cosmetology community because it interferes with the metalloproteinases that contribute to skin wrinkling
- Black raspberry *(Rubus occidentalis)* may have a role in preventing oral cancer.
- Boophone (*Boophone disticha*) This highly toxic plant has been used in South African traditional medicine for treatment of mental illness. Research demonstrate *in vitro* and *in vivo* effect against depression.
- Butterbur *(Petasites hybridus)*
- Calendula *(Calendula officinalis)* has been used traditionally for abdominal cramps and constipation. In animal research an aqueous-ethanol extract of *Calendula officinalis* flowers was shown to have both spasmolytic and spasmogenic effects, thus providing a scientific rationale for this traditional use. There is "limited evidence" that calendula cream or ointment is effective in treating radiation dermatitis.
- Cannabis, see also medical cannabis.
- Cranberry *(Vaccinium oxycoccos)* may be effective in treating urinary tract infections in women with recurrent symptoms.
- Echinacea (*Echinacea angustifolia, Echinacea pallida, Echinacea purpurea*) extracts may limit the length and severity of rhinovirus colds; however, the appropriate dosage levels, which might be higher than is available over-the-counter, require further research.
- Elderberry (*Sambucus nigra*) may speed the recovery from type A and B influenza. However it is possibly risky in the case of avian influenza because the immunostimulatory effects may aggravate the cytokine cascade.

- Feverfew (*Chrysanthemum parthenium*) is sometimes used to treat migraine headaches. Although many reviews of Feverfew studies show no or unclear efficacy, a more recent RTC showed favorable results Feverfew is not recommended for pregnant women as it may be dangerous to the fetus.
- Gawo (*Faidherbia albida*), a traditional herbal medicine in West Africa, has shown promise in animal tests
- Garlic (*Allium sativum*) may lower total cholesterol levels

  German Chamomile (*Matricaria chamomilla*) has demonstrated antispasmodic, anxiolytic, antiinflammatory and some antimutagenic and cholesterol-lowering effects in animal research. *In vitro* chamomile has demonstrated moderate antimicrobial and antioxidant properties and significant antiplatelet activity, as well as preliminary results against cancer. Essential oil of chamomile was shown to be a promising antiviral agent against herpes simplex virus type 2 (HSV-2) *in vitro*.
- Ginger (*Zingiber officinale*), administered in 250 mg capsules for four days, effectively decreased nausea and vomiting of pregnancy in a human clinical trial.
- Grapefruit (Naringenin) components may prevent obesity.
- Green tea (*Camelia sinensis*) components may inhibit growth of breast cancer cells and may heal scars faster.
- Purified extracts of the seeds of *Hibiscus sabdariffa* may have some antihypertensive, antifungal and antibacterial effect. Toxicity tested low except for an isolated case of damage to the testes of a rat after prolonged and excessive consumption.
- Honey may reduce cholesterol. May be useful in wound healing.
- Lemon grass (*Cymbopogon citratus*), administered daily as an aqueous extract of the fresh leaf, has lowered total cholesterol and fasting plasma glucose levels in rats, as well as increasing HDL cholesterol levels. Lemon grass administration had no effect on triglyceride levels.
- Magnolia
- Marshmallow Root (althaea officinalis L.), a mucilage used for various inflammitory diseases including bronchitis and peptic ulcers.
- Meadowsweet (*Filipendula ulmaria, Spiraea ulmaria*) can be used for a variety of anti-inflammatory and antimicrobial purposes due to presence of salicylic acid. Effective for fevers and inflammations, pain relief, ulcers and bacteriostatic. Listed as therapeutical in 1652 by Nicholas Culpeper. In 1838, salicylic acid was isolated from the plant. The word Aspirin is derived from spirin, based on Meadowsweet's synonym name Spiraea ulmaria.
- Milk thistle (*Silybum marianum*) extracts have been recognized for many centuries as "liver tonics.". Research suggests that milk thistle extracts both prevent and repair damage to the liver from toxic chemicals and medications.
- Morinda citrifolia (noni) is used in the Pacific and Caribbean islands for the treatment of inflammation and pain. Human studies indicate potential cancer preventive effects.
- Nigella sativa (Black cumin) has demonstrated analgesic properties in mice. The mechanism for this effect, however, is unclear. In vitro studies support antibacterial, antifungal, anticancer, anti-inflammatory and immune modulating effects. However few randomized double blind studies have been published.
- Ocimum gratissimum and tea tree oil can be used to treat acne.
- Oregano (*Origanum vulgare*) may be effective against multi-drug resistant bacteria.
- Pawpaw can be used as insecticide (killing lice, worms).

- Peppermint oil may have benefits for individuals with irritable bowel syndrome.
- Phytolacca or Pokeweed can be applied topically or taken internally. Topical treatments have been used for acne and other ailments. It is used as a treatment for tonsilitis, swollen glands and weight loss.
- Pomegranate contains the highest percentage of ellagitannins of any commonly consumed juice. Punicalagin, an ellagitannin unique to pomegranate, is the highest molecular weight polyphenol known. Ellagitannins are metabolized into urolithins by gut flora, and have been shown to inhibit cancer cell growth in mice.
- Rauvolfia Serpentina, high risk of toxicity if improperly used, used extensively in India for sleeplessness, anxiety, and high blood pressure.
- Rooibos (*Aspalathus linearis*) contains a number of phenolic compounds, including flavanols, flavones, flavanones, flavonols, and dihydrochalcones. Rooibos has traditionally been used for skin ailments, allergies, asthma and colic in infants. In an animal study with diabetic mice, aspalathin, a rooibos constituent improved glucose homeostasis by stimulating insulin secretion in pancreatic beta cells and glucose uptake in muscle tissue.
- Rose hips – Small scale studies indicate that hips from *Rosa canina* may provide benefits in the treatment of osteoarthritis. Rose hips show anti COX activity.
- Salvia lavandulaefolia may improve memory
- Saw Palmetto can be used for BPH. Supported in some studies, failed to confirm in others.
- Shiitake mushrooms (*Lentinus edodes*) are edible mushrooms that have been reported to have health benefits, including cancer-preventing properties. In laboratory research a shiitake extract has inhibited the growth of tumor cells through induction of apoptosis. Both a water extract and fresh juice of shiitake have demonstrated antimicrobial activity against pathogenic bacteria and fungi in vitro.
- Soy and other plants that contain phytoestrogens (plant molecules with estrogen activity) (black cohosh probably has serotonin activity) have some benefits for treatment of symptoms resulting frommenopause.
- St. John's wort, has yielded positive results, proving more effective than a placebo for the treatment of mild to moderate depression in some clinical trials. A subsequent, large, controlled trial, however, found St. John's wort to be no better than a placebo in treating depression. However, more recent trials have shown positive results or positive trends that failed significance. A 2004 meta-analysis concluded that the positive results can be explained by publication bias but later analyses have been more favorable. The Cochrane Database cautions that the data on St. John's wort for depression are conflicting and ambiguous.
- Stinging nettle In some clinical studies effective for benign prostatic hyperplasia and the pain associated with osteoarthritis. In-vitro tests show antiinflammatory action. In a rodent model, stinging nettle reduced LDL cholesterol and total cholesterol. In another rodent study it reduced platelet aggregation.
- Umckaloabo (*Pelargonium sidoides*): an extract of this plant showed efficacy in the treatment of acute bronchitis in a controlled trial and is approved for this use in Germany.
- Valerian root can be used to treat insomnia. Clinical studies show mixed results and researchers note that many trials are of poor quality.
- Vanilla

- Willow bark (*Salix alba*) can be used for a variety of anti-inflammatory and antimicrobial purposes due to presence of salicylic acid and tannins. Has been in use for aprox. 6000yrs and was described in the 1st century AD by Dioscorides.

3. Herbals and diabetes

Using herbal remedies and plant derivatives to help in the treatment of diabetes should certainly not be discounted. Although numerous 'miracle herbal cure' companies exist, and champion the ability of herbal compounds to supplement insulin as a treatment, these should not be taken at face value without thorough research and consultation with experts.That is not to say that some of the following herbs do not have properties that some diabetics will find beneficial.The herbs and plant derivatives listed below have been employed traditionally by native people in the treatment of diabetes, in the areas in which they grow. Many suffer from an inadequate knowledge base.Allium sativum is more commonly known as garlic, and is thought to offer antioxidant properties and micro-circulatory effects. Although few studies have directly linked allium with insulin and blood glucose levels, results have been positive.Allium may cause a reduction in blood glucose, increase secretion and slow the degradation of insulin. Limited data is available however, and further trials are needed. Further herbs that have been studied and may have positive effects for diabetic patients include berberine, Cinnamomym tamala, curry, Eugenia jambolana, gingko, Phyllanthus amarus, Pterocarpus marsupium, Solanum torvum, Vinca rosea, Trigonella foenum graecum, Silybum marianum, Opuntia streptacantha (nopal), Ocimum sanctum, Ginseng, Gymnema sylvestre, Coccinia indica, Bauhinia forficate, Myrcia uniflora and Aloe vera.

3.1 Ginger (Zingiber officinale)

3.1.1 Scientific classification

Kingdom: Plantae
Clade: Angiosperms, Monocots, Commelinids
Order: Zingiberales
Family: Zingiberaceae
Genus: Zingiber
Species: Z.officinale
Binominal name: Zingiber officinale

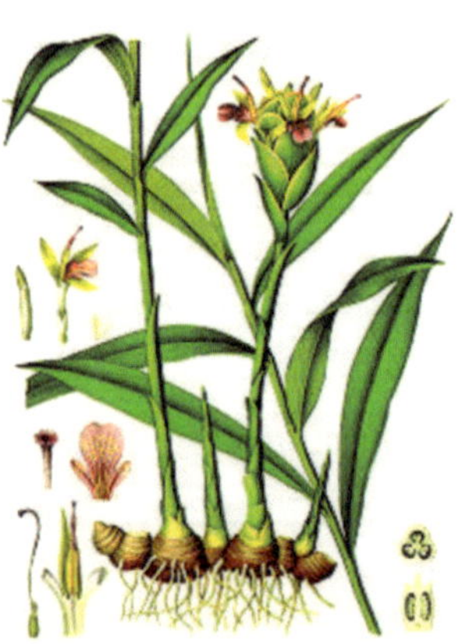

3.1.2 Medical properties and research

The Zingiber officinale plant, common ginger, has medicinal properties. Traditionally used as a digestive aid, ginger also helps fight diabetes, cancer and anxiety. The roots of this plant, sold at grocery stores, can affect the reproductive system as well. A 2010 article in "Food and Chemical Toxicology" looked at the impact of ginger on hormone levels in an animal model of diabetes. Rats were given extracted ginger or no treatment for 65 days. The results indicated that ginger enhanced testosterone levels relative to controls. It also reduced diabetic lesions. No adverse events appeared, but long-term treatment may have a different effect.

Ginger have been claimed to decrease the pain from arthritis, though studies have been inconsistent. It may also have blood thinning and cholesterol lowering properties that may make it useful for treating heart disease.

Preliminary research also indicates that nine compounds found in ginger may bind to human serotonin receptors, possibly helping to affect anxiety.

Advanced glycation end-products are possibly associated in the development of several pathophysiologies, including diabetic cataract for which ginger was effective in preliminary studies, apparently by acting through antiglycating mechanisms.

Ginger compounds are active against a form of diarrhea which is the leading cause of infant death in developing countries. Zingerone is likely to be the active constituent against enterotoxigenic *Escherichia coli* heat-labile enterotoxin-induced diarrhea.

Ginger has been found effective in multiple studies for treating nausea caused by seasickness, morning sickness and chemotherapy, though ginger was not found superior over a placebo for pre-emptively treating post-operative nausea. Ginger is a safe remedy for nausea relief during pregnancy. The television program *Mythbusters* performed an experiment using one of their staff who suffered from severe motion sickness. The staff member was placed in a moving device which, without treatment, produced severe nausea. Multiple treatments were administered. None, with the exception of the ginger and the two most common drugs, were successful. The staff member preferred the ginger due to lack of side effects. Several studies over the last 20 years were inconclusive with some studies in favor of the herb and some not.

3.1.3 Folk medicine

The traditional medical form of ginger historically was called *Jamaica ginger*; it was classified as a stimulant and carminative and used frequently fordyspepsia, gastroparesis, slow motility symptoms, constipation, and colic. It was also frequently employed to disguise the taste of medicines.

Tea brewed from ginger is a common folk remedy for colds. Ginger ale and ginger beer are also drunk as *stomach settlers* in countries where the beverages are made.

- In Burma, ginger and a local sweetener made from palm tree juice (*htan nyat*) are boiled together and taken to prevent the flu.
- In China, ginger is included in several traditional preparations. A drink made with sliced ginger cooked in water with brown sugar or a cola is used as a folk medicine for the common cold."Ginger eggs" (scrambled eggs with finely diced ginger root) is a

common home remedy for coughing. The Chinese also make a kind of dried ginger candy that is fermented in plum juice and sugared, which is also commonly consumed to suppress coughing. Ginger has also been historically used to treat inflammation, which several scientific studies support, though one arthritis trial showed ginger to be no better than a placebo or ibuprofen for treatment of osteoarthritis.

- In Congo, ginger is crushed and mixed with mango tree sap to make tangawisi juice, which is considered a panacea.
- In India, ginger is applied as a paste to the temples to relieve headache, and consumed when suffering from the common cold. Ginger with lemon and black salt is also used for nausea.
- In Indonesia, ginger (*jahe* in Indonesian) is used as a herbal preparation to reduce fatigue, reducing "winds" in the blood, prevent and cure rheumatism and control poor dietary habits.
- In Nepal, ginger is called *aduwa*, अदुवा and is widely grown and used throughout the country as a spice for vegetables, used medically to treat cold and also sometimes used to flavor tea.
- In the Philippines, ginger is known as *luya* and is used as a throat lozenge in traditional medicine to relieve sore throat. It is also brewed into a tea known as *salabat*.
- In the United States, ginger is used to prevent motion and morning sickness. It is recognized as safe by the Food and Drug Administration and is sold as an unregulated dietary supplement. Ginger water was also used to avoid heat cramps in the United States.
- In Peru, ginger is sliced in hot water as an infusion for stomach aches as *infusión de Kión*.

3.2 Onion (Alluim Cepa)

3.2.1 Scientific classification

Kingdom: Plantae
Clade: Angiosperms, Monocots
Order: Asparagales
Family: Amaryllidaceae
Subfamily: Allioideae
Genus: Allium
Species: A.cepa
Binominal name: Allium cepa

The onion (*Allium cepa*), also known as the bulb onion, common onion and garden onion, is the most widely cultivated species of the genus *Allium*. The genus *Allium* also contains a number of other species variously referred to as onions and cultivated for food, such as the Japanese bunching onion (*A. fistulosum*), Egyptian onion (A. *proliferum*), and Canada onion (*A. canadense*). The name "wild onion" is applied to a number of *Allium*species.

The vast majority of cultivars of *A. cepa* belong to the 'common onion group' (*A. cepa* var. *cepa*) and are usually referred to simply as 'onions'. The 'Aggregatum group' of cultivars (*A. cepa* var. *aggregatum*) includes both shallots and potato onions.

Allium cepa is known only in cultivation, but related wild species occur in Central Asia. The most closely related species include *Allium vavilovii* (Popov & Vved.) and *Allium asarense*

(R.M. Fritsch & Matin) from Iran. However, Zohary and Hopf warn that "there are doubts whether the *A. vavilovii* collections tested represent genuine wild material or only feral derivatives of the crop.

3.3 Possible medicinal properties and health effects of onion

Wide-ranging claims have been made for the effectiveness of onions against conditions ranging from the common cold to heart disease, diabetes,osteoporosis, and other diseases. They contain chemical compounds believed to have anti-inflammatory, anticholesterol, anticancer, and antioxidantproperties, such as quercetin. Preliminary studies have shown increased consumption of onions reduces the risk of head and neck cancers.

Raw Onions	
Nutritional value per 100 g (3.5 oz)	
Energy	166 kJ (40 kcal)
Carbohydrates	9.34 g
Sugars	4.24 g
Dietary fiber	1.7 g
Fat	0.1 g
saturated	0.042 g
monounsaturated	0.013 g
polyunsaturated	0.017 g
Protein	1.1 g
Water	89.11 g
Vitamin A equiv.	0 µg (0%)
Thiamine (Vit. B_1)	0.046 mg (4%)
Riboflavin (Vit. B_2)	0.027 mg (2%)
Niacin (Vit. B_3)	0.116 mg (1%)
Vitamin B_6	0.12 mg (9%)
Folate (Vit. B_9)	19 µg (5%)
Vitamin B_{12}	0 µg (0%)
Vitamin C	7.4 mg (9%)
Vitamin E	0.02 mg (0%)
Vitamin K	0.4 µg (0%)
Calcium	23 mg (2%)
Iron	0.21 mg (2%)
Magnesium	0.129 mg (0%)
Phosphorus	29 mg (4%)
Potassium	146 mg (3%)
Sodium	4 mg (0%)
Zinc	0.17 mg (2%)
Percentages are relative to US recommendationsfor adults. Source: USDA Nutrient database	

Table 1. Possible medicinal properties of onions

Among all varieties, Asian white onions have the most eye irritating chemical reaction. Regular use of white onion, if eaten raw, is good for male sexual power due to its antioxidant and anti-inflammatory properties.

In India some sects do not eat onions as they believe them to be an aphrodisiac; various schools of Buddhism also advise against eating onions and other vegetables of the Allium family.

In many parts of the undeveloped world, onions are used to heal blisters and boils. A traditional Maltese remedy for sea urchin wounds is to tie half a baked onion to the afflicted area overnight. A similar traditional cure is known in Bulgaria. Half-baked onion with sugar is placed over the finger and fingernail in case of inflammation.

An application of raw onion is also said to be helpful in reducing swelling from bee stings. In the United States, products that contain onion extract are used in the treatment of topical scars; some studies have found their action to be ineffective, while others found that they may act as an anti-inflammatory or bacteriostatic and can improve collagen organization in rabbits

Onions may be beneficial for women, who are at increased risk for osteoporosis as they go through menopause, by destroying osteoclasts so they do not break down bone.

An American chemist has stated the pleiomeric chemicals in onions have the potential to alleviate or prevent sore throat. Onion in combination withjaggery has been widely used as a traditional household remedy for sore throat in India.

Shallots have the most phenols, six times the amount found in Vidalia onion, the variety with the lowest phenolic content. Shallots also have the mostantioxidant activity, followed by Western Yellow, pungent yellow (New York Bold), Northern Red, Mexico, Empire Sweet, Western White, Peruvian Sweet, Texas 1015, Imperial Valley Sweet, and Vidalia. Western Yellow onions have the most flavonoids, eleven times the amount found in Western White, the variety with the lowest flavonoid content.

The Allium cepa plant also affects the reproductive system. Bulbs from this plant, onions, are used as a vegetable and as a condiment. Yet, onions may treat erectile dysfunction as well. The underlying cause of these benefits remains unclear, but it could involve sex steroids. In a 2009 study conducted by Arash Khaki and colleagues that was published in the journal of "Folia Morphologica," researchers evaluated the impact of onion on sperm production in subjects. They discovered that animals consuming fresh onion juice for three weeks experienced significant improvements in testosterone production compared to the control groups. Scientists suggest that onion boosts testosterone levels by increasing the output of luteinizing hormone, which signals to the testes to stimulate testosterone production. Our previous study since 2005 up to 2011 showed onion and Ginger can regulate nephropathy disorders by their anti-oxidant capacity.

For all varieties of onions, the more phenols and flavonoids they contain, the more reputed antioxidant and anticancer activity they provide. When tested against liver and colon cancer cells in laboratory studies, 'Western Yellow', pungent yellow (New York Bold) and shallots were most effective in inhibiting their growth. The milder-tasting cultivars (i.e., 'Western White,' 'Peruvian Sweet,' 'Empire Sweet,' 'Mexico,' 'Texas 1015,' 'Imperial Valley Sweet' and 'Vidalia') showed little cancer-fighting ability.

Shallots and ten other onion (*Allium cepa* L.) varieties commonly available in the United States were evaluated: Western Yellow, Northern Red, pungent yellow (New York Bold), Western White, Peruvian Sweet, Empire Sweet, Mexico, Texas 1015, Imperial Valley Sweet, and Vidalia. In general, the most pungent onions delivered many times the effects of their milder cousins.

The 3-mercapto-2-methylpentan-1-ol in onion was found to inhibit peroxynitrite-induced mechanisms *in vitro*.

While members of the onion family appear to have medicinal properties for humans, they can be deadly for dogs and cats.

4. Syzygium jambolanum

4.1 Scientific classification:

Kingdom: Plantae
Order: Myrtales
Family: Myrtaceae
Genus: Syzygium
Species: S.cumini
Binominal name: Syzygium cumini
Synonyms: Eugenia cumini(L.) Druce
    Eugenia jambolana Lam.
    Syzygium jambolanum DC.

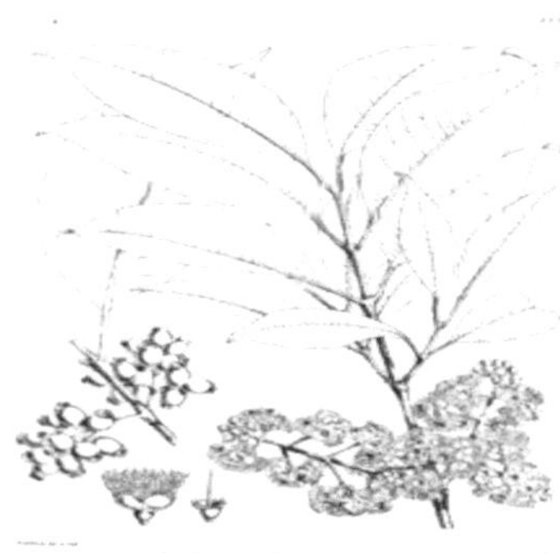

Syzygium jambolanum (Lam.) DC (henceforth to be denoted as SJ) tree belongs to Myrtaceae family and consists of about 90 genera and 2800 species, commonly called Jamun, Jambol fruit in India and Rose apple in English. Jambol is also known as jambu/jambula/jamboola, Javaplum, jamun, jaam/kalojaam, jamblang, jambolan, black plum , Damson plum , Duhat plum , Jambolan plum or Portuguese plum. Malabar plum may also refer to other species of Syzygium. In Tamil, this fruit is called Naaval Pazham or Navva Pazham.

It is a large, evergreen tree found primarily in India, Pakistan, Southern Asia and Brazil. The leaves and bark are used for controlling blood pressure and gingivitis. It has a high source in vitamin A and vitamin C. The powdered seeds of Syzygium Jambolanum are a well known Indian folk medicine for treatment of diabetes mellitus. They also have anti-bacterial and anti-inflammatory activities.

Syzygium jambolanum seeds are used by the village people to treat illnesses caused by bacterial, fungal and viral pathogens. The seed extract of Syzygium jambolanum is used to treat cold, cough, fever and skin problems such as rashes and the mouth, throat, intestines and genitourinary tract ulcers (infected by Candida albicans).

The chemical composition of the seed extract has only been recently reported by a lone study to contain glycoside (jamboline), tannin, ellagic acid and gallic acid as principal ingredients. The seeds are sweet, astringent to the bowels and good for diabetes. It also stops urinary discharges.

In recent years, in view of toxic side-effects of most of the modern medicines, there is a growing popularity of scientifically validated natural products as alternative medicines. Though ethanolic extract of SJ (EESJ) has long been used as a good anti-diabetic drug in various traditional and folk medicines (Samadder et al, 2011).

Achrekar et al in 1991 have described that the seeds or fruit of this tree, in which various methods were used to prepare the medicine and administer it to normal and diabetic animals, the following effects were observed: reduction of glycaemia and glycosuria, anti-oxidant activity and partial restoration of altered liver and skeletal muscle glycogen content and liver glucokinase, hexokinase, glucose-6-phosphate and phosphofructokinase levels. In India, it has been used, in a mix with honey or milk, to treat diabetes and digestive diseases and the fresh fruits has been taken orally to treat stomachache.

4.2 Nutrients and phytochemicals

Java Plum, raw	
Nutritional value per 100 g (3.5 oz)	
Energy	251 kJ (60 kcal)
Carbohydrates	15.56 g
Fat	0.23 g
Protein	0.72 g
Water	83.13 g
Vitamin A	3 IU
Thiamine (Vit. B_1)	0.006 mg (1%)
Riboflavin (Vit. B_2)	0.012 mg (1%)
Niacin (Vit. B_3)	0.260 mg (2%)
Pantothenic acid (B_5)	0.160 mg (3%)
Vitamin B_6	0.038 mg (3%)
Vitamin C	14.3 mg (17%)
Calcium	19 mg (2%)
Iron	0.19 mg (1%)
Magnesium	15 mg (4%)
Phosphorus	17 mg (2%)
Potassium	79 mg (2%)
Sodium	14 mg (1%)
Percentages are relative to US recommendationsfor adults. Source: USDA Nutrient database	

Table 2. Some nutrients of Java Plum

The leaf composition is shown in the tables below.

Java Plum Leaf	
Compound	**Percent**
Crude Protein	9.1
Fat	4.3
Crude Fiber	17.0
Ash	6.0
Calcium	1.3
Phosphorus	0.19

Table 3. The leaf composition of Java Plum

5. Antioxidants

An antioxidant is a molecule capable of inhibiting the oxidation of other molecules. Oxidation is a chemical reaction that transfers electrons or hydrogen from a substance to an oxidizing agent. Oxidation reactions can produce free radicals. In turn, these radicals can start chain reactions. When the chain reaction occurs in a cell, it can cause damage or death to the cell. When the chain reaction occurs in a purified monomer, it produces a polymer resin, such as a plastic, a synthetic fiber, or an oil paint film. Antioxidants terminate these chain reactions by removing free radical intermediates, and inhibit other oxidation reactions. They do this by being oxidized themselves, so antioxidants are often reducing agents such as thiols, ascorbic acid, or polyphenols.

Antioxidants are important additives in gasoline. These antioxidants prevent the formation of gums that interfere with the operation of internal combustion engines. Although oxidation reactions are crucial for life, they can also be damaging; hence, plants and animals maintain complex systems of multiple types of antioxidants, such as glutathione, vitamin C, and vitamin E as well as enzymes such as catalase, superoxide dismutase and various peroxidases. Low levels of antioxidants, or inhibition of the antioxidant enzymes, cause oxidative stress and may damage or kill cells.

As oxidative stress appears to be an important part of many human diseases, the use of antioxidants in pharmacology is intensively studied, particularly as treatments for stroke and neurodegenerative diseases. However, it is unknown whether oxidative stress is the cause or the consequence of disease.

Antioxidants are widely used as ingredients in dietary supplements and have been investigated for the prevention of diseases such as cancer, coronary heart disease and even altitude sickness. Although initial studies suggested that antioxidant supplements might promote health, later large clinical trials did not detect any benefit and suggested instead that excess supplementation is harmful. (Concerning the previous studies cited the first only shows that antioxidant supplements were not effective in helping against "mountain sickness", and in the second study showed that the supplements beta carotene, vitamin A , and vitamin E, "singly or combined, significantly increased mortality." Though it says that "Most trials investigated the effects of supplements administered at higher doses than those commonly found in a balanced diet" whereas it says "Vitamin C and selenium had no significant effect on mortality.") In addition to these uses of natural antioxidants in medicine, these compounds have many industrial uses, such as preservatives in food and cosmetics and preventing the degradation of rubber and gasoline.

6. Measurement and levels of antioxidants in food

Measurement of antioxidants is not a straightforward process, as this is a diverse group of compounds with different reactivities to different reactive oxygen species. In food science, the oxygen radical absorbance capacity (ORAC) has become the current industry standard for assessing antioxidant strength of whole foods, juices and food additives. Other measurement tests include the Folin-Ciocalteu reagent, and the Trolox equivalent antioxidant capacity assay.

Antioxidants are found in varying amounts in foods such as vegetables, fruits, grain cereals, eggs, meat, legumes and nuts. Some antioxidants such as lycopene and ascorbic acid can be destroyed by long-term storage or prolonged cooking. Other antioxidant compounds are more stable, such as the polyphenolic antioxidants in foods such as whole-wheat cereals and tea. The effects of cooking and food processing are complex, as these processes can also increase the bioavailability of antioxidants, such as some carotenoids in vegetables. In general, processed foods contain fewer antioxidants than fresh and uncooked foods, since the preparation processes may expose the food to oxygen.

Antioxidant compounds	**Foods containing high levels of these antioxidants**
Vitamin C (ascorbic acid)	Fresh Fruits and vegetables
Vitamin E (tocopherols, tocotrienols)	Vegetable oils
Polyphenolic antioxidants (resveratrol, flavonoids)	Tea, coffee, soy, fruit, olive oil, chocolate, cinnamon, oregano and red wine
Carotenoids (lycopene, carotenes, lutein)	Fruit, vegetables and eggs.

Table 4. Antioxidant compounds of some food

Other antioxidants are not vitamins and are instead made in the body. For example, ubiquinol (coenzyme Q) is poorly absorbed from the gut and is made in humans through the mevalonate pathway. Another example is glutathione, which is made from amino acids. As any glutathione in the gut is broken down to free cysteine, glycine and glutamic acid before being absorbed, even large oral doses have little effect on the concentration of glutathione in the body. Although large amounts of sulfur-containing amino acids such as acetylcysteine can increase glutathione, no evidence exists that eating high levels of these glutathione precursors is beneficial for healthy adults. Supplying more of these precursors may be useful as part of the treatment of some diseases, such as acute respiratory distress syndrome, protein-energy malnutrition, or preventing the liver damage produced by paracetamol overdose.

Other compounds in the diet can alter the levels of antioxidants by acting as pro-oxidants. Here, consuming the compound causes oxidative stress, which the body responds to by inducing higher levels of antioxidant defenses such as antioxidant enzymes. Some of these compounds, such as isothiocyanates and curcumin, may be chemopreventive agents that either block the transformation of abnormal cells into cancerous cells, or even kill existing cancer cells.

7. Health effects of antioxidants

7.1 Disease treatment

The brain is uniquely vulnerable to oxidative injury, due to its high metabolic rate and elevated levels of polyunsaturated lipids, the target of lipid peroxidation. Consequently, antioxidants are commonly used as medications to treat various forms of brain injury. Here, superoxide dismutase mimetics, sodium thiopental and propofol are used to treat reperfusion injury and traumatic brain injury, while the experimental drug NXY-059 and ebselen are being applied in the treatment of stroke. These compounds appear to prevent oxidative stress in neurons and preventapoptosis and neurological damage. Antioxidants are also being investigated as possible treatments for neurodegenerative diseases such as Alzheimer's disease, Parkinson's disease, and amyotrophic lateral sclerosis, and as a way to prevent noise-induced hearing loss. Targeted antioxidants may lead to better medicinal effects. Mitochondria-targeted ubiquinone, for example, may prevent damage to the liver caused by excessive alcohol.

7.2 Disease prevention

People who eat fruits and vegetables have a lower risk of heart disease and some neurological diseases, and there is evidence that some types of vegetables, and fruits in general, protect against some cancers. Since fruits and vegetables happen to be good sources of antioxidants, this suggested that antioxidants might prevent some types of diseases. This idea has been tested in clinical trials and does not seem to be true, as antioxidant supplements have no clear effect on the risk of chronic diseases such as cancer and heart disease. This suggests that these health benefits come from other substances in fruits and vegetables (possibly flavonoids), or come from a complex mix of substances.

It is thought that oxidation of low density lipoprotein in the blood contributes to heart disease, and initial observational studies found that people taking Vitamin E supplements had a lower risk of developing heart disease. Consequently, at least seven large clinical trials were conducted to test the effects of antioxidant supplement with Vitamin E, in doses ranging from 50 to 600 mg per day. None of these trials found a statistically significant effect of Vitamin E on overall number of deaths or on deaths due to heart disease. Further studies have also been negative. It is not clear if the doses used in these trials or in most dietary supplements are capable of producing any significant decrease in oxidative stress. Overall, despite the clear role of oxidative stress in cardiovascular disease, controlled studies using antioxidant vitamins have observed no reduction in either the risk of developing heart disease, or the rate of progression of existing disease.

While several trials have investigated supplements with high doses of antioxidants, the "Supplémentation en Vitamines et Mineraux Antioxydants" (SU.VI.MAX) study tested the effect of supplementation with doses comparable to those in a healthy diet. Over 12,500 French men and women took either low-dose antioxidants (120 mg of ascorbic acid, 30 mg of vitamin E, 6 mg of beta carotene, 100 µg of selenium, and 20 mg of zinc) or placebo pills for an average of 7.5 years. The study concluded that low-dose antioxidant supplementation lowered total cancer incidence and all-cause mortality in men but not in women. Supplementation may be effective in men only because of their lower baseline status of certain antioxidants, especially of beta carotene.

Many nutraceutical and health food companies sell formulations of antioxidants as dietary supplements and these are widely used in industrialized countries. These supplements may include specific antioxidant chemicals, like the polyphenol, resveratrol (from grape seeds or knotweed roots), combinations of antioxidants, like the "ACES" products that contain beta carotene (provitaminA), vitamin C, vitamin E and Selenium, or herbs that contain antioxidants - such as green tea and jiaogulan. Although some levels of antioxidant vitamins and minerals in the diet are required for good health, there is considerable doubt as to whether these antioxidant supplements are beneficial or harmful, and if they are actually beneficial, which antioxidant(s) are needed and in what amounts. Indeed, some authors argue that the hypothesis that antioxidants could prevent chronic diseases has now been disproved and that the idea was misguided from the beginning. Rather, dietary polyphenols may have non-antioxidant roles in minute concentrations that affect cell-to-cell signaling, receptor sensitivity, inflammatory enzyme activity or gene regulation.

For overall life expectancy, it has even been suggested that moderate levels of oxidative stress may increase lifespan in the worm Caenorhabditis elegans, by inducing a protective response to increased levels of reactive oxygen species. The suggestion that increased life expectancy comes from increased oxidative stress conflicts with results seen in the yeast Saccharomyces cerevisiae, and the situation in mammals is even less clear. Nevertheless, antioxidant supplements do not appear to increase life expectancy in humans.

7.3 Adverse effects

Relatively strong reducing acids can have antinutrient effects by binding to dietary minerals such as iron and zinc in the gastrointestinal tract and preventing them from being absorbed. Notable examples are oxalic acid, tannins and phytic acid, which are high in plant-based diets. Calcium and iron deficiencies are not uncommon in diets in developing countries where less meat is eaten and there is high consumption of phytic acid from beans and unleavened whole grain bread.

Foods	Reducing acid present
Cocoa bean and chocolate, spinach, turnip and rhubarb.	Oxalic acid
Whole grains, maize, legumes.	Phytic acid
Tea, beans, cabbage.	Tannins

Table 5. Some acid reducing foods

Nonpolar antioxidants such as eugenol—a major component of oil of cloves—have toxicity limits that can be exceeded with the misuse of undiluted essential oils. Toxicity associated with high doses of water-soluble antioxidants such as ascorbic acid are less of a concern, as these compounds can be excreted rapidly in urine. More seriously, very high doses of some antioxidants may have harmful long-term effects. The beta-Carotene and Retinol Efficacy Trial (CARET) study of lung cancer patients found that smokers given supplements containing beta-carotene and vitamin A had increased rates of lung cancer. Subsequent studies confirmed these adverse effects.

These harmful effects may also be seen in non-smokers, as a recent meta-analysis including data from approximately 230,000 patients showed that β-carotene, vitamin A or vitamin E supplementation is associated with increased mortality but saw no significant effect from vitamin C. No health risk was seen when all the randomized controlled studies were examined together, but an increase in mortality was detected only when the high-quality and low-bias risk trials were examined separately. However, as the majority of these low-bias trials dealt with either elderly people, or people already suffering disease, these results may not apply to the general population. This meta-analysis was later repeated and extended by the same authors, with the new analysis published by the Cochrane Collaboration; confirming the previous results. These two publications are consistent with some previous meta-analyzes that also suggested that Vitamin E supplementation increased mortality, and that antioxidant supplements increased the risk of colon cancer. However, the results of this meta-analysis are inconsistent with other studies such as the SU.VI.MAX trial, which suggested that antioxidants have no effect on cause-all mortality. Overall, the large number of clinical trials carried out on antioxidant supplements suggest that either these products have no effect on health, or that they cause a small increase in mortality in elderly or vulnerable populations.

While antioxidant supplementation is widely used in attempts to prevent the development of cancer, it has been proposed that antioxidants may, paradoxically, interfere with cancer treatments. This was thought to occur since the environment of cancer cells causes high levels of oxidative stress, making these cells more susceptible to the further oxidative stress induced by treatments. As a result, by reducing the redox stress in cancer cells, antioxidant supplements could decrease the effectiveness of radiotherapy and chemotherapy. On the other hand, other reviews have suggested that antioxidants could reduce side effects or increase survival times.

8. Acknowledgments

We thank our student, Dr. Elham Ghadamkheir from the Faculty of Medicine, for her valuable help, and especially thanks to my Adviser, Professor Dr. Iraj Sohrabi Haghdoust

9. References

Acharya, D. & Shrivastava, A. (2008). *Indigenous Herbal Medicines: Tribal Formulations and Traditional Herbal Practices*, p.440, Aavishkar Publishers Distributor, ISBN 978-81-7910-252-7,Jaipur, India

Achrekar, S.; Kaklij, G.S.; Pote, M.S. & Kelkar, S.M. (1991). Hypoglycemic activity of *Eugenia jambolana* and ficus bengalensis. Mechanism of Action. *In vivo*, Vol.5, pp.143-148

Aggarwal, B.B. & Shishodia, S. (2006). Molecular targets of dietary agents for prevention and therapy of cancer. *Biochemical Pharmacology,* Vol.71, No.10, (February 2006), p. 1397–421

Aggarwal, B.B.; Sundaram, C.; Malani, N. & Ichikawa, H. (2007). Curcumin: the Indian solid gold. *Advances in Experimental Medicine and Biology,* Vol.595, p.1–75

American Diabetes Association. (2010). Standards of medical care in diabetes. *Diabetes Care,* Vol.33, No.1, (January 2010), pp. s11- s61

Aviram, M. (2000). Review of human studies on oxidative damage and antioxidant protection related to cardiovascular disease. *Free Radical Research,* Vol.33, (November 2000), p. S85–97

Baillie, J.K.; Thompson, A.A.R.; Irving, J.B.; Bates, M.G.D.; Sutherland, A.I.; MacNee, W.; Maxwell, S.R.J. & Webb, D.J. (2009). Oral antioxidant supplementation does not prevent acute mountain sickness: double blind, randomized placebo-controlled trial. *QJM,* Vol.102, No.5, (May 2009), p. 341–8

Beecher, G. (2003). Overview of dietary flavonoids: nomenclature, occurrence and intake. *Journal of Nutrition,* Vol.133, No.10, (October 2003), p.3248S–3254S

Benzie, I. (2003). Evolution of dietary antioxidants.*Comparative Biochemistry and Physiology,* Vol.136, No.1, (September 2003), p.113–26

Bjelakovic, G.; Nikolova, D.; Gluud, L.L.; Simonetti, R.G. & Gluud, C. (2008). Antioxidant supplements for prevention of mortality in healthy participants and patients with various diseases. *Cochrane Database of Systematic Reviews,* Issue.2

Bloom, B.S.; Retbi A.; Dahan, S. & Jonsson, E. (2000) . Evaluation Of Randomized Controlled Trials On Complementary And Alternative Medicine. *International Journal of Technology Assessment in Health Care,* Vol.16, No.1, p. 13–21

Castleman, M.(2001). *The New Healing Herbs: The Classic Guide to Nature's Best Medicines Featuring the Top 100 Time-Tested Herbs,* p. 15, Rodale, ISBN 1579543049, 97815795430,Emmaus, Pennsylvania, USA

Chandrasekaran, M. & Venkatesalu, V. (2004). Antibacterial and antifungal activity of *Syzygium jambolanum* seeds. *Ethnopharmacology,* Vol.91, pp. 105–108

Davies, K.J. (1995). Oxidative stress: The paradox of aerobic life. *Biochemical Society Symposia,* Vol.61, p.1–31

Duraipandiyan, V.; Ayyanar, M. & Ignacimuthu, S. (2006). Antimicrobial activity of some ethnomedicinal plants used by Paliyar tribe from Tamil Nadu, India. *BMC Complementary and Alternative Medicine,* Vol.6, (October 2006), p.35

Elvin-Lewis, M. (2001). Should we be concerned about herbal remedies. *Journal of Ethnopharmacology,* Vol.75, No.2–3, (May 2001),p.141–164

E number index. *UK food guide,* 05.03.2007, Available from http://www.ukfoodguide.net/enumeric.htm#antioxidants

Fabricant, D.S. & Farnsworth, N.R. (2001). The value of plants used in traditional medicine for drug discovery. *Environmental Health Perspectives,* Vol.109, No.1, (March 2001), p. 69–75

Fahd, T. (1996). Botany and agriculture, In: *Encyclopedia of the History of Arabic Science,* M.Régis & R.Roshdi, p.815, Routledge, ISBN 0415124107, London

Finkel, T. & Holbrook, N.J. (2000). Oxidants, oxidative stress and the biology of ageing. *Nature,* Vol.408, No.6809,(November 2000), p. 239–47

Girish, D. & Shridhar, D.(2007). History of Medicine: Sushruta – the Clinician – Teacher par Excellence. *Indian Journal of Chest Disease and allied sciences*, Vol.49, p.243-244

Grover, J.K.; Yadav, S. & Vats, V. (2002). Medicinal plants of India with anti-diabetic potential. *Journal of Ethnopharmacology*, Vol.81, pp. 81–100

Helmut, S. (1997). Oxidative stress: Oxidants and antioxidants. *Experimental physiology* , Vol.82, No.2, (March 1997), pp. 291–5

Hirst, J.; King, M.S. & Pryde, K.R. (2008). The production of reactive oxygen species by complex I. *Biochemical Society Transactions*, Vol.36, No.5,(October 2008), p. 976–80

Huffman, M.A. (2003). Animal self-medication and ethno-medicine: exploration and exploitation of the medicinal properties of plants (in hindi). *Proceedings of the Nutrition Society*, Vol.62, No.2, (May 2003), p. 371–81

Inzucchi, S.E. & Sherwin, R.S. (2007). Diabetes Mellitus, In: *Cecil Textbook of Medicine* (23rd ed.), L.Goldman , D.Ausiello,(eds.), chap 248. Pa: Saunders Elsevier, Philadelphia

Khaki, A.; Nouri, M.; Fathiazad, F.; Ahmadi-Ashtiani, H.R.; Rastgar, H & Rezazadeh, Sh.(2009a). Protective Effects of Quercetin on Spermatogenesis in Streptozotocin-induced Diabetic Rat. *iranian journal of medical plants*, Vol. 8, No. 4, (March 2009), pp. 57-64

Khaki, A.; Fathiazad, F.; Nouri, M.; Khaki, A.A.; Jabbari–kh, H. & Hammadeh, M. (2009b). Evaluation of Androgenic Activity of Allium cepa on Spermatogenesis in Rat. *Folia Morphologica*, Vol. 68, No. 1, (February 2009), pp. 45-51

Khaki, A.; Fathiazad, F.; Nouri, M.; Khaki, A.A.; Ozanci, C.C.; Ghafari-Novin, M. & Hamadeh M. (2009c). The Effects of Ginger on Spermatogenesis and Sperm parameters of Rat. *Iranian Journal of Reproductive Medicine*, Vol.7, No.1, pp.7-12

Khaki, A.; Fathiazad, F.; Nouri, M.; Khaki, A.A.; Abassi-maleki, N.; Ahmadi, P. & Jabari-kh, H. (2010a). Beneficial Effects of Quercetin on sperm parameters in streptozotocin - induced diabetic male rats. *Phytotherapy Research journal*, Vol. 24, No. 9, (September 2010), pp. 1285-1291

Khaki, A. (2010b). Protective effect of quercetin against necrosis and apoptosis induced by experimental ischemia and reperfusion in rat liver. *AJPP*, Vol. 4, No. 1, (January 2010), pp. 022-026

Khaki, A.; Fathiazad, F.; Ahmadi-ashtiani, H.R.; Rezazadeh, Sh.; Rastegar, H.; Imani, A.M. (2010c). Comparatment of Quercetin & Allium cepa on blood glucose in diabetics rats. *Iranian Journal of Medical Plants*, Vol.9, No.6,(February 2010), pp.107-113

Khaki, A. (2011a). Effect of Rosmarinic acid on LH, FSH and Estrogen in Female Diabetic rats. *African Journal of Pharmacy and Pharmacology*,2011 up to publish

Khaki, A.; Fathiazad, F.; Nouri, M.; khaki, A.A.; Ghanbari, Z.; Ghanbari, M.; Ouladsahebmadarek, E. & Farzadi, L. (2011b). Anti-oxidative Effects of Citro_flavonoids on Spermatogenesis in Rat. *African Journal of Pharmacy and Pharmacology*,Vol.5, No.6, (June 2011), pp.721-725

Khaki, A.; Ghadamkheir, E.; Farzadi, L.; Khaki, A.A.; shojaee, S. & Ahmadi, S.(2011c). Recovery of Spermatogenesis by Allium cepa in Toxoplasma gondii infected Rats. *African Journal of Pharmacy and Pharmacology*, Vol.5, No.7, (July 2011), pp.903-907

Khaki, A.A.; Khaki, A.; Nouri, M.; Ahmadi-Ashtiani, H.R.; Rastega, H.; Rezazadeh, Sh.; Fathiazad, F. & Ghanbari, M. (2009). Evaluation Effects of Quercetin on Liver Apoptosis in Streptozotocin-induced Diabetic Rat. *iranian journal of medical plants*, Vol. 8, No. 5, (March 2009), pp. 70-78

Khaki, A.A.; khaki, A.; Ahmadi-Ashtiani, H.R.; Rezazadeh, Sh.; Rastegar, H.; Babazadeh, D. & Ghanbari, Z. (2010a).Treatment effects of Ginger rhizome & Carrot seed on Diabetic Nephropathy in Rat. *Iranian journal of medical plants*, Vol. 9, No. 6, (March 2010), pp. 75-81

Khaki, A.A. & Khaki, A. (2010b). Antioxidant effect of ginger to prevents lead-induced liver tissue apoptosis in rat. *Journal of Medicinal Plants Research,* Vol. 4, No. 14, (July 2010), pp. 1492-1495

Lai, P.K. & Roy, J. (2004). Antimicrobial and chemopreventive properties of herbs and spices. *Current Medicinal Chemistry,* Vol.11, No.11 (June 2004), p.1451–60

Lee, I.M.; Cook, N.R. & Gaziano, J.M. (2005). Vitamin E in the primary prevention of cardiovascular disease and cancer: the Women's Health Study: a randomized controlled trial. *the Journal of the American Medical Association, Vol.* 294, No.1, (July 2005), p. 56–65

Lees, K.; Davalos, A.; Davis, S.; Diener, H.; Grotta, J.; Lyden, P.; Shuaib, A.; Ashwood, T.; Hardemark, H.; Wasiewski, W.; Emeribe, U. & Zivin, J. (2006). Additional outcomes and subgroup analyses of NXY-059 for acute ischemic stroke in the SAINT I trial. *Stroke,* Vol.37, No.12, (October 2006), p. 2970–8

Lenaz, Giorgio (2001). The Mitochondrial Production of Reactive Oxygen Species: Mechanisms and Implications in Human Pathology. *IUBMB Life,* Vol.52, No.3–5,(September 2001), p.159–64

Maiani, G.; Periago Castón, M.J. & Catasta, G. (2009). Carotenoids: Actual knowledge on food sources, intakes, stability and bioavailability and their protective role in humans. *Molecular Nutrition & Food Research,* Vol.53, No.2, (September 2009), p.S194-218

Market Study: Antioxidants. *Ceresana Research,* Available from http://www.ceresana.com/en/market-studies/additives/antioxidants

Mattill, H.A. (1947). Antioxidants. *Annual Review of Biochemistry* , Vol.16, p.177–92

Miller, R.A. & Britigan, B.E. (1997). Role of oxidants in microbial pathop. *Clinical Microbiology Reviews,* Vol.10, No.1,(January 1997), p.1-18

Morton, J. (1987). Jambolan, In: *Fruits of warm climates,* F.J. Morton, 375–378, Miami, FL

Nakabeppu, Y.; Sakumi, K.; Sakamoto, K.; Tsuchimoto, D.; Tsuzuki, T. & Nakatsu, Y. (2006). Mutagenesis and carcinogenesis caused by the oxidation of nucleic acids. *Biological Chemistry* , Vol.387, No.4, (April 2006), p. 373–9

Nassiri ,M.; Khaki, A.; Gharachurlu, Sh.; Ashtiani, H.R. & Rastegar, H. & Rezazadeh, Sh. (2009). Effects of Ginger on spermatogenesis in Streptozotocin-induced Diabetic Rat. *iranian journal of medical plants,* Vol.8, No.31, (June 2009), pp.118-125

Neumann, C.; Krause, D.; Carman, C.; Das, S.; Dubey, D.; Abraham, J.; Bronson, R.; Fujiwara, Y.; Orkin, S. & Van Etten, R. (2003). Essential role for the peroxiredoxin Prdx1 in erythrocyte antioxidant defence and tumour suppression. *Nature,* Vol.424, No.6948, (July 2003), p. 561–5

Noomrio, M.H. & Dahot, M.U. (1996). Nutritive value of Eugenia jambosa fruit. *Medical Journal of the Islamic World Academy of Sciences,* Vol. 9, No.1, pp. 9–12

Parsonage, D.; Youngblood, D.; Sarma, G.; Wood, Z.; Karplus, P. & Poole, L. (2005). Analysis of the link between enzymatic activity and oligomeric state in AhpC, a bacterial peroxiredoxin. *Biochemistry,* Vol.44, No.31, (August 2005), p.10583–92

Parving, H.; Mauer, M. & Ritz, E. (2007). Diabetic Nephropathy, In: *Brenner and Rector's The Kidney* (8th ed), B.M.Brenner, chap 36. Pa: Saunders Elsevier, Philadelphia

Prior, R.; Wu, X. & Schaich, K. (2005). Standardized methods for the determination of antioxidant capacity and phenolics in foods and dietary supplements. *Journal of Agricultural and Food Chemistry,* Vol.53, No.10, (May 2005), p. 4290–302

Raha, S. & Robinson, B.H. (2000). Mitochondria, oxygen free radicals, disease and ageing. *Trends in Biochemical Sciences,* Vol.25, No.10, (October 2000), p. 502–8

Schneider, C. (2005). Chemistry and biology of vitamin E. *Molecular Nutrition & Food Research,* Vol.49, No.1, (January 2005), p 7–30

Seifried, H.; McDonald, S.; Anderson, D.; Greenwald, P. & Milner, J. (2003). The antioxidant conundrum in cancer .*Cancer Reserch,* Vol.63, No.15, (August 2003), p.4295–8

Shahreari, Sh.; Khaki, A.; Ahmadi-Ashtiani, H.R.; Rezazadeh, Sh. & Rastegar, H. (2010). Effects of Danae racemosa on Testosterone Hormone in Experimental Diabetic Rats. *Iranian journal of medical plants,* Vol. 9, No. 35, (September 2010), pp. 114-119

Shanbhag, D.A. & Khandagale, A.N. (2011). Application of HPTLC in the standardization of a homoeopathic mother tincture of Syzygium jambolanum. *Journal of Chemical and Pharmaceutical Research,* Vol.3, pp. 395–401

Smirnoff, N. (2001). L-Ascorbic acid biosynthesis. *Vitamins and hormones,* Vol.61, p. 241–66

Shenkin, A. (2006). The key role of micronutrients. *Clinical Nutrition,* Vol.25, No.1, (February 2006), p 1–13

Sohal, R. (2002). Role of oxidative stress and protein oxidation in the aging process. *Free Radical Biology & Medicine,* Vol.33, No.1, (July 2002), p. 37–44

Sridhar, S.B.; Sheetal, U.D.; Pai, M.R.S.M. & Shastri, M.S. (2005). Proclinical evaluation of the anti diabetic effect of Eugenia jambolana seed powder in streptozotocin diabetes rats. *Brazilian Journal of Medical and Biological Research,* Vol. 38, pp. 463–468

Stadtman, E. (1992). Protein oxidation and aging. *Science,* Vol.257, No.5074,(Agust 1992), p. 1220–4

Stohs, S. & Bagchi, D. (1995). Oxidative mechanisms in the toxicity of metal ions. *Free Radical Biology and Medicine,* Vol.18, No.2,(February 1995), p. 321–36

Szabó, I.; Bergantino, E. & Giacometti, G.M. (2005). Light and oxygenic photosynthesis: Energy dissipation as a protection mechanism against photo-oxidation. *EMBO reports,* Vol.6, No.7, (July 2005), p. 629–34

Talalay, P. & Talalay, P. (2001). The importance of using scientific principles in the development of medicinal agents from plants. *Academic Medicine,* Vol.76, No.3,(March 2001), p.238–47

Tapsell, L.C.; Hemphill, I. & Cobiac, L. *et al.* (2006). Health benefits of herbs and spices: the past, the present, the future. *The Medical Journal of Australia,* Vol.185, No.4, (August 2004), p.S4–24

Tschanz, D.W. (2003). Arab Roots of European Medicine .*Heart Views,* Vol.4, No.2, (June 2003), p.9

Valko, M.; Izakovic, M.; Mazur, M.; Rhodes, C.J. & Telser, J. (2004). Role of oxygen radicals in DNA damage and cancer incidence. *Molecular and Cellular Biochemistry,* Vol.266, No.1–2, (November 2004), p.37–56

Valko, M.; Leibfritz, D.; Moncol, J.; Cronin, M.; Mazur, M. & Telser, J. (2007). Free radicals and antioxidants in normal physiological functions and human disease. *The International Journal of Biochemistry & Cell Biology* , Vol.39, p. 44–84

Venturi, S.; Donati, F.M.; Venturi, A. & Venturi, M. (2000). Environmental Iodine Deficiency: A Challenge to the Evolution of Terrestrial Life?.*Thyroid*, Vol.10, No.8, (August 2000), p. 727-9

Vertuani, S.; Angusti, A. & Manfredini, S. (2004). The Antioxidants and Pro-Antioxidants Network: An Overview. *Current Pharmaceutical Design*, Vol.10, No.14, p.1677-94

Wolf & George .(2005). The discovery of the antioxidant function of vitamin E: The contribution of Henry A. Mattill. *The Journal of nutrition*, Vol.135 , No.3, (March 2005), p. 363-6

10

Potential Genotoxic and Cytotoxic Effects of Plant Extracts

Tülay Askin Celik
Adnan Menderes University, Faculty of Art and Science, Department of Biology, Aydin, Turkey

1. Introduction

The medicinal use of plants is probably as old as human kind itself. The World Health Organization (WHO) estimates that up to 80% of the world's population relies on traditional medicinal system for some aspect of primary health care (Farnsworth et al., 1985) and the traditional medicines are generally more acceptable from a cultural and spiritual perspective. Many of the plants species used for this purpose have been found to contain therapeutic substances which can be extracted and used in preparation of drugs, but the plant itself can also be used either directly or as an extract for medication, a practice that is particularly popular in developing countries (Ishii et al., 1984; Hoyos et al., 1992). Two hundred and fifty years ago there were few or no synthetic medicines and species of higher plants were the main source of medicines for the World (Duke, 2003). The method of discovery of medicines was probably trial and error that related the cause-and effect-relationship to the use of the plant or animal part and a desired result. People used to the whole plant or some part of the plant (leaves, bark, roots, seeds and fruits), animals, their organs and glands for the therapeutic purpose, e.g., cinchona bark, digitalis leaf, ephedra aerial parts, poppy capsule, hog testes, etc (http:/www.mosby.com/MERLIN/drug_card_update/history_drug_development.htm.)

Many of the drugs, which we use today are based on folk remedies and subsequent ethnopharmacological studies. There are more than 100 drugs of known structure that are extracted from higher plants and used in allopathic medicine (Cox, 1994; Fransworth, 1990). More than hundred years old drugs like morphine, digitalis and atropine are the time honoured remedies. Further, pharmaceutical preparations were discovered that were solid or aqueous, alcoholic or hydroalcoholic fluid extracts of soluble plant or animal constituents. During this period, the use of plants and animals or their parts were abandoned for the more concentrated extracts. Plant extracts can be used for scientific testing, to find out which nutrients or chemicals are present in the plant. Plant extracts are also used in some beauty products (shampoos, soaps, perfumes), medicines, or food flavoring (like vanilla extract). Different pharmaceutical dosage forms or preparations were originally designed to extract and concentrate the active drug principles like alkaloids, glycosides and volatile oils primarily from plants and used for therapy (http:/www.mosby.com/MERLIN/drug_card_update/history_drug_development.htm.) These preparations greatly decreased the dosage amount and showed increased therapeutic effects. These preparations were in the crude forms of plant or animal material and the main types of these preparations are described as below (Koul et al., 2005).

Plant extract preparations:

Aromatic waters: Saturated solutions of volatile plant oils or other volatile substances in water, e.g., rose water.

Decoctions: Soluble principles ofplant or animal parts extracted with boiling water, e.g., Terminalia decoction.

Elixirs: Aromatic and sweetened hydroalcoholic liquids that contain one or more ingredients, e.g., cinchona alkaloid elixir.

Extracts: These are primarily semisolids or solids obtained by extracting the active principles from plant or animal parts with a suitable solvent and allowing the solvent to evaporate, e.g., belladonna and liver extract.

Fluid extracts: Alcoholic or hydroalcoholic extracts from plant principles in which 1 ml of fluid extract is obtained from 1g of plant, e.g., gelsemium fluid extract.

Infusions: Soluble plant principles extracted by soaking the plant in hot water, e.g., digitalis infusion.

Liniments: Liquid preparations containing drug(s) applied to the skin with rubbing, e.g., camphor and belladonna liniment.

Mixtures: Aqueous suspensions intended for oral administration that contain insoluble drug(s).

Ointments: Semisolid preparations of drug(s) in a greasy base that liquefy after application to the skin.

Powders: Solid mixtures of finely powdered drugs intended for oral use.

Tinctures: Alcoholic or hydroalcoholic extracts made from 10 to 20 g of dried plant per 100 ml, e.g., tincture of belladonna (http:/www.mosby.com/MERLIN/drug_card_update/history_drug_development.htm.)

For safety, do not ingest any extract you make, since you do not know which chemicals are present in the plant and many plant chemicals are poisonous.

In the last years, the use of plant extracts, as well as other alternative forms of medical treatments, is enjoying great popularity all over the world. Aromatic plants have been used for generations not simply as food ingredients but also to treat a plethora of ailments and, in recent times, scientific data are accumulating that demonstrate for many herbs and related essential oils medicinal properties useful in the prevention of diseases or in the relieve of their symptoms (Tognolini et al., 2006). Essential oils, mixtures of natural volatile compounds deriving from plant secondary metabolism, mainly monoterpenes, sesquiterpenes, and their oxygenated derivatives (alcohols, aldehydes, esters, ethers, ketones, phenols and oxides), are isolated by steam distillation and have been known since antiquity to possess antibacterial and antifungal properties (Lopes-Lutz et al., in press).

Generally, the oil composition is a balance of various compounds, although in many species one constituent may prevail over all others. Changes in the essential oil compositions might arise from several environmental, chemical, seasonal, geographical and genetic differences (Delamare et al., 2007). Essential oils antimicrobial, antioxidant, anti-inflammatory, antispasmodic and relaxing properties have been described both in animals and humans (Tognolini et al., 2006).

Research laboratories worldwide have found literally thousands of phytochemicals which have *in vitro* inhibitory effects on all types of organisms. These *in vitro* screening programs, using the ethnobotanical approach, are important in validating the traditional use of herbal remedies and for providing leads in the search for new active substances. Whereas activity identified by an *in vitro* test does not necessarily confirm that a plant extract is an effective medicine, nor a suitable candidate for drug development, it does provide basic understanding of a plant efficacy and in some cases toxicity. However, more of these compounds should be subjected to animal and human studies to determine their effectiveness in whole organism systems, including particular toxicity studies as well as an evaluation of their effects on normal microbiota. The non prescription use of medicinal plants is cited today as an important health problem, in particular their toxicity to the kidneys (Mendonça-Filho, 2006).

A number of aromatic medicinal plants used for treating infectious diseases have been mentioned in different phytotherapy manuals due to their availability, fewer side effects, and reduced toxicity (Almeida et al., 2006).

Although, essential oil of oregano and its component carvacrol slightly increased the incidence of apoptotic cell death, they showed extensive antimicrobial activity even at lower concentrations (Dusan et al., 2006). Relatively high cytotoxicity was demonstrated by thyme oil, which increased both apoptotic and necrotic cell death incidence.

2. Crude extracts

Traditional medicines differ from the modern medicines in that the starting point is a history of observation of the effects of plant or animal materials on humans, and it uses crude extracts that are complex mixtures of naturally- occurring compounds, as opposed to single pure compounds of synthetic origin. Now there is increasing evidence that many current chemically synthesized medicines simply suppress symptoms of the diseases and ignore the underlying causes. In contrast traditional medicines, including herbal and glandular products, appear to address the cause of many diseases and yield superior clinical results. Therefore, crude plant extracts in the form of decoction, infusion or tincture are traditionally more used by the population for the treatment of several diseases, as well as an antiinflammatory and healing agent (Holetz et al., 2005). As a general rule crude therapeutic products are less toxic than their synthetic counterparts because they contain the total family of medicinal compounds (known and unknown) just as they are found in their natural source and hence offer less risk of side effects. In crude preparations, perhaps, the other components that are present in addition to the active components may be affecting the effects of the active components. These known and unknown components might be acting as synergists for the therapeutic effects and antagonists for the side effects of the active components as well as the other toxic components in the crude preparation (Koul et al.,

2005). They may be involved in the gastrointestinal absorption and determination of target sites for the active components too. Also it has been reported that most of botanical dietary supplements often contain complex mixtures of phytochemicals that have additive or synergistic interactions. For example, the tea catechins include a group of related compounds with effects that are demonstrable beyond those that are seen with epigallocatechin gallate, the most potent catechin. The metabolism of families of related compounds may be different than the metabolism of purified crystallized compounds (Heber, 2003).

It is generally accepted that the active principles (whether natural or synthesized) may be more toxic than the whole extract or its crude form (Saxena, 1985). Perhaps other ingredients present in the crude extract modulate the toxicity of the active principle. The Ayurvedic remedy worked almost as well as the conventional drug but with fewer side effects (Brown, 1995).Sharma et al., (2000) have reported the protective effect of crude, *Emblica myrobalan, Emblica officinalis* Gaertn. (Hindi: Amla) extract and its major active component ascorbic acid on the in vivo clastogenicity of two chemicals namely Benzo(a)pyrene (a well-known carcinogen) and Cyclophosphamide (an anticancer drug) in mice. The extent of chromosomal aberrations (CAs) and the frequencies of micronucleated polychromatic erythrocytes (MnPCEs) were taken as an index of clastogenecity in their investigation. They observed that the crude extract of amla showed a higher protection than its principle component, ascorbic acid. Ascorbic acid alone did not show any significant inhibitory effect on CAs or MnPCEs induced either by Benzo(a)pyrene or Cyclophosphamide.

This clearly reflected that the inhibitory effects are related to the total activity of the crude extract, rather than that of a single major component (Sarkar et al., 1996). In fact, purified form of ascorbic acid has been reported to enhance the clastogenic and carcinogenic effects of some chemicals (Dhir et al., 1990). Rossner et al., (1988) observed ascorbic acid to be ineffective in reducing CAs in occupationally exposed workers. It has been reported that ascorbic acid has a non-significant effect on the antioxidant defense system in mice, whereas the crude amla extract do enhance the reduced glutathione contents as well as the activities of glutathione-S-transferase, glutathione reductase and glutathione peroxidase, suggesting that the anti- oxidant activity is mainly due to the presence of other compounds present in amla (Jeena et al., 1999; Sharma et al., 2000). Ascorbic acid has also been shown to antagonize the toxic effects of certain metallic salts in mammalian systems as well as (Chakrabarty, 1977). However, studies performed with equivalent amount of synthetic ascorbic acid as present in crude fruit extract showed that it was not as effective as the extract in reducing the metal toxicity in mice (Dhir et al.,1990, 1991).

3. Toxicity risk of plant extract

The belief that natural medicines are much safer than synthetic drugs has caused exceptional growth in human exposure to natural products, as plants, phytotherapeutic agents, and phytopharmaceutical products. This fact has lead to a resurgence of scientific interest in their biological effects. In most countries there is no universal regulatory system insuring the safety and activity of natural products and they had not been sufficiently investigated analytically or toxicologically (Valerio Jr.&Gonzales, 2005). Herbal medicines can be potentially toxic to human health. In this way, scientific research has shown that many plants used in traditional and folk medicine are potentially toxic, mutagenic, and carcinogenic (Mengs, 1988., Ferreira-Machado et al, 2004).

Based on their long-term use by humans, one might expect herbs used in traditional medicine to have low toxicity. Nevertheless, some of them can cause adverse effects or have the potential to interact with other medications (Zink&Chaffin, 1998); moreover, there is little information on the potential risk to health of such herbs (Basaran et al., 1996). Recent investigations have revealed that many plants used as food or in traditional medicine have mutagenic, cytotoxic and genotoxic effects in vitro and in vivo assays (Plewa&Wagner, 1993; Higashimoto et al., 1993; Schimmer et al., 1994; Zink&Chaffin, 1998). This raises concern about the potential mutagenic or genotoxic hazards resulting from the long-term use of such plants and their use has been correlated with high rate of tumor formation in some human populations (Schimmer et al., 1994; Askin Celik&Aslanturk, 2007a; Ames, 1986; De Śa Ferreira & Ferrãro Vargas, 1999; Wynder et al., 1983). Assessment of the potential genotoxicity of traditional medicines is indeed an important issue as damage to the genetic material may lead to critical mutations and therefore also to an increased risk of cancer and other diseases. Direct interaction between a DNA-reactive agent and DNA is one of several pathways that may lead to primary DNA damage, because major end-points measured in the comet assay such as DNA strand breaks (which could also reflect repair incisions) and alkali-labile sites may also follow from other more indirect events such as cytotoxicity. A situation where DNA damage appears without concomitant cytotoxicity is then obviously of greater concern than a situation where DNA damage only occurs when there are simultaneous overt signs of cytotoxicity (Galloway et al., 1998; Galloway, 2000), and this is true also when evaluating the potential DNA damaging effects of plant extracts containing a plethora of more or less potent bioactive compounds (Demma et al., 2009).

The continuing growth in human exposure to natural products originating from traditional medicines has led to a resurgence of the scientific interest in their biological effects. Its scientific perspective deals with the search for various active components and understanding its mechanism of action to encourage the medicinal use. Under certain conditions, plant products may induce mutagenic, genotoxic and cytotoxic effects, due to the presence of multiple biological properties. Specific biological action of a drug is due to its specific binding to a functional molecular receptor. In complex plant extracts, the variable observed effects can be attributed to the many chemically reactive species that are formed during the processing and ingestion of the extract, which could act as non-specific redox agents, scavengers of free radicals, and ligands for binding to toxicants. The final effects are obviously the outcome of interactions between the components and their individual and collective interaction with the toxicant. The specificity and efficacy of such responses will be influenced also by the physiological factors influencing the plants and the process of administration of the extract.

4. Plant extracts as genotoxic agents

In screening for genotoxic and cytotoxic effects, extracts of different plant parts have been used, ranging from leafy vegetables, fruits, and underground storage organs to whole plants. The extracts were prepared mainly in water or organic solvents. Several of these assays have indicated the involvement of certain factors that are intrinsic components of the extracts, ranging from specific compounds like ascorbic acid to vegetable fibres which could act as nonspecific redox agents, free radical scavengers, or ligands for binding metals or toxic principles. The possible ways in which inhibitors of genotoxic agents can act include the inhibition of interaction between genes and biochemically reactive genotoxic agent and the inhibition of metabolic activation of indirectly acting toxicants. Human cells are continuously subjected to physiological and external influences which can give rise to cytotoxic, genotoxic and oxidative damage. However, cells have sophisticated mechanisms for counteracting and minimizing these types of damage. In recent years there has been increasing understanding that dietary patterns and constituents can modulate these forms of toxicity in cells. A considerable body of epidemiological evidence indicates that diets high in fruit and vegetables are inversely related to risk of chronic, degenerative diseases such as coronary heart disease and certain cancers. Much research effort has focused on the identification of phytochemicals in fruit and vegetables that exert beneficial effects and elucidation of the mechanisms by which they inhibit cellular injury and degeneration (Sarkar et al., 2008).

Various experimental systems (e.g. membrane systems, plant test systems, cell culture, animal models, human (clinical trials) are used to study the bioactivity of these plant derived compounds. The assessment of the efficacy and safety profiles of the medicinal plants should be based on scientific evidence-based approaches including, for example, different types of well established short-term tests when evaluating the genotoxic profile of such plants. The short term tests for genotoxicity and cytotoxicity are typically used to identify potential mutagens and carcinogens, but the same methods can also be used to identify anti-genotoxic agents. The effects of toxicants can be observed at the level of chromosomes (clastogenesis) through alterations in chromosome structure (chromosomal aberrations) and number (aneuploidy, polyploidy). A wide range of short-term and long-term screening procedures is available. The most common ones use higher plants or rodents in vivo as test systems for monitoring chromosomal aberrations. Experiments with a number of crude vegetable and fruit extracts have demonstrated their anticlastogenic activities against known genotoxic agents. The individual components of the extracts—e.g., sulfhydryl and flavonoid compounds, gallic acid, ellagic acid, mucic acid, citric acid, reducing sugars, tannin—are observed to have an additive interaction with the major constituents chlorophyll and ascorbic acid, when modulating the effects of the clastogens (Leme&Marin-Morales, 2009).

An increase in chromosomal aberrations may result from interactions of a great variety of chemical agents with DNA. According to Ishidate et al. (1988), the agents which induce an increase in the chromosomal aberrations (CA) frequency by direct or indirect mechanism may also be cytotoxic, for damage to both DNA and other cell targets (enzymes, membranes, structural proteins). CA and SCE are extremely valuable and highly relevant endpoints for the detection of potential carcinogens (Swierenga et al., 1991). Chromosomal aberrations are changes in chromosome structure resulting from a break or exchange of chromosomal material. Most of the CA observed in cells are lethal, but there are many corresponding aberrations that are viable and can cause genetic effects, either somatic or inherited (Swierenga et al., 1991).

Mitotic and replication indexes are used as indicators of adequate cell proliferation biomarkers. MI measures the proportion of cells in the M-phase of the cell cycle and its inhibition could be considered as cellular death or a delay in the cell proliferation kinetics

(Rojas et al., 1993). A cytotoxic effect of both medicinal herbs was observed, evidenced by the decrease of the MI (Gadano et al., 2006).

5. Plant extracts as cytotoxic agents

Low concentrations of tobacco leaf extract exerted a stimulating effect, whereas high concentration acted as a mitodepressant, on root-tip cells of *Allium sativum* L. (Sopova et al., 1983). Stronger concentrations of extract of immature *Solanum nigrum* L. fruits reduced the intensity of mitosis in *A. sativum* L., whereas weaker concentrations stimulated it. The presence of a cytokinin-like substance in the extract has been suggested to be responsible (Krivokapic et al., 1970). Extracts of leaves and inflorescences of male spinach and aster plants increased the frequency of chromosomal aberrations and mutations in Welsh onion and barley, respectively, whereas the female plants inhibited the processes (Sidorskii, 1984). Cellular damage including heavy pycnosis, clumping of chromosomes, fragmentation, and spindle disturbances in *Allium cepa* L. root meristem were induced by the leaf extract of *Ricinus communis* L. (George & Geethamma, 1990). Abraham and Cherian (1978) investigated the cellular changes produced by extracts of betel leaves on root tip cells of onion and demonstrated the cytotoxicity of such extracts. Chromosome-breaking activity has been exhibited by aqueous extract of mushroom (*Paxillus involutus*) in dry and pre-soaked seeds of *Nigella damascena* L. (Gilot-delhalle et al., 1991).

Extracts of *Vicia faba* L. roots and leaves and *Zea mays* L. leaves were compared for their ability to induce chromosomal aberrations and sister-chromatid exchanges in *Chinese hamster* ovarian cells and human lymphocytes. Both the extracts induced CAs in both systems; however, maize extract was more potent than *Vicia* extract (Kanaya et al., 1992). Aqueous extract of *Heliotropium curassavicum* L., though employed widely in therapeutics, has been found to induce chromosomal aberrations and anaphase delay in CHO cell line. This toxic effect was associated with the pyrrolidizing alkaloids and the N- oxides, which are changed into pyrrolic derivatives through a process of in vitro metabolism (Carballo et al., 1992).

As mentioned earlier, extensive use is made of plant products in traditional systems of medicine and as part of life style. A limited screening of some of these products indicates a combination of effects. Chili and its pure alkaloid capsaicin, and ginger and its phenolics gingerol and shogaol are mutagenic. Turmeric (*Curcuma longa* L.) and its pure components are non-mutagenic and suppress the mutagenicity of chili and capsaicin and also of several mutagens and carcinogens such as tobacco, cigarette, and benzo(a)anthracene. A diet that included 1% turmeric reduced BaP-and DMBA-induced stomach tumours and spontaneous mammary tumours in mice (Nagabhushan & Bhide, 1985; Nagabhushan et al., 1987a, 1987b). Crude aqueous extracts of *Areca catechu* L. and *Nicotiana tabacum* L. leaf given separately were mitogenic and also increased nuclear DNA content. Tobacco, in any combination of chewing mixture, induced duration-dependent clastogenicity. The addition of high lime and betel leaf (*Piper betel* L.) to the quid reduced the degree of mitogenicity and induction of aneuploidy but was ineffective when both tobacco and areca nut were added to the quid (Sen et al., 1987, 1991).

Higher plants, even showing low concentrations of oxidase enzymes and alimitation in the substrate specification in relation to other organism groups, present consistent results that may serve as a warning to other biological systems, since the target is DNA, common to all organisms. Among the plant species, *Alium cepa and Vicia faba* have been used to evaluate DNA damages, such as chromosome aberrations and disturbances in the mitotic cycle. The mitotic index and some nuclear abnormalities are used to evaluate cytotoxicity, genotoxicity and analyze micronucleus to verify mutagenicity, of different chemicals. The mitotic index (MI), replication index (RI), and micronucleus (MN) analysis methods are cytogenetic tests that are used both in vivo and in vitro. MI measures the proportion of cells in the M-phase of the cell cycle and its inhibition could be considered as cellular death or delay in the cell proliferation kinetics (Rojas et al. 1993). RI measures cell division kinetics by counting the percent of cells in first, second, third or more metaphase (Holland et al. 2002). MI frequencies and RI values decreased with increasing extracts of *H. pallasii*, *H. plicatum* subsp. *polyphyllum*, *H. plicatum* subsp. *pseudoplicatum*, *H. goulandriorum (*Eroğlu et al., 2010*)*. This state can explain with two different mechanisms: cellular death and decreasing of cell divisions. The results point to cytotoxic as well as antiproliferative effects and suggest that extracts of these species. MN is a small extra nucleus separated from the main one, generated during cellular division by lagging chromosomes or by chromosome fragments. A negative correlation was observed between MN induction and cell proliferation; the higher the MN frequency detected in exposed individuals, the lower the values of nuclear division progression expressed as RI. In living creatures, which are exposed to a mutagen factor, the probability of formation of mitotic and meiotic defects is increased and the rate of MN could increase due to this increase (Ramalho et al. 1988). This may mean that cells with greater chromosomal damage may die before cell division or may be less capable to enter this phase (Santos-Mello *et al.*, 1974). Multiple MN as the result of the loss of large part of the genome impairs or even prevents cell division (Nath & Ong, 1990).

6. Plant extracts as clastogenic agent

Genotoxins can induce mutations in chromosomes (*clastogenesis*) or in a small number of base pairs (*mutagenesis*). Genotoxic agents include X-rays, natural carcinogens, some man-made products (e.g. acridine and vinyl chloride), and viruses. The effects of toxicants can be observed at the level of chromosomes (clastogenesis) through alterations in chromosome structure (chromosomal aberrations or CA) and number (aneuploidy, polyploidy). The clastogenic effects caused by the extracts from plant extracts species included anaphase/telophase bridges, chromosome fragments and sticky chromosome. Babich et al. (1997) reported that metaphases with sticky chromosomes lose their normal appearance and appear to have a sticky "surface" which causes chromosome agglomeration, possibly due to effects on chromatin and chromosome organization. Singh (2003) states that the presence of chromosome fragments is an indication of chromosome breaks, and can be a consequence of anaphase/telophase bridges.Many plant extracts and their active principles have been described and utilized as therapeutic agents. There is considerable interest in determining the risks that these products may pose to health, because many of these plants contain compounds which are known to cause diseases or even death in animals and humans. Thus, an assessment of their cytotoxic and mutagenic potential is necessary to ensure a relatively safe use of medicinal plants (Surh & Ferguson, 2003).

Plant test system is widely used for monitoring genotoxicity of chemicals because of many advantages such as low cost, easily available throughout the year, ease to handle, good chromosome condition for the study of chromosome damage and above all good correlation with other test systems. A wide range of short-term and long-term screening procedures is available. The most common ones use higher plants (*Allium cepa, Allium sativum, Vicia faba, Tradescantia virginiana)* or rodents (mice, rats) in vivo as test systems for monitoring chromosomal aberrations (Hsu, 1982; Kihlman, 1971; Levan, 1949; Naismith, 1987; Sharma & Sharma, 1989). Root tip cells of *V. faba* constitute an excellent system for such cytogenetic tests (Abraham & John 1989; Gowrisankar et al., 1993; John & Abraham 1991; Upadhya et al., 1996; Wuu & Grant 1967). However WHO (1971) and Committee 17 (1975) argued that a single test system is not sufficient to come to the conclusion that a particular agent is mutagenic or not. Moreover all these plants are internally used for treatment of various diseases (Sinha, 1996) posing definite risk if they contain toxic substances. Therefore further tests of these plants using mammalian test system were conducted. For examples, fifty percent ethanol extracts of *N. odorum* and S. *indicum,* dried and dissolved in PBS, induced significant increase in frequencies of bone marrow micronuclei, bone marrow chromosome aberrations and synaptonemal complex damages when given as i.p. injection to mice (in preparation) (Sobita & Bhagirath., 2005) . Confirmed mutagenicity on the one hand and medicinal importance on the other hand these plants have made it necessary to isolate the active priciples.

Human cells are continuously subjected to physiological and external influences which can give rise to cytotoxic, genotoxic and oxidative damage. However, cells have sophisticated mechanisms for counteracting and minimizing these types of dam age. In recent years there has been increasing understanding that dietary patterns and constituents can modulate these forms of toxicity in cells. A considerable body of epidemiological evidence indicates that diets high in fruit and vegetables are inversely related to risk of chronic, degenerative diseases such as coronary heart disease and certain cancers.Much research effort has focused on the identification of phytochemicals in fruit and vegetables that exert benefcial effects and elucidation of the mechanisms by which they inhibit cellular injury and degeneration. Various experimental systems (e.g. membrane systems, cell culture, animal models, human clinical trials) are used to study the bioactivity of these plant- derived compounds. There are, of course, advantages and limitations to all of these systems. Cell-culture models have a number of advantages over other experimental systems, including avoidance of ethical issues relating to animal or human studies, ability to cryopreserve cell lines, ability to conduct mechanistic studies at molecular level, ease of control of the experimental environment and cost (Walum et al, 1990).

However, cell-culture systems cannot replicate conditions found in the body, e.g. systemic functions such as the nervous and endocrine systems are missing. Thus control of cellular metabolism may be more constant in vitro and the cultured cells will not be fully representative of the tissue from which they were derived. Provided the limits of the model are appreciated, cell culture is a valuable, if not the most valuable, tool in biomedical science (O'Brien et al, 2000).

In vitro studies using leukocytes or cell lines are relatively rare. The genotoxicity of *P. granantum* has also been reported by Settheetham & Ishida (1995), who, using in vitro assays, showed that the administration of an aqueous pomegranate fruit peel extract induced apoptosis in human cells. On the contrary, Amorin (1995) did not observe genotoxic effect using MN assay in mouse treated orally with fruit aqueous extracts of this plant at dose of 1000 and 2000mg/kg b.w. The data presented here show that the *P. granatum* L. fruit hydroalcoholic extract can induce genetic damage at different expression levels: recombinogenic, mutagenic and clastogenic. These results indicate that the use of this extract carries a genetic risk and an analysis of the risk-benefit balance appears to be crucial (S´anchez-Lamar et al., 2008).

Carthamus lanatus L. (Asteraceae) is known as a plant of phytopharmaceutical importance with sedative, anti-tumor and interferon-inducing activities (Benedi et al., 1986; Yasuhuko et al., 1979). Recently, a variety of biological activities of *C. lanatus,* including antioxidant, antibacterial, anti- fungal activity and cytotoxicity were shown (Taskova et al., 2002, 2003; Mitova et al., 2003). Some data about the closely related *C. tinctorius* were reported. Ames test and Salmonella microsome reversion assay (Morimoto et al., 1982) showed a mutagenic effect of the water extract of *C. tinctorius* flowers, which was confirmed by Esmaili-rad et al. (1995). Yin et al. (1991) demonstrated that the water extract was negative in the Ames test but positive in the chromosomal aberration and micronucleus assay in mice. The results of Nobakht et al. (2000) indicated harmful effects on cellular growth and differentiation during the embryonic development.The clastogenic effect of total dichloromethane, methanol and water extracts, four bioactive fractions and three individual constituents from *Carthamus lanatus* aerial parts were evaluated in mice by bone marrow chromosome aberration assay with mitomycin C as positive control. Significant differences in the percentage of aberrant mitosis of the extracts were observed. The dichloromethane extract exhibited a considerable clastogenic effect and the water extract a negligible one. Different types of chromosome aberrations and time-dependant effects for the active fractions and individual compounds were found (Topashka-Ancheva et al., 2003).

Clastogenic i.e. chromosome damaging substances are present in the plasma of patients with a variety of pathological conditions accompanied by oxidative stress (Emerit, 2007). The formation of clastogenic factors (CF) and their damaging effects are mediated by superoxide, since superoxide dismutase is regularly protective. CF are produced via superoxide and stimulate the production of superoxide by monocytes and neutrophils. These results in a selfsustaining and longlasting process of clastogenesis, which may exceed the DNA repair system and ultimately lead to cancer (Emerit, 1994). An increased cancer risk is indeed observed in conditions accompanied by CF formation. These include irradiated persons, patients with chronic inflammatory diseases, HIV-infected persons and the chromosomal breakage syndromes ataxia telangiectasia, Bloom's syndrome and Fanconi's anemia. Biochemical analysis has identifi ed lipid peroxidation products, arachidonic acid metabolites, nucleotides of inosine and cytokines, in particular tumor necrosis factor alpha, as the clastogenic and also superoxide stimulating components of CF. Due to their chromosome damaging effects, these oxidants can be detected with classical cytogenetic techniques (Emerit, 2007).

When testing the potential DNA-damaging effects by pharmaceutical drugs and other chemicals, the test systems are generally based on experimental animals, bacteria or various kinds of transformed cells. The major objective of our in vitro studies is to improve the risk assessment regarding exposures to genotoxic agents. From point of view of risk assessment, it is important to differ between genotoxic carcinogens and other substances that increase the risk of cancer by other mechanisms. In the case of drug-induced oxidative DNA-changes, for instance, one can distinguish two different main groups of substances: those who cause various types of reactive oxygen radicals in the cells directly and those who cause oxidative stress indirectly, as a consequence of general cytotoxicity. The research of recent years has also shown that the DNA repair has a great impact on whether the DNA-damage is manifested as a mutation or not, and there is reason to believe that there is a great variation in individual sensitivity to genotoxic agents, due to individual differences in DNA repair, metabolic bioactivation/detoxification pattern and/or other defense mechanisms in the cells.

Specific biological action of a drug is due to its specific binding to a functional molecular receptor. In complex plant extracts, the variable observed effects can be attributed to the many chemically reactive species that are formed during the processing and ingestion of the extract, which could act as non-specific redox agents, scavengers of free radicals, and ligands for binding to toxicants. The final effects are obviously the outcome of interactions between the components and their individual and collective interaction with the toxicant. The specificity and efficacy of such responses will be influenced also by the physiological factors influencing the plants and the process of administration of the extract (Sarkar et al., 1996).

Much research effort has focused on the identification of phytochemicals in fruit and vegetables which exert beneficial effects. In a recent project, we are currently also evaluating the genotoxic and antigenotoxic effects of some plant extracts used in traditional medicine in Turkey, and in these studies we also include fractions of extracts and/or pure compounds from extracts. Our researches has focused on the cytoprotective, antioxidant and o cytotoxic and antigenotoxic effects of plant extracts in meristematic cell systems and human peripheral lymphocytes which is important in helping to understand the fundamental mechanisms of action of these compounds. Our data add to the body of evidence supporting dietary guidelines to increase fruit and vegetable intake. First, the potential beneficial effects of phytochemicals are demonstrated. For example, lycopene are reported to exhibit a wide variety of biological effects, including antioxidant and free-radical scavenging activities (Aslanturk & Aşkın Çelik, 2005, 2006). Secondly, we illustrate the use of meristematic cellular models to study plant extracts-induced genotoxicity and cytotoxicity (Aşkın Çelik & Aslanturk, 2007b, 2009a, 2009b, 2010; Özmen & Çelik Aşkın, 2007). However, working with crude extracts, also means working with complex mixtures of biologically active compounds. Some of the compounds in such a mixture can be cytotoxic and/or genotoxic, others can be cytoprotective and/or anti-genotoxic.

Our findings show that plant extracts evaluated have a genotoxic potential in vitro which calls for a more thorough safety evaluation. Such evaluation should include other endpoints of genotoxicity apart from DNA damage, and possibly also pure compounds. The inhibitory action tends to lower the active dose of genotoxic agents and the accelerating action raises it. The ultimate load of mutations is the result of interaction between these opposing forces, modified by a large number of exogenous and endogenous factors. Therefore, a comprehensive overview is needed before arriving at conclusions regarding the environmental safety of any new chemical. The determination of genetic biomarkers would help estimate the potential toxicity of medicinal herbs in order to regulate medicinal plant consumption, which would be an important measure of public health protection. Thus, caution regarding the indiscriminate use of medicinal plants by the population remains a necessity.

7. Acknowledgements

The author wish to thank Research Asisstant Dr. Özlem Sultan ASLANTÜRK for her helpful advice in this chapter.

8. References

Abraham, S. & Cherian,V. D. (1978). Studies on cellular damage by extracts of betel leaves used for chewing. *Cytologia*, 43, 203-208.

Abraham, S. & John, A.T. (1989). Clastogenic effects produced by black pepper in mitotic cells of *Vicia faba*. *Mut. Res.*, 224, 281-285.

Agarwal, K., Dhir, H., Sharma, A. & Talukder, G. (1989). Comparison of the modification of Ni and Pb clastogenicity by plant extract and essential metals. pp 1303-1311 in Anke, M., Baumann,W., Braunlick, H., Brauckner,C., Grappel,B.& Grun,M.eds., *Proceedings of the 6th International Trace Element Symposium*. Vol. 4. Friedrich-Schieler Universitat, Jena.

Almeida, C.F.C.B.R., Amorim, E.L.C.; Albuquerque, U.P. & Maia, M.B.S. (2006). Medicinal plants popularly used in the Xingó region - a semi-arid location in Northeastern Brazil. *J. Ethnobiol Ethnomed.*, 2, 1-7.

Amonkar, A. J. & Bhide, S.V. (1987a). Mutagenicity of gingerol and shagaol and antimutagenicity of zingerone in *Salmonella* microsome assay. *Cancer Lett.*, 36, 221-233.

Amorin, A. (1995). Test of mutagenesis in mice treated with aqueous extracts from *Punica granatum* L. *Revista Brasilena de Farmacia*, 74, 110–111.

Ames, B. N. (1986). Food constituents as a source of mutagens, carcinogens and anticarcinogens. in Genetic Toxicology of the Diet, I. *Knudsen, Ed.*, 55–62, Alan R. Liss, New York, NY, USA.

Askin Celik, T. & Aslanturk, O.S. (2007a). Cytotoxic and genotoxic effects of *Lavandula stoechas* aqueous extracts. *Biologia*, 62 (3), 292–296.

Aslantürk, Ö.S. & Çelik, T. (2005). Preventive effect of lycopene on chromosome aberrations in *Allium cepa*. *Pakistan Journal of Biological Sciences*, 8 (3), 482-486.

Aslantürk, Ö.S., & Çelik, T. (2006). Protective effect of lycopene on Ethyl Methane Sulfonate induced chromosome cberrations in *Allium cepa*. *Caryologia*, 59 (3), 220-225.

Aslantürk, Ö.S. & Aşkın Çelik, T. (2009b). Genotoxic and antimutagenic effects of *Capparis spinosa* L. on the *Allium cepa* L. root tip meristem cells. *Caryologia*, 62 (2), 114-123.

Aşkın Çelik, T. & Aslantürk, Ö.S. (2007b). Cytotoxic and genotoxic effects of *Lavandula stoechas* aqueous extracts. *Biologia*, 62(3), 292-296

Aşkın Çelik, T. & Aslantürk, Ö.S. (2009a). Investigation of cytotoxic genotoxic effects of *Ecballium elaterium* Juice based on Allium Test. *Methods and Findings in Experimental and Clinical Pharmacology*, 31 (9), 591-596.

Aşkın Çelik, T. & Aslantürk, Ö.S. (2010). Evaluation of Cytotoxicity and Genotoxicity of *Inula viscosa* Leaf Extracts with Allium Test. *Journal of Biomedicine and Biotechnology*, (doi: 10.1155/2010/189252).

Babich H, Segall MA.,Fox KD. (1997). The Allium test - A simple, eukaryote genotoxicity assay. *Am Biol Teach.*, 59:580-583.

Basaran, A. A., Yu, T.W., Plewa, M. J. & Anderson, D. (1996). An investigation of some Turkish herbal medicines in *Salmonella typhimurium* and in the COMET assay in human lymphocytes. *Teratogenesis Carcinogenesis and Mutagenesis*, 16 (2), 125–138.

Benedi J., Iglesias I., Manzanares J., & Zaragoza F.(1986). Preliminary pharmacological studies of *Carthamus lanatus* L. *Plant. Med. Phytother.*, 20,25-30.

Brito, M. T., Martinez, A. & Cadavid, N. F. C. (1990). Mutagenic activity in regional foods and beverages from the Venezuelan Andean region. *Mutation Research*, 243 (2), 115–120.

Brown, S.J. (1995) Mental health researchers explore Hindu herbs, Clin Psychiat News, 15.

Carballo, M., Mudry, M. D., Villamil, I. B. L. & Mo D'aquino. (1992). Genotoxic action of an aqueous extract of Heliotropium curassavicum vat. argentinum. *Mutation Res.*, 279, 245-253.

Chan, K. (2003). Some aspects of toxic contaminants in herbal medicines. *Chemosphere*, 52, 1361-1371.

Chakrabarty, D., Bhattacharya, A., Majumdar, K. & Chatterjee, G.C. (1977). Effect of chronic vanadium pentoxide administeration on L- ascorbic acid supplementation. Int *J Vit Nutr Res.*, 47, 81-86.

Committee-17, 1975. History and rationale of genetic toxicity testing: An impersonal, and sometimes personal view. *Science*, 187, 503-514.

Cox, P.A. (1994) Ciba Foundation Symposium, Chichester, John Wiley & Sons, 184, 25-44. Fransworth NR, *Ciba Foundation Symposium*, Chichester, John Wiley & Sons, 1990, 154, 221.

Delamare, A.P.L. Moschen-Pistorello, I.T., Artico, L., Atti- Serafini, L. & Echeverrigaray, S. (2007). Antibacterial activity of the essential oils of *Salvia officinalis* L. and *Salvia triloba* L. cultivated in South Brazil. *Food Chem.*,100, 603- 608.

Demma, J., Engidawork, E. & Hellman, B.(2009). Potential genotoxicity of plant extracts used in Ethiopian traditional medicine. *Journal of Ethnopharmacology*, 122(1), 136-142.

Dusan, F., Marián, S., Katarína, D. & Dobroslava, B. (2006). Essential oils--their antimicrobial activity against *Escherichia coli* and effect on intestinal cell viability. *Toxicology*, 20, 1435-1445.

Dhir, H., Roy, A. K., Sharma, A. & Talukder, G. (1990). Modification of clastogenicity of lead and aluminium in mouse bone marrow cells by dietary ingestion of *Phyllanthus emblica* fruit extract. *Mutation Res.*, 241, 305-312.

Dhir, H., Agarwal, K., Sharma, A. & Talukder, G. (1991). Modifying role of *Phyllanthus emblica* and ascorbic acid against nickel clastogenicity in mice. *Cancer Lett.*, 59, 9-18.

Duke, J.A. (1990). Promising phytomedicinals In: Advances in new crops, [J Janick and JE Simon (eds)] Timber Press, Portland, OR, 191 198.

D'Souza, A. V. & Bhide, S. V. (1987b). In vitro antimutagenicity of curcumin against environmental mutagens. *Food Chem. Toxicol.*, 25, 545-547.

Emerit, I. (1994). Reactive oxygen species, chromosome mutation and cancer: possible role of clastogenic factors in carcinogenesis. *Free Radic. Biol. Med.*, 16, 99–9.

Emerit, I. (2007). Clastogenic factors as potential biomarkers of increased superoxide production. *Biomarker Insights*, 2, 429- 438.

Eroğlu, H.E., Budak, Ü., Hamzaoğlu, E.,Aksoy, A., Albayrak, S. (2010). *In vitro* cytotoxıc effects of methanol extracts of sıx *Helichrysum* taxa used in traditional medicine. *Pak. J. Bot.*, 42(5), 3229-3237.

Esmaili-rad, S., Daneshvar, N., Rastegar-Lati, A. & Mahmoudian, M. (1995). Mutagenicity screening of food coloring agents (herbal and synthetic) with Ames test. In: *Proceedings of the 12th Iranian Congress of Physiology and Pharmacology*. IUMS Press. Teheran, 414.

Farnsworth, N.R., Akerele, O.O., Bingel, A.S., Soejarta, D.D. & Eno, Z. (1985). Medicinal plants in therapy. *Bulletin World Health Organisation*, 63, 965–981.

Fernandes De S´a Ferreira, I. C. Ferraro Vargas, V. M. 1999. Mutagenicity of medicinal plant extracts in *Salmonella*/microsome assay. Phytotherapy Research. 13(5), 397–400.

Ferreira-Machado, S. C., Rodrigues, M. P., Nunes, A. P. M., et al.(2004). "Genotoxic potentiality of aqueous extract prepared from *Chrysobalanus icaco* L. leaves," *Toxicology Letters*, 151(3), 481–487.

Galloway, S.M., Miller, J.E., Armstrong, M.J., Bean, C.L., Skopek, T.R., Nichols, W.W., (1998). DNA synthesis inhibition as an indirect mechanism of chromosome aberrations: comparison of DNA-reactive and non-DNA-reactive clastogens. *Mutation Research*. 400, 169 -186.

Gadano, A.B., Gurni, A.A., Carballo, M.A. (2006). Argentine folk medicine: Genotoxic effects of *Chenopodiaceae* family. *Journal of Ethnopharmacology*. 103, 246–251.

Galloway, S.M. (2000). Cytotoxicity and chromosome aberrations in vitro: Experience in industry and the case for an upper limit of toxicity in the aberration assay. *Environmental and Molecular Mutagenesis* 35, 191–201.

George, K. & Geethamma, S. (1990). Effects of leaf extract of *Ricinus communis* on *Allium cepa*. *Cytologia*, 55, 391-394.

Gilot-delhalle, J., Moutschen, J.& Moutschen-dahmen, M. (1991). Chromosome-breaking activity of extracts of the mushroom *Paxillus involutus* Fries ex Batsch. *Experientia*, 47, 282-284.

Gowrishanker, B. & Vivekananda, O.S. (1993). Cytotoxic effects of whisky on *Vicia faba* in vivo. *Nucleus*, 36 (1, 2), 62-65.

Heber, D. (2003). Herbal preparations for obesity: are they useful? *Prim Care*, 30 , 441-463.

Higashimoto, M., Purintrapiban, J., Kataoka, K et al., (1993). Mutagenicity and antimutagenicity of extracts of three spices and a medicinal plant in Thailand. *Mutation Research*, 303 (3), 135–142.

Holland, N., Duramad, P., Rothman, N. et al (2002). Micronucleus frequency and proliferation in human lymphocytes after exposure to herbicide 2, 4-dichlorophenoxyacetic acid in vitro and in vivo. *Mutat Res*, 521: 165–178

Holetz, R.B., Nakamura, T.U., Filho, B.P.D., Melllo, J.C.P., Diaz, J. A .M., Toledo, C.E.M. & Nakamura, C.V. (2005). Biological effects of extracts obtained from *Stryphnodendron adstringens on Herpetomonas samuelpessoai. Mem. Inst. Oswaldo Cruz*, v. 100, 4, 397-401.

Hoyos, L.S., Au, W.W., Heo, M.Y., Morris, D.L. & Legator, M.S. (1992). Evaluation of the genotoxic effects of a folk medicine, *Petiveria alliacea* (anamu). *Mutation Research*, 280, 29- 34.

Hsu, T. C., ed. (1982). Cytogenetic assays of environmental mutagens. Osmun Publ.

Ishii, R., Yoshikawa, H., Minakata, N.T., Komura, K. & Kada, T. (1984). Specificity of bioantimutagens in the plant kingdom. *Agricultural and Biological Chemistry*, 48, 2587-2591.

Ishidate, M., Hammois, M.C., Sofuni, T., (1988). A comparative analysis of data on the clastogenicity of 951 chemical substances tested in mammalian cell cultures. *Mutation Research*, 195, 151–213.

Ito, Y., Maeda, S., Souno, K., Ueda, N.& Sugiyama, T. (1984). Induction of hepatic glutathione S-transferase and suppression of 7,12-dimethybenz(a)anthracene-induced chromosome aberrations in rat bone marrow cells by Sudan III and related azo dyes. *J. Natl. Cancer Inst.*, 73, 177-183.

Jeena, K.J., Joy, K.L. & Kuttan, R. (1999). Effect of *Emblica officinalis, Phyllanthus amarus* and *Picrorrhiza kurroa* on N- nitroso-diethylamine induced hepato-carcinogenesis, *Cancer Lett.*, 136, 11-16.

John, A.T. & Abraham, S. (1991). Cytological changes produced by red pepper in mitotic cells of *Vicia faba* L. *Caryologia*, 44(3, 4), 325-331.

Joseph, A.A. Mosby's Nursing Drug Cards: The History of Drug Development, http://www.mosby.com/MERLIN/drug_card_update/history_drug_developmen t.htm.

Kanaya, N., Takehisa, S., Nicoloff, H., Nikolova, T. & Damianova, V. (1992). Plant extracts induce chromosome aberrations and sister-chromatid exchanges in Chinese hamster ovary cells and human lymphocytes. *Mutation Res.*, 281, 47-54.

Kassie, F., Parzefall, W., Musk, S et al., (1996). Genotoxic effects of crude juices from *Brassica* vegetables and juices and extracts from phytopharmaceutical preparations and spices of cruciferous plants origin in bacterial and mammalian cells. *Chemico-Biological Interactions*, 102 (1), 1–16.

Kihlman, B. A. (1971). Root tips for studying the effects of chemicals on chromosomes. Pp. 484-514 in A. Holleander, ed., *Chemical mutagens: Principles and methods for their detection*.Plenum, New York.

Kong, J.M., Goh, N.K., Chia, L.S. & Chia, T.F. (2003) Recent advances in traditional plant drugs and orchids. *Acta Pharmacol Sin.*, 24, 7-21.

Koul, A., Gangar, S.C. & Sandhir, V. (2005). Pitfalls in Journey from Traditional to Modern Medicine. *Natural Product Radiance*, 4 (1), January-February.

Krivokapic, K., Hadziselimovic, R.& Sofradzija, A. (1970). Effect of the extract from immature fruits of *Solanum nigrum* L.on the intensity of mitosis in *Allium sativum*. *Iugosl. Physiol. Pharmacol. Acta*, 6, 363-367.

Levan, A. (1949). The influence on chromosomes and mitosis of chemicals, as studied by the Allium test. Eighth International Congress on Genetics. *Hereditas* (suppl. vol.), 325-337.

Lopes-Lutz, D., Alviano, D.S., Alviano, C.S. & Kolodziejczyc, P.P. (2008). Screening of chemical composition, antimicrobial and antioxidant activities of *Artemisia* essential oils. *Phytomedicine*, 69 (8), 1732-1738

Mendonça-Filho, R.R. (2006). In: *Modern phytomedicine: turning medicinal plants into drugs Bioactive Phytocompounds: New Approaches in the Phytosciences*. (Ahmad, I., Aqil, F. and Owais, M., Eds.), WILEY-VCH Verlag GmbH & Co. KGaA, Weinheim, 1-24.

Mengs, U. (1988). "Toxiceffects of sennosides in laboratory animals and in vitro," *Pharmacology*, 36(1).180–187,

Morimoto, I., Watanabe, F., Osawa, T., Okitsu, T. & Kada, T. (1982). Mutagenicity screening of crude drugs with *Bacillus subtilis* resassay and *Salmonellas* micro-study on mutagenicity of microsome reversion assay. *Mutat. Res.*, 97, 81-102.

Nagabhushan, M. & Bhide, S. V. (1985). Mutagenicity of chilli extract and capsaicin in short-term tests. *Environm.Mutagen*, 7, 881-888.

Nagao, M., Wakabayashi, K., Fujita, Y., Tahira, T., Ochiaia, T. & Sugimura, T. (1986). Mutagenic compounds in soy sauce, Chinese cabbage, coffee and herbal teas. In: *Genetic Toxicology of theDiet*, I. Knudsen, Ed., 55–62, Alan R. Liss, New York, NY, USA.

Naismith, R. W. (1987). Guidelines for minimal criteria of acceptability for selected short-term assays for genotoxicity. *Mutation Res.*, 189, 181-183.

Nath, C.J. & T. Ong. (1990). Micronuclei assay in cytokinesis-blocked binucleated and conventional mononucleated methods in human peripheral lymphocytes. *Teratogen Carcin Mutagen.*, 10, 273-279.

Nguyen, T., Fluss, L., Hodej, R., Ginther, G. & Leighton, T. (1989). The distribution of mutagenic activity in red rose and White wines. *Mutation Research*, 223, 205–212.

Nobakht, M., Fattahi, M., Hoormand, M., Milanian, I., Rahbar, N. & Mahmoudian M. (2000). A study on the teratogenic and cytotoxic effects of safflower extract. J. *Ethnopharmacol.*, 73, 453- 459.

O'Brien, N.M., Woods, J. A., Aherne S. A., O'Callaghan, Y. C. (2000). Cytotoxicity, genotoxicity and oxidative reactions in cell-culture models: modulatory effects of phytochemicals. *Biochemical Society Transactions.*, 28 (2), 22-26.

Özmen, A. & Çelik Aşkın, T. (2007). Cytotoxic Effects of Peel Extracts from *Citrus Limon* and *Citrus sinensis*. *Caryologia*, 60 (1-2), 48-51.

Plewa, M. J. & Wagner E. D. 1993. Activation of promutagens by green plants. *Annual Review of Genetics*, 27, 93–113.

Ramalho, A., Sunjevaric. I., Natarajan, A.T.(1988). Use of the frequencies of micronuclei as quantitative indicators of X-ray-induced chromosomal aberrations in human peripheral blood lymphocytes: comparison of two methods. *Mutat Res*, 207:141–146

Rojas, E., Herrera, L.A., Sordo, M., Gonsebatt, M.E., Montero, R., Rodriguez, R., Ostrosky-Wegman, P., (1993). Mitotic index and cell proliferation kinetics for the identification of antineoplastic activity. *Anticancer Drugs*, 4, 637–640.

Rossner, P., Cerna, M., Pokorna, D., Hajek, V. & Petr, J. (1988). Effect of ascorbic acid prophylaxis on the frequency of chromosome aberrations, urine mutagenicity and nucleolus test in workers occupationally exposed to cytostatic drugs. *Mutat Res.*, , 208 (3-4), 149-153.

S´anchez-Lamar, A., Fonseca, G., Luis Fuentes, J ., Cozzi, R., Cundari, E., Fiore,M., Degrassi, F., Ricordy,R., Perticone R. & De Salvia, D. (2008) Assessment of the genotoxic risk of *Punica granatum* L. (*Punicaceae*) whole fruit extracts. *Journal of Ethnopharmacology*, 115, 416–422.

Santos-Mello, R., D. Kwan and A. Norman. (1974). Chromosome aberrations and T-cell survival in human lymphocytes. *Radiat Res.*, 60, 482-488.

Sarkar, D. (1992). Protective effect of crude extract of *Phyllanthus emblica* L. against the cytotoxicity of chlordane in mice in vivo. *Perspect. Cytol.Genet.*, 7, 1035-1042.

Sarkar, D., Sharma, A. & Talukder, G. (2008). Plant extracts as modulators of genotoxic effects. *The Botanical Review*, 62(4), 275-300.

Saxena, R.C. (1985). Drug reactions with herbal drugs, *Indian J Pharmacol.*, 17, 165-169.

Schimmer, O., Kruger, A., Paulini, H. & Haefele, F. (1994). An evaluation of 55 commercial plant extracts in the Ames mutagenicity test. *Pharmazie*, 49 (6), 448–451.

Sen, S., Talukder, G. & Sharma, A. (1987). Potentiation of betel-induced alterations of mouse glandular stomach mucosa by tobacco in studies simulating betel addiction. *Intl. J. Crude Drug Res.*, 25, 209-215.

Sen, S., Talukder, G. & Sharma, A. (1991). Betel cytotoxicity: further evidence from mouse bone marrow cells. *Intl. J. Pharmacog.*, 29, 130-140.

Sharma, A., & A. K. Sharma. (1989). Genetic toxicology testing of hazardous materials and wastes. Pages 281-293 In: Majumdar, S. K., Miller, E. W. & Schmalz, R. F., eds., *Management of hazardous materials and wastes: treatment, minimization and environmental effects*. Pennsylvania Academy of Sciences, Harrisburg.

Sharma, N., Trikha, P., Athar, M. & Raisuddin, S. (2000). Inhibitory effect of *Emblica officinalis* on the in vivo clastogenicity of benzo[a]pyrene and cyclophosphamide in mice. *Hum Exp Toxicol.*, 19, 377-384.

Sidorskii, A. G. (1984). Effects of extracts from vegetative and generative organs of dioecious plants on the frequency of mutagen-induced chromosome aberrations and mutagenesis in plants. *Genetika*, 20, 1507-1510.

Singh, R.J. (2003). *Plant cytogenetics*. Pp. 463, CRC Press, Boca Raton,.

Sobita, K. & Bhagirath, T.H. (2005). Effects of some medicinal plant extracts on *Vicia faba* root tip chromosomes. *Caryologia*, 58(3), 255-261.

Sopova, M., Sekovski, Z.& Jovanovska, M. (1983). Cytological effects of tobacco leaf extract on root-tip cells of *Allium sativum*. *Acta Biol. Med. Exp.*, 8, 49-56.

Surh, Y. & Ferguson, L.R. (2003). Dietary and medicinal antimutagens and anticarcinogens: Molecular mechanisms and chemopreventive potential - highlights of a symposium. *Mutat. Res.*, 523-524, 1-8.

Swierenga, S.H.H., Heddle, J.A., Sigal, E.A., Gilman, J.P.W., Brillinger, R.L., Douglas, G.R., Nestmann, E.R. (1991). Recommended protocols based on a survey of current practice in genotoxicity testing laboratories. IV. Chromosome aberrations and sister-chromatid exchange in Chinese hamster ovary, V79 Chinese hamster lung and human lymphocyte cultures. Mutation Research, 246, 301–322.

Taskova, R., Mitova, M., Najdenski, H., Tzvetkova, I. & Duddeck, H. (2002). Antimicrobial activity and cytotoxicity of *Carthamus lanatus*. *Fitoterapia*, 73, 540-543.

Tognolini, M., Barocelli, E., Ballabeni, V., Bruni, R., Bianch, A.,Chiavarini, M. & Impecciatore, M. (2006). Comparative screening of plant essential oils: Phenylpropanoid moiety as basic core for antiplatelet activity. *Life Science*, 78, 1419-1432.

Topashka-Anchevaa, M., Taskovab, R., Handjievac, N., Mikhovac, B., Duddeckd, H. (2003). Clastogenic Effect of *Carthamus lanatus* L. (Asteraceae).*Verlag der Zeitschrift für Naturforschung*, Tübingen http://www.znaturforsch.com

Upadhya, T.T., Daniel, T., Sudalai, A., Ravindraanthan, T., and Sabu, K.R. (1996) Natural kaolinitic clay: A mild and efficient catalyst for the tetrahydropyranylation and trimethylsilylation of alcohols. *Synthetic FCommunications*, 26, 4539-4544.

Valerio Jr, G., Gonzales, G. F. (2005). "Toxicological aspects of the South American herbs cat's claw (*Uncaria tomentosa*) and maca (*Lepidium meyenii*): a critical synopsis," Toxicological Reviews, 24(1), 11–35.

Walum, E., Stenberg, K. and Jenssen, D. (1990). Understanding Cell Toxicology, Ellis Horwood, London

World Health Organization. (1971).Technical report no. 482.

Wuu, K.D. & Grant, W.F. (1967). Chromosomal aberrations induced in somatic cells of *Vicia fava* by pesticides. *Nucleus*, 10(1), 37-46.

Wynder, E. L., Hall, N. E. L. & Polansky, M. (1983). Epidemiology of coffee and pancreatic cancer. *Cancer Research*, 43 (8), 3900–3906.

Yasuhuko, K., Kanagawa, Y., Seishi, K., & Takashii H. (1979). Wasserlöslicher Interferoninduktor, Verfahren zu seiner Gewinnung und dessen Verwendung. Ger Offen 3,004,018 Appl. 07 Feb.

Yin, X. J., Liu, D., Wang, H. C. & Zhou, Y. (1991). A study on mutagenicity of 102 raw pharmaceuticals used in Chinese traditional medicine. *Mutat. Res.*, 260, 73-82.

Zink, T. & Chaffin, J. (1998). Herbal health products: what family physicians need to know. *American Family Physician.*, 58 (5), 1133–1140.

http://herbalgram.org/naturemade/herbclip/review.asp?i=41574.

11

Searching for Analogues of the Natural Compound, Caffeic Acid Phenethyl Ester, with Chemprotective Activity

José Roberto Macías-Pérez[1], Olga Beltrán-Ramírez[2] and Saúl Villa-Treviño[1]
[1]*Department of Cell Biology, Cinvestav-IPN,*
[2]*Dirección de Investigación, Hospital Juárez de México,*
México, D.F.

1. Introduction

Cancer is a disease characterized by uncontrolled growth and division of genetically altered cells and its emergence requires several elements, including self-sufficiency in growth signals, insensitivity to growth-inhibitory signals, evasion of apoptosis, limitless replicative potential, tissue invasion and metastasis, and sustained angiogenesis (Hanahan and Weinberg, 2011). Cancer is thought to evolve along a multi-step process, cancer cells are the descendants of a normal cell in which some kind of internal or external stress causes a change in its genetic code. This event is said to "initiate" the cell to a precancerous state. In a second stage, this precancerous cell divides in response to a promoting agent to produce daughter cells, and these daughter cells divide to produce more daughter cells, and so on. The genetic instabilities passed down through the generations finally result in one cell that no longer requires the promoting agent to stimulate its proliferation, and a cancer cell is born with the ability to make proteins such as growth factors that stimulate proliferation. Finally in the third stage of carcinogenesis, progression, this cancer cells divides to produce daughter cells, these cells also divide, and soon there is a population of cancer cells with the ability to invade and metastasize (Vincent & Gatenby, 2008).

The study of liver cancer has been intensified in recent years. Hepatocellular carcinoma (HCC) is the most common hepatic cancer responsible for over one million deaths annually worldwide, the percentage of affected men compared to affected women varies between 2:1 and 4:1, depending on the geographic region (Naugler & Schwartz, 2008). The cause of HCC in most cases is the ongoing liver cell damage, so HCC occurs in persons with chronic liver disease, most often in the setting of cirrhosis but other risk factors are the infection with hepatitis type C and type B, consumption of mycotoxins such as aflatoxin, genetic and hormonal factors, obesity, and exposure to chemical carcinogens such as nitrosamines.

Early detection of HCC plays an important role to have more treatment options and chances of survival. Survival of lately diagnosed individuals is poor, surgical resection provides the only chance of cure, but it is not suitable for the majority of patients. For most patients, nonsurgical treatment is the only option. Therefore, the study of the origin of the disease and at the early stages of HCC is still of great interest to find methods of prevention, early diagnosis and treatment.

Chemoprotection involves the use of synthetic or natural compounds to inhibit slow or reverse carcinogenesis, is based on the hypothesis that the disruption of biological events involved in carcinogenesis will inhibit this process and can be applied to any stage of carcinogenesis. Chemoprotective compounds can act at any of the various stages of carcinogenesis. Those that block mutagenesis prior to tumor development can be considered antimutagens and by its mechanism are classified in four groups: **Bioantimutagens** are naturally occurring substances that reduce mutant yield by acting on the DNA repair or replicative processes. These compounds act after a DNA adduct has formed but before the DNA lesion is fixed into a mutation. An example of a bioantimutagen is vanillin, present in vanilla beans, which appears to enhance post-replication recombinational repair under certain conditions. **Desmutagens** encompass all agents that affect mutagenicity through mechanisms other than DNA repair or replication. These mechanisms include enzyme induction, mutagen scavenging, and blocking of mutagen activation. **Chemical Inactivaters and Enzymatic Modulators** are agents that prevent the formation of mutagens or their activation to more potent forms. And a final group, **Antioxidants and Free Radical Scavengers,** scavengers bond with mutagens to render the mutagen incapable of reacting with DNA, one class of chemicals that forms complexes with mutagenic compounds is the porphyrins, including chlorophyllin. Chlorophyllin inhibits the mutagenicity of a variety of dietary mixtures as well as individual large planar mutagens as aflatoxin B1 and benzo[a]pyrene. Antioxidants exert their effect by donating electrons to unstable oxygen species generated from endogenous processes or formed as a result of radiation or chemical exposure. Ascorbic acid (vitamin C) is an example of a water-soluble extracellular antioxidant with intriguing dual properties. On one hand, it quenches singlet oxygen and assorted free radicals; on the other hand, it preserves the function of reducing them back to active form after they have quenched free radicals. Carotenoids such as 5-carotene and lycopene illustrate lipid-based antioxidants (Kohlmeier et al., 1995).

2. Natural products with biological activities

Medicinal herbs have been used to treat diseases and this practice continues today worldwide. Chemoprotectors have often been detected when studying the effect of substances purified from extracts of natural products to which folk medicine has attributed therapeutic properties.

An example is Rhoeo discolor is a plant with extended use for treatment of commonly used to treat cancer, venereal diseases and superficial mycoses in Mexican traditional medicine. Rhoeo extract is antimutagenic for S. typhimurium strain TA102 pretreated with ROS generating mutagen norfloxacin in the Ames test, and protects liver cell cultures against N-diethylnitrosamine (DEN) induction of unscheduled DNA synthesis. Rhoeo extract showed similar radical scavenging effect to that of α-tocopherol and more than ascorbic acid. It is important to note that this extract was neither mutagenic in S. typhimurium nor genotoxic in liver cell culture, even at concentrations as high as 4 and 166 fold of those needed for maximal antimutagenic or chemoprotective activities (Gonzalez-Avila et al., 2003; Rosales-Reyes et al., 2008).

Sprague Dawely rats injected with methylnitrosourea MNU produced a variety of alterations ranging from severe inflammatory reaction in lung and skin to colon adenocarcinoma. There are an elevation of malondialdehyde (MDA) and nitric oxide (NO) in serum obtained from these rats. When is given to this rats a daily dose of Nigella grains with honey from bees after one week of MNU administration and for six months, this compounds protected 100% against MNU-induced oxidative stress, carcinogenesis and abolished the NO and MDA elevations (Mabrouk et al., 2002).

As in the case of honey, propolis has been known to mankind from the remotest of ancient times and has been widely used by many cultures for different purposes, among which its long history of use in herbal medicine traditions is included. Propolis is a complex resinous mixture gathered from plants and used by honeybees in their hives as a general-purpose sealer and antibiotic. This is a product of interest as much in the field of medicine as the pharmaceutical industry. It is attributed with numerous properties: it is an anti-flammatory agent, an immunostimulant, a hepatoprotector, a carcinostatic, it has anti-microbial, anti-viral, anti-fungal, antiprotozoan properties, and it is an anesthetic and a tissue regenerator. It has been demonstrated that Korean propolis, like the commercial type, induces apoptosis of human hepatoma cell lines. The ethanolic extract of propolis is a good inhibitor of mutagenicity and the methanolic extract presents cytotoxicity against murine colon 26-L5 carcinoma and human HT-1080 fibrosarcoma. It is suggested that propolis exerts a protective effect in colonic carcinogenesis, preventing the development of preneoplastic lesions, given that ethanolic extract administered after exposure to a cancerous agent (1,2 dimethylhydrazine), is strongly associated with a reduction in the number of aberrant crypts in the distal colon (Farré, 2004).

2.1 Active compounds in propolis

Patients are experimenting with natural compounds in their efforts to heal themselves of cancer, in different regions of the world is estimated that from 10 to 80 percent of cancer patients use some form of complementary medicine as part of their overall therapy. For many of these patients, a part of the complementary approach is the use of natural compounds, without the guidance of their oncologist or any real guidance from scientific studies. This is the reason to study natural compounds that can be used properly in the treatment of cancer (Boik, 2001).

Polyphenolic compounds are widely distributed in the plant kingdom and display a variety of biological activities, including chemoprevention and tumor growth inhibition. Propolis is made up of a variety of polyphenolic compounds, several of its isolated compounds have shown anti-carcinogenic activity, associated with the inhibition of the cellular cycle and the induction of apoptosis, as in the case of 3-2 acid (2-dimethyl 8.3 methyl 2-butenyl) benzopyran-6-propenoic or induced apoptosis without affecting the cellular cycle of cancerous cells, such as prenyl flavanone propolin A, which also shows antioxidant activity. It has been shown that the carbon prenylates of p-cummaric acid in Brazilian propolis act against hepatocarcinoma. Caffeic acid (CA) and caffeic acid phenethyl ester (CAPE), members of the polyphenolic compounds, are present in high concentrations in medicinal plants and propolis. CA and CAPE have been investigated for direct antitumor activity in vivo and in vitro. Orsolic et al, found that the local presence of CA and CAPE, by subcutaneous injection in the tumoral tissue, caused a significant delay in tumor formation and increased life span 29.3 to 51.73%, respectively. CA and CAPE, significantly suppressed human HeLa cervical carcinoma cell proliferation in vitro (Orsolic et al., 2005).

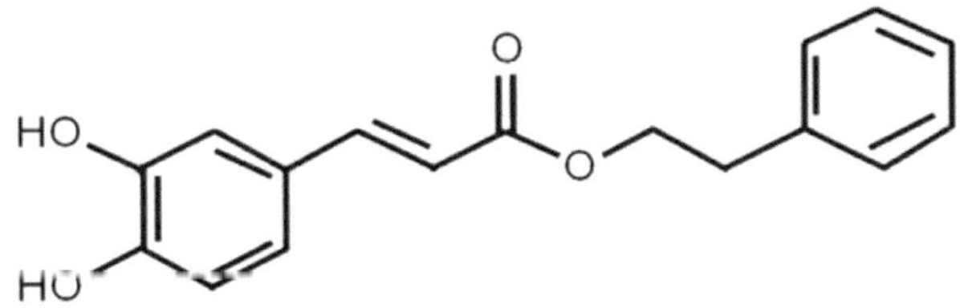

Fig. 1. CAPE

The CAPE [2-propenoic acid, 3-(3,4-dihydroxyphenyl)-, 2-phenethyl ester] is an active component of propolis with a wide variety of biological activities at non-toxic concentrations in mammals organisms. It has shown activities as antibacterial, anti-inflammatory, antioxidant, antitumor and antiproliferative. CAPE is chemopreventive against intestinal, colon and skin cancer, and has shown to decreases the formation of preneoplastic hepatic lesions when is administered on a rat model of liver carcinogenesis (Carrasco-Legleu et al., 2004; Carrasco-Legleu et al., 2006) but the mechanism for these properties is not completely known. Besides CAPE, other caffeic acid esters in propolis may have biological effects; here we focus on CAPE and structurally related compounds.

2.2 Analogues and derivatives

As well as CAPE, its analogues are widely distributed in the plant kingdom as in coffee, fruit and propolis. Analogue is a drug whose structure is related to another, but its chemical and biological properties may be different. The term "analogue" refers to chemical compounds with a close structural relationship to the parent compound. It includes compounds having a structural similarity, but one or more atoms in its structure have been replaced by others (Fischer & Ganellin, 2006; Nill, 2002; Wermuth, 2006).

Crude propolis itself is not an ideal source of CAPE because the concentration can vary greatly depending on the source of the propolis, CAPE is commonly present at 1 to 5 percent, but some propolis samples appear to contain none and such a standardized extract is not yet available commercially. Propolis can cause allergic dermatitis after topical contact in sensitive individuals, and oral administration may sensitize a person to this (Boik, 2001). One impediment to the widespread use of CAPE is that its extraction from natural products, is complex and with very low yields. In a similar way, by chemical synthesis, reaction together with purification methods require prolonged purification procedures and the yields range between 35 and 50%. And currently is commercially available only at high cost.

For this reason, molecules with structure related to the CAPE have been studied, seeking to obtain compounds that retain biological activity, as well as showing advantages of being cheap, and obtained quickly and easily. Currently the research for compounds with biological activity is supported on methodologies such as quantitative structure- activity relationship (QSAR) that aims to predict and optimize the biological activity, suggest a mode of action, classified according to biological activity, determine structural features of the molecule important for biological activity and reduce the experimental part. It is based in that biological activity is a function of chemical structure, chemical structure implies given properties that can be quantified using physicochemical parameters and there is always a function relating biological activity with changes in the properties. The QSAR methodology starts with a compound showing activity in relation to the desired therapeutic goal. Later in the learning phase is necessary to test an exploration series, which consists of a set of products with similar structure to the original compound but with variable substituents or fragments, which allows observation of the changes produced in their biological activity depending on the substituents. In the optimization phase, from data collected it is possible get a function that allows design the best combination of substituents to achieve optimal biological activity (Kubinyi, 1990).

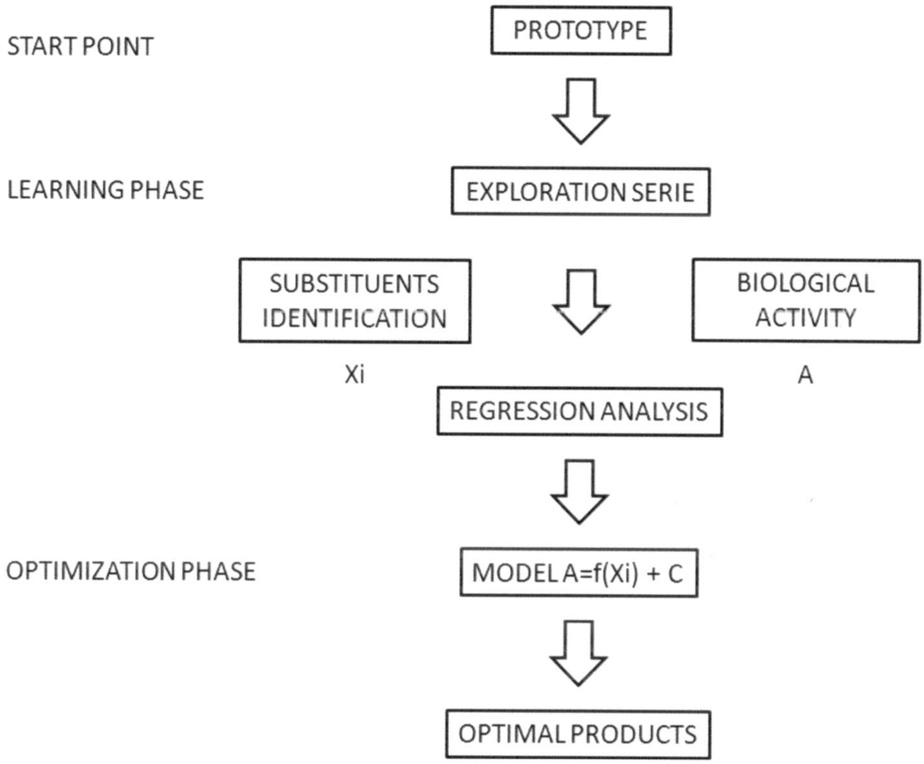

Fig. 2. QSAR methodology diagram

Several compounds structurally related to CAPE are simple derivatives including cinnamic acid amides, sugar esters and glycosides, or in more complex forms such as rosmarinic acid (caffeic acid dimer), litospermic acid (caffeic acid trimer), verbascoside (ester and glycoside heterosidic of dihydroxyphenetylethanol and caffeic acid) and derivatives linked to flavonoids (Jiang et al., 2005; Lin et al., 2005). Several publications have shown that many compounds structurally related to CAPE, preserve in different degree its biological activity, and these compounds are known by properties like antibacterial, anti-inflammatory, immunostimulatory, anti-atherosclerotic, neuroprotective, antiproliferative, antiviral and antioxidative (Chang et al., 2007; Natarajan et al., 1996; Son & Lewis, 2002; Uwai et al., 2008).

To obtain information about the molecular mechanism of CAPE chemoprevention, Natarajan et al. test the effect of CAPE on this transcription factor. U-937 cells were stimulated with Tumor Necrosis Factor-α (TNF-α), to induce Nuclear Factor Kappa B (NF-κB) activation and by Electrophoretic Mobility-Shift Assays (EMSA) of nuclear proteins they found that the activation of NF-κB by TNF-α is completely blocked by 2h preincubation with CAPE (25 μg/ml), and this effect was similar in an *in vivo* rat model (Carrasco-Legleu et al., 2004; García-Román et al., 2007; García-Román et al., 2008). It's worth mentioning that the role of the NF-κB in activities as antibacterial, anti-inflammatory, antioxidant, antitumor and antiproliferative, has been documented. Normally NF-κB is found in the cytoplasm in an inactive state held by an inhibitory subunit called NF-κB Inhibitor (IκB), with a steric impediment which stop the translocation to the nucleus. Several stimuli as cytokines IL 1 and TNF-α act over the membrane receptors, and activate a series of enzymes and proteins kynasa that fosforilate IκB. Fosforilated IκB and its subsequent degradation allow translocation of NF-κB to the nucleus, and triggers the transcription of widely gamma of genes. Following this line of thought, also were examined structural analogues of CAPE, these analogues have been previously characterized for their ability to inhibit human HIV integrase and cell growth (Burke et al., 1995), and although all the compounds were active in inhibiting NF-κB activation, there were marked variations in their inhibitory ability, they found that compounds 1 and 6 (Fig. 3) inhibited NF-κB translocation to the nucleus more efficiently that CAPE (line P) (Natarajan et al., 1996).

As result of structure activity relationship analysis they found that alteration of the hydroxyl group placement from 3,4-dihydroxy (CAPE) to 2,5-dihydroxy (compound 1) increased the potency of inhibition over that resulting from replacement of the hydroxyl groups of CAPE with two methyl ethers (compound 2) and the addition of a third hydroxyl group (compound 3) resulted in a loss of potency, with these analysis they suggest that the number and the placement of hydroxyl groups is a critical determinant of the extent of inhibition. In the ester group of analogues, the caffeic acid portion was held constant and the phenylethyl side chain was varied. An increase in the length of the alkyl chain (compound 4) resulted in a significant loss of inhibition. Bicyclic analogues of the two isomers of CAPE that differed in the placement of hydroxyl substituents showed a drastic change in the inhibitory potency of the two analogues; the isomer 5 was completely ineffective, whereas the isomer 6 completely abolished the binding, once again indicating that the placement of the hydroxyl groups played a critical role in inhibiting NF-κB activation. In the saturated amide analogues, the analogue with three additional hydroxyls (compound 7) and the reverse amide analogue (compound 8), which lacked an additional hydroxyl group, were less active than CAPE. Thus it is possible to find structural analogues of CAPE that are more active than CAPE (compound 6), as active as CAPE (compound 1), and less active than CAPE (compounds 2-5, 7, and 8).

The analogues that were maximally active in inhibiting NF-κB activation were different from those with maximum inhibitory activity for either HIV integrase or cell growth, suggesting a difference in the mechanism. For instance, compound 6, one of the conformationally constrained CAPE variants (5, 6 dihydroxy derivative), was more potent than native CAPE for NF-κB activation but less potent than the parent compound for inhibition of HIV integrase and cell growth (Burke et al., 1995).

The antibacterial activity of cinnamic acid derivates has been reported (Ramanan & Rao, 1987), and some QSAR studies have been done, and they reported that the introduction of halogen onto the benzene ring of cinnamic acid enhance the antimicrobial activity against gram negative bacteria (Ramanan et al., 1987). The reactive αβ-unsaturated carbonyl is a common factor in compounds showing antimutagenic activity, it is speculated that αβ-unsaturated carbonyl systems react with nucleophiles and exert their antimutagenic activity by trapping thiol groups of target proteins (Kakinuma, 1986). Structure-activity analysis suggests that 3', 4' catechol ring is important for the antioxidant potential, metal chelation and free radical captures (Kerry & Rice-Evans, 1998), although both groups hydroxyl decrease its lipophilicity and thus their ability to cross cell membranes. On the other hand, it has been reported that increasing the length of the carbon chain reduces the fungitoxic activity of CAPE analogues (Jun ZHU, 2000).

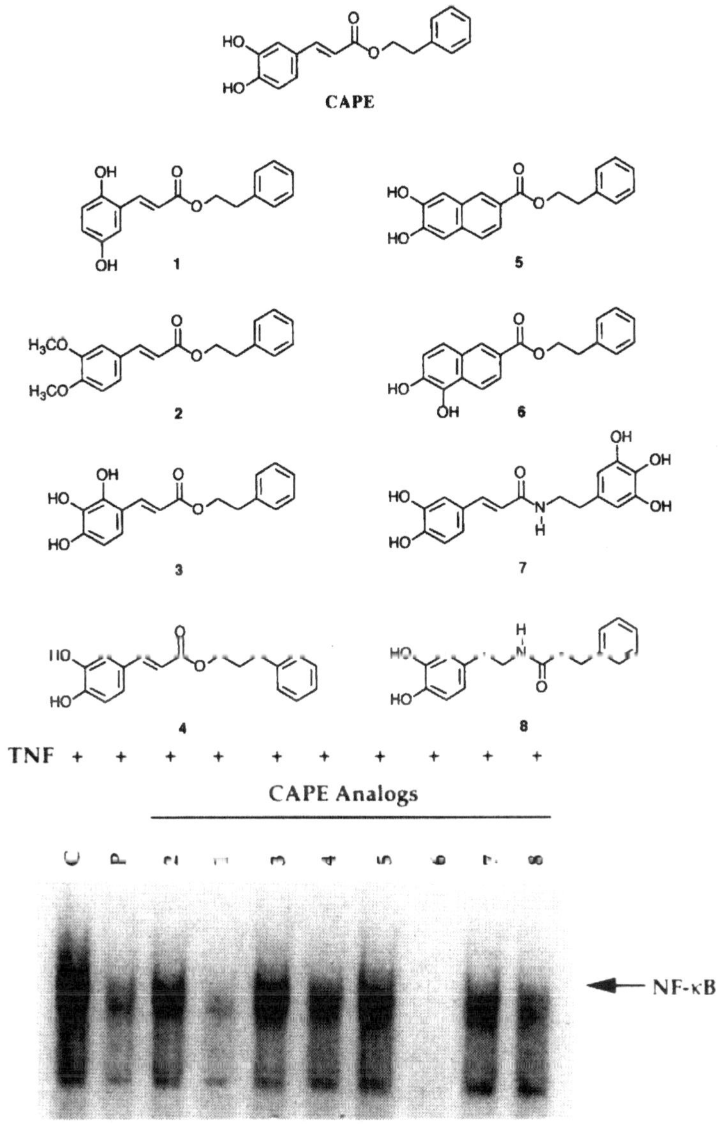

Fig. 3. Structure-activity relationship studies: several analogues of CAPE were synthesized including ring substituents (compounds 1 to 3), ester groups (compound 4), rotationally constrained Variants (compounds 5 and 6), and saturated amide analogues (compounds 7 and 8). Taken from Natarajan et al 1996.

Jun ZHU et al. tested the biological activity of several cinnamato and cinnamide derivatives in a fungitoxicity test in which *Pythium sp.* and *C. rolfsii*, were used as test plant pathogenic fungi. They were cultured in potato dextrose agar for 4-5 days at 27 °C, was added and the test compunds and fungitoxic activity was expresed as % inhibition of mycelial growth diameter.

They work too with a Phytotoxicity test in which the test compound in solution was poured into a filter paper, ten seeds of *Brassica rapa* var. *amplexicaulis* were sown on the filter paper in petri dishes. After three day incubation at 27 °C, inhibitory activity on the length of the plant's radicle and hypocotyl was measured and compared with the control. The cinnamic acid analogues remain in varying degrees phytotoxic and cytotoxic effect, they reported that cinnamic acid derivatives having methyl, propyl or isopropyl group as the substituent R2 showed the highest fungitoxic activity. Derivatives of 4-Isopropylcinnamamide showed high fungitoxic activity and derivatives of 4-Chlorocinnamamide showed relatively high fungitoxic activity, the introduction of two chlorine atoms at 2 and 4 positions of cinnamic acid decreased activity against both pathogenic fungi and plant growth (Jun ZHU et al., 2000).

Compound	R	EC_{50}	
		Cytotoxicity (μM)	NO Inhibition (μM)
1	H	3406.000 ± 714	165.295 ± 16.05
2	CH_3	367.500 ± 133	3.199 ± 0.27
3	C_2H_5	121.700 ± 17.16	3.183 ± 0.27
4	C_3H_7	26.420 ± 4.38	0.440 ± 0.08
5	C_4H_9	7.419 ± 0.93	0.240 ± 0.06
6	C_6H_{13}	2.677 ± 0.96	0.340 ± 0.05
7	C_7H_{15}	4.594 ± 1.12	0.236 ± 0.02
8	C_8H_{17}	1.588 ± 0.22	0.060 ± 0.01
9	C_9H_{19}	1.658 ± 0.02	0.052 ± 0.02
10	$C_{10}H_{21}$	1.542 ± 0.18	0.045 ± 0.09
11	$C_{11}H_{23}$	1.188 ± 0.06	0.018 ± 0.02
12	$C_{12}H_{25}$	1.000 ± 0.08	0.556 ± 0.05
13	$C_{14}H_{29}$	1.256 ± 0.07	0.292 ± 0.03
14	$C_{16}H_{33}$	3.200 ± 0.36	0.713 ± 0.13
15	$C_{18}H_{37}$	2.671 ± 0.29	0.573 ± 0.04
16	$(CH_3)_2CH$	42.200 ± 5.97	0.302 ± 0.03
17	$C_2H_3(CH_3)_2$	13.000 ± 1.81	0.303 ± 0.08
18	*cyclo*-Hexyl	28.700 ± 3.88	1.655 ± 0.36
19	Benzyl	38.800 ± 3.57	0.347 ± 0.04
20	Prenyl	30.000 ± 1.61	0.578 ± 0.04
21	Geranyl	3.054 ± 0.16	0.223 ± 0.01
22	Farnesyl	2.658 ± 0.16	0.258 ± 0.03
	Phenethyl	4.518 ± 0.04	0.193 ± 0.04

Table 1. Effect of Caffeic acid derivatives on NO production in RAW264.7 macrophage. Obtained from Uwai et al., 2008.

As shown in table 1, a structure activity relationship analysis showed that caffeic acid esters in different degrees preserved their activity to inhibit nitric oxide (NO) production induced by lipopolysaccharide in murine RAW264.7 macrophages, which is reflected in the median effective concentration (EC50) of each compound. The inhibitory effect of these derivatives on NO production in RAW264.7 macrophage was dependent on the length and size of the alkyl moiety, and undecyl caffeate was the most potent inhibitor of NO production (Uwai et al., 2008).

Additionally, these authors showed that the connection between caffeic acid and the alkyl chain is critical for activity. Amide and ketone derivatives showed that not only the ester functional group but also the amide and ketone functional groups exhibit an inhibitory effect on NO production (Uwai et al., 2008).

These examples suggest that compounds with similar structure to CAPE Could keep on varying degrees the chemoprotective effect that CAPE has shown on in vivo models like is the resistant hepatocyte modified model.

2.3 *In vivo* assays on the resistant hepatocyte modified model

It has been possible to study the chemical carcinogenesis and the chemoprotective effect of some chemical compounds using experimental animal's models. In the animal models, the chemical carcinogenesis is reproducible, and has advantages over cell culture and clinical biopsies as the possibility of study the carcinogenesis from the initiation trough the different stages until the tumor establishment, also is possible to obtain information of the participation of cell not belonging to the tumor, or test the secondary effect of these compounds, while human precancerous lesions such as dysplastic nodules are rather difficult to obtain because of their small size, difficult detection, and coexistence with other liver pathologies. The models of chemical carcinogenesis require chemical compounds able to alter the DNA, so they are mutagenics, many of them need a metabolic bioactivation and they showed a direct relation in its ability to form adducts, produce mutations and lead to cancer. The modified Semple-Roberts model in rats, allow the study of hepatocarcinogenesis (Semple-Roberts et al., 1987; Solt & Farber, 1976), providing valuable information about the changes that occur throughout the process.

On the initiation, produced by the carcinogen diethylnitrosamine (DEN) in the resistant hepatocyte modified model, Fischer 344 male adult rats weighing between 180 and 200 g are administrated with the carcinogen DEN at dose of 200 mg/kg i.p. at day 0 of treatment, as promotion stimulus is administered a daily dose of 20 mg/kg o.p. of 2-acetyl-aminofluorene (2-AAF) at days 7, 8 and 9, and is performed a partial hepatectomy at 10th day. In addition, using histoenzimatic staining for gamma-glutamyl-tranpeptidasa (GGT) and Glutation-S-transferasa (GST-p) as markers of preneoplastic lesions (Carrasco-Legleu et al., 2004; Carrasco-Legleu et al., 2006) was determined that the highest number of preneoplastic lesions in rat liver is reached between 25 and 30 days after start the treatment, and lead to tumor after one year of the treatment.

Mutations in DNA and hepatocyte proliferation are common to models of hepatocarcinogenesis, DEN is a genotoxic and mutagenic alkylating agent, its metabolic bioactivation by cytochromes P-450 produce oxidative stress and reactive chemical species such as ethyl carbonium ion, producing ethylated and oxidized adducts with macromolecules as DNA and proteins, both of them have an important role in the carcinogenesis (Sánchez-Pérez et al., 2005; Takabe et al., 2001). As example of the adducts formed by DEN are the N-7-ethylguanine and the O6-ethylguanine because the nitrogenated base more likely to be ethylated by DEN is guanine in the N7 and O6 positions, due to the electrophilic character of the ethyl carbonium ion, it react covalently with nucleophilic sites of the cell components to produce ethylated adducts (Verna et al., 1996). As result of cell damage DEN is necrogenic and cellular death is a stimulus to restore the lost tissue, inducing a cell division that fixes mutations in cells with unrepaired adducts on its genetic material. Hepatocyte regeneration have been implicated in the development of HCC, 2-AAF has a mitoinhibitory effect on the uninitiated hepatocytes, while allow the selective proliferation of initiated hepatocytes as consequence of the proliferative stimulus of partial hepatectomy (Ohlson et al., 2004), it means, only proliferate the hepatocytes resistan to the mitoinhibitory effect of 2-AAF.

The resistant hepatocyte model modified allows the study of the chemopreventive properties observed in various compounds such as the anti-inflammatory drug (NSAID) celecoxib (Arellanes-Robledo et al., 2006; Arellanes-Robledo et al., 2010) and antioxidants quercetin (Vasquez-Garzon et al., 2009) and CAPE (Beltrán-Ramírez et al., 2008), these compounds decreased the percentage of GGT+ area in rat liver, used as a marker of preneoplastic lesions, compared to the livers of rats receiving carcinogen treatment only. Each chemopreventive compound can be studied under different conditions in the model, such as a different stage (Three main steps: initiation, promotion, and progression), dose or route of administration, given that many chemicals possess multiple modes of action. CAPE has shown anticarcinogenic properties on initiation and in progression stages in the modified resistant hepatocyte model.

When given during promotion, CAPE decreased the expression of number and area of altered hepatic foci (GGT+ AHF) by 91% and 97%, respectively at 25 d of carcinogenic treatment. Glutathione S-transferase placental (GST-P), another protein marker for preneoplastic lesions was decreased 82%. Additionally, were evaluated the effect of CAPE on the expression of nuclear factor NF-κB and found an 85% decrease in nuclear localization of NF-κB (Carrasco-Legleu et al., 2004).

When is given 12 h before initiation, CAPE prevents preneoplastic lesions, as were shown by GGT histoenzymatic staining of liver sections, showing that CAPE decrease 84% the number and 91% the area GGT+ AHF in the liver rats at 25 days with respect to the group that received only the carcinogenic treatment as see in Figure 4, and in case of the GSTp the protein level was reduced by 90% (Carrasco-Legleu et al., 2006).

On initiation stage the mechanism of action were further investigated testing the effect of CAPE during the early stages of liver carcinogenesis. When CAPE is administered at dose of 20 mg/kg to the rats 12 h before initiation, the hematoxylin-eosin histological staining of liver sections showed that CAPE prevents necrosis at 24 h after DEN administration, in relation to the group of rats that received only DEN; indicating that CAPE administration reduces the toxicity of DEN.

DEN requires metabolic activation by CYP to lead to the formation of diazoalkanes or carbocations and ultimately to the alkylation of nucleophiles, reactive species are known to induce cancer in mammals. With the research in this model were reported that CAPE modifies the enzymatic activity of CYP isoforms involved in the activation of DEN, such CYP1A1, CYP1A2, CYP2B1/2, and CYP2E1 (Beltrán-Ramírez et al., 2008). Suggesting that CAPE may modify the enzyme activity of CYP isoforms involved in DEN activation, and the modification of DEN metabolism could lead to a detoxification without the formation of reactive chemical species.

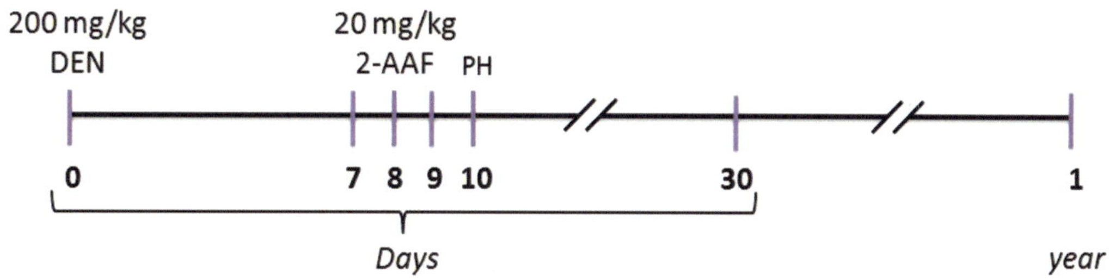

A

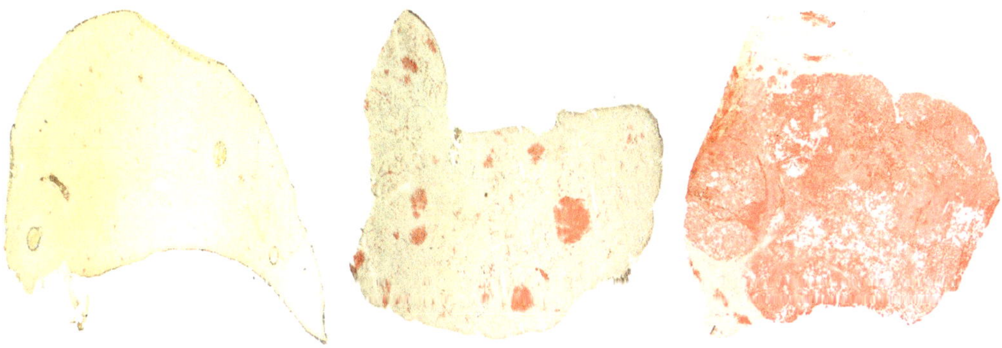

B C D

Fig. 4. A) Resistant hepatocyte modified model. DEN: Diethylnitrosamine, 2AAF: 2-acetyl-aminofluorene, HP: Partial hepatectomy. B) Untreated liver. C) preneoplastic lesions on liver 1 month after carcinogenic treatment. D) Liver tumor 1 year after carcinogenic treatment.

Increased concentrations of active oxygen, organic peroxides and free radicals can promote initiated cells to neoplastic growth, inducing alterations in DNA structure or producing epigenetic mechanisms. It has been reported antioxidant activity for catechol rings, like in CAPE related compounds (Bors et al., 2004), and the effect of CAPE on lipid peroxidation (LPX) was measured by the tiobarbituric acid reactive species assay (TBARS), 12 h after DEN administration was detected a 68% increase of (TBARS). When CAPE was administered before DEN, it completely protected from liver TBARS induction (Carrasco-Legleu et al., 2006).

This model has been analyzed by DNA microarray methodologies at different stages, for the gene expression profile of preneoplastic nodules and hepatocellular carcinomas (HCC) to define the genes implicated in cancer progression (Pérez-Carreón et al., 2006), as a result we have a big database of genes that will allow to investigate the mechanism by which the cancer evolve, with the option of inquiring how this genes participate in carcinogenesis and how could be modulated. Among the main possibilities it also allows to search for possible early markers, that is important to prevention or to design a treatment. Gene expression profiles induced by DEN have been compared with those obtained from rats previously administered with a single dose of CAPE, as example of the results obtained by microarrays, it has been found that CAPE alone did not alter the expression profile, DEN treatment modified the expression of 665 genes, and CAPE plus DEN changes 1371 genes in the expression profile. Some of the genes found decreased in its expression on CAPE plus DEN treatment were Glutation reductasa, *GST-k*, *GST-0*, *p53* and CYP2b1, the last one involved in DEN bioactivation. The database obtained will help to elucidate the mechanism by which CAPE exert its chemoprotective activity (Beltrán-Ramírez et al., 2010).

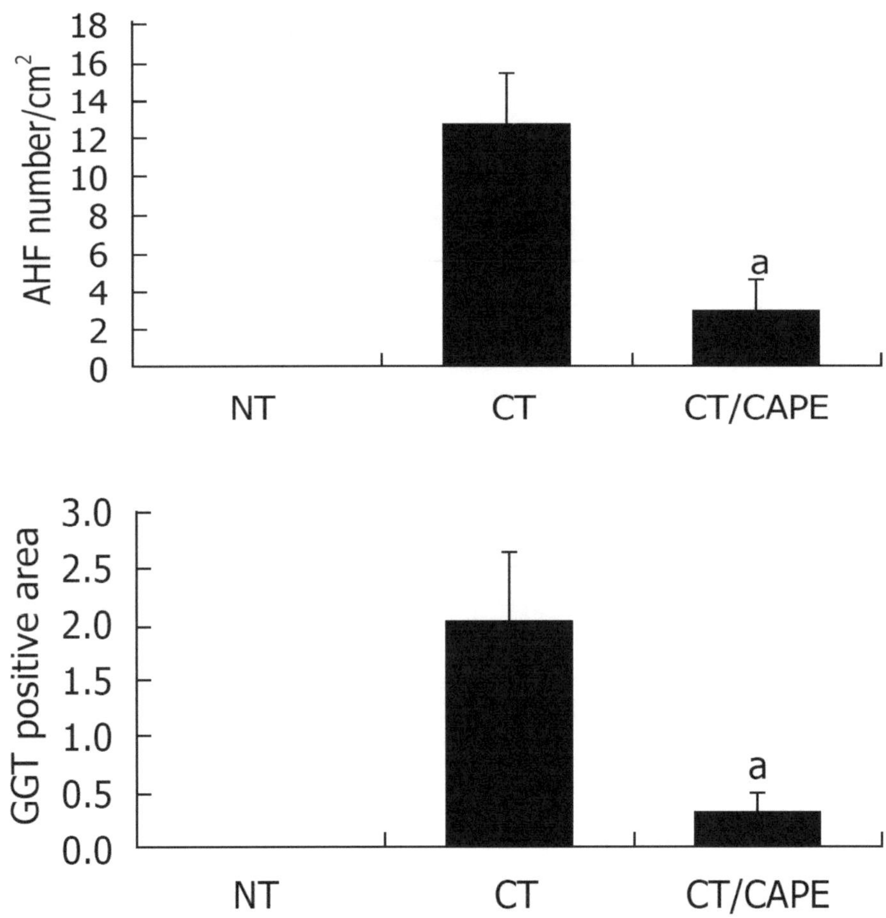

Fig. 5. Effect CAPE pretreatment on number/cm^2 of AHF and percentage of GGT+ area/tissue. Taken from Carrasco-Legleu et al 2006.

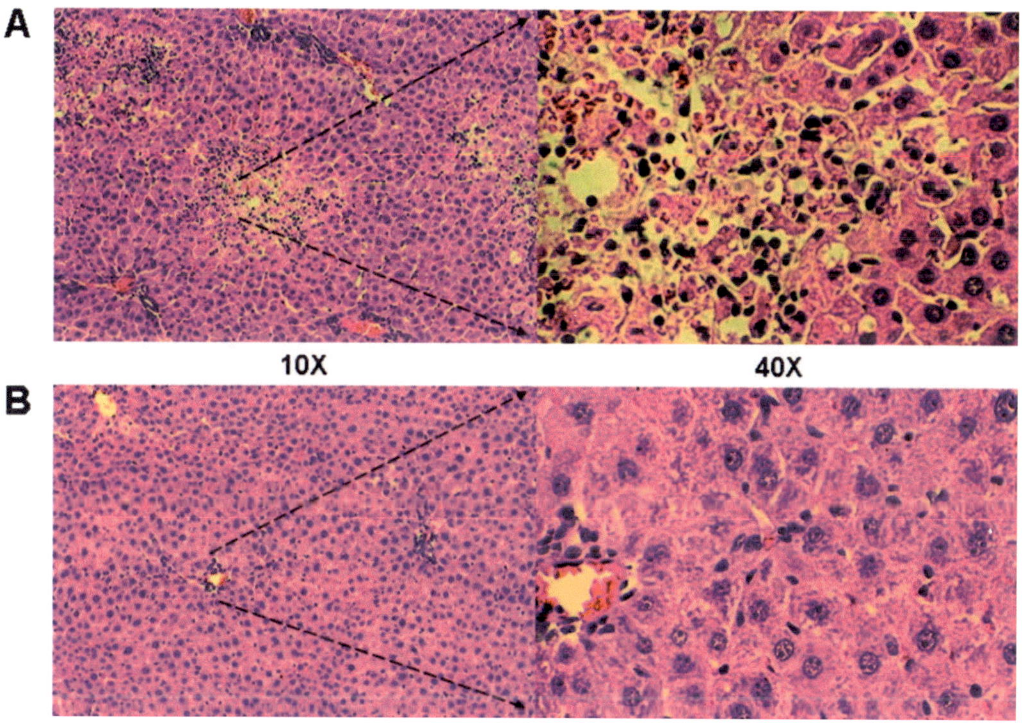

Fig. 6. Effect of CAPE on Necrosis induced by DEN. A) Necrosis produced by DEN 24h after administration. B) Diminution of necrosis produced by DEN 24h after administration by effect of CAPE. Taken from Beltrán-Ramírez et al., 2008

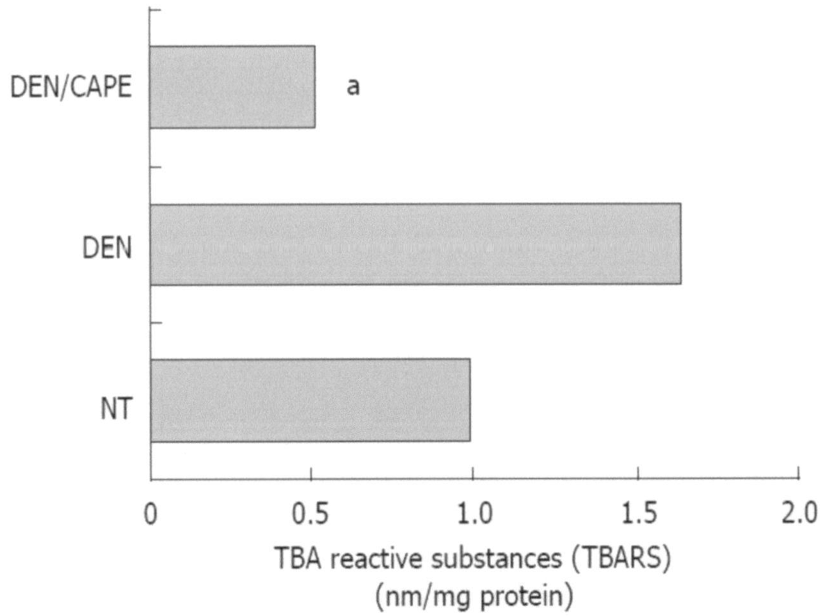

Fig. 7. Effect of CAPE on LPX levels induced by DEN. Tiobarbituric acid reactive substances in group NT: Not treated; DEN: 12h After DEN administration; DEN/CAPE: CAPE pretreatment 12h before DEN. Taken from Carrasco-Legleu 2006.

3. Conclusions

The standardization of natural products is necessary as well as the study of its components, given that substances with biological activity often have been found while studying substances purified from natural products to which folk medicine has attributed therapeutic properties. Many natural products are chemopreventive, several of them as dietary constituents, and experiments with cultured cells and animal models are revealing their potential mechanisms of action, and mainly these mechanism are related with the capability of prevent or greatly reduce initiation of carcinogenesis, or cell proliferation.

Honey and propolis are rich in phenolic compounds, and are becoming increasingly popular because of their potential role in contributing to human health. Data from laboratory studies indicate that CAPE has important effects on cancer chemoprevention and many mechanisms of action have been identified for CAPE and related compounds. First were reported that the antitumor activity of polyphenolic compounds like CAPE includes direct cytotoxic effects on tumor cells on in vitro experiments, this effect have been tested with positive results in several kinds of tumors in vivo, the effect on initiation was tested in an rat hepatocarcinogenesis model, were CAPE show a protective effect when a single dose was given before initiation, decreasing the induction of area and number of GGT+ AHF. As chemoprotection mechanism of CAPE was proposed it is due to its anti-oxidative and free-radical scavenging activities, and now have been added to chemoprotection mechanism on initiation stage that CAPE modifies the CYP-dependent DEN bioactivation and decreases reactive chemical species, inhibiting the initiation stage of carcinogenesis.

Although, the biological activities of caffeic acid esters and other analogues have been studied by analyzing their structure, the detailed mechanisms of their activities remain unclear. The research of mechanism-based compound can contribute to a greater understanding of cancer and a faster development of successful therapies, as suggested by the experiments analyzed here, compounds with similar structure to CAPE could keep or enhance the chemoprotective effect that CAPE has shown. Is of special importance that many protective effects of CAPE and related compounds could have common mechanisms for chemoprotection, by this reason is needed to test on *in vivo* models the effect of modifications on the structure of CAPE that let us know the participation of properties like lipophilicity, anti-oxidative and free radical scavenging among others on the chemoprotection. If the CAPE analogues compounds share one of more of the mechanism of action and his preparation is easy, quick and inexpensive, these compounds may be promising anticancer agents as well as CAPE.

HCC is an aggressive tumor with a high fatality rate, early detection likely will be based on characterization of the molecular pathogenesis of this disease, and a successful treatment should be developed with this knowledge together with the understanding of the mechanism of action of drugs.

4. References

Arellanes-Robledo, J., L. Márquez-Rosado, J. I. Pérez-Carreón, S. Fattel-Fazenda, J. Aguirre-García & S. Villa-Treviño (2006) Celecoxib induces regression of putative preneoplastic lesions in rat liver. *Anticancer Res,* 26, 1271-80.

Arellanes-Robledo, J., M. E. Salcido-Neyoy, A. Márquez-Quiñones, R. García-Román, O. Beltrán-Ramírez, V. Le Berre, S. Sokol, J. M. Francois & S. Villa-Treviño (2010) Celecoxib activates Stat5 and restores or increases the expression of growth hormone-regulated genes in hepatocarcinogenesis. *Anticancer Drugs,* 21, 411-22.

Beltrán-Ramírez, O., L. Alemán-Lazarini, M. Salcido-Neyoy, S. Hernández-García, S. Fattel-Fazenda, E. Arce-Popoca, J. Arellanes-Robledo, R. García-Román, P. Vázquez-Vázquez, A. Sierra-Santoyo & S. Villa-Treviño (2008) Evidence that the anticarcinogenic effect of caffeic acid phenethyl ester in the resistant hepatocyte model involves modifications of cytochrome P450. *Toxicol Sci,* 104, 100-6.

Beltrán-Ramírez, O., S. Sokol, V. Le-Berre, J. M. Francois & S. Villa-Treviño (2010) An approach to the study of gene expression in hepatocarcinogenesis initiation. *Transl Oncol,* 3, 142-8.

Boik, J. (2001) Natural Compounds in Cancer Therapy. *Oregon Medical Press,* 275-278.

Bors, W., C. Michel, K. Stettmaier, Y. Lu & L. Y. Foo (2004) Antioxidant mechanisms of polyphenolic caffeic acid oligomers, constituents of Salvia officinalis. *Biol Res,* 37, 301-11.

Burke, T. R., Jr., M. R. Fesen, A. Mazumder, J. Wang, A. M. Carothers, D. Grunberger, J. Driscoll, K. Kohn & Y. Pommier (1995) Hydroxylated aromatic inhibitors of HIV-1 integrase. *J Med Chem,* 38, 4171-8.

Carrasco-Legleu, C. E., L. Márquez-Rosado, S. Fattel-Fazenda, E. Arce-Popoca, J. I. Pérez-Carreón & S. Villa-Treviño (2004) Chemoprotective effect of caffeic acid phenethyl ester on promotion in a medium-term rat hepatocarcinogenesis assay. *Int J Cancer,* 108, 488-92.

Carrasco-Legleu, C. E., Y. Sánchez-Pérez, L. Márquez-Rosado, S. Fattel-Fazenda, E. Arce-Popoca, S. Hernández-García & S. Villa-Treviño (2006) A single dose of caffeic acid phenethyl ester prevents initiation in a medium-term rat hepatocarcinogenesis model. *World J Gastroenterol,* 12, 6779-85.

Chang, Y. C., F. W. Lee, C. S. Chen, S. T. Huang, S. H. Tsai, S. H. Huang & C. M. Lin (2007) Structure-activity relationship of C6-C3 phenylpropanoids on xanthine oxidase-inhibiting and free radical-scavenging activities. *Free Radic Biol Med,* 43, 1541-51.

Farré, R. (2004) Propolis and human health. *Ars Pharmaceutica,* 45, 21-43.

Fischer, J. & C. R. Ganellin. 2006. *Analogue-based drug discovery*. Weinheim: Wiley-VCH.

García-Román, R., J. I. Pérez-Carreón, A. Márquez-Quiñones, M. E. Salcido-Neyoy & S. Villa-Treviño (2007) Persistent activation of NF-kappaB related to IkappaB's degradation profiles during early chemical hepatocarcinogenesis. *J Carcinog,* 6, 5.

García-Román, R., D. Salazar-González, S. Rosas, J. Arellanes-Robledo, O. Beltrán-Ramírez, S. Fattel-Fazenda & S. Villa-Treviño (2008) The differential NF-kB modulation by S-adenosyl-L-methionine, N-acetylcysteine and quercetin on the promotion stage of chemical hepatocarcinogenesis. *Free Radic Res,* 42, 331-43.

González-Avila, M., M. Arriaga-Alba, M. de la Garza, M. del Carmén Hernández Pretelin, M. A. Dominguez-Ortiz, S. Fattel-Fazenda & S. Villa-Treviño (2003) Antigenotoxic, antimutagenic and ROS scavenging activities of a Rhoeo discolor ethanolic crude extract. *Toxicol In Vitro,* 17, 77-83.

Hanahan, D. & R. A. Weinberg (2011) Hallmarks of cancer: the next generation. *Cell,* 144, 646-74.

Jiang, R. W., K. M. Lau, P. M. Hon, T. C. Mak, K. S. Woo & K. P. Fung (2005) Chemistry and biological activities of caffeic acid derivatives from Salvia miltiorrhiza. *Curr Med Chem,* 12, 237-46.

Jun ZHU, H. Z., Naotada KABAMOTO, Masaaki YASUDA & Shinkichi TAWATA (2000) Fungitoxic and Phytotoxic Activities of Cinnamic Acid Esters and Amides. *J. Pesticide Sci.,* 263-266.

Kakinuma, K. (1986) [Perspectives in microbial secondary metabolism]. *Seikagaku,* 58, 167-75.

Kerry, N. & C. Rice-Evans (1998) Peroxynitrite oxidises catechols to o-quinones. *FEBS Lett,* 437, 167-71.

Kohlmeier, L., N. Simonsen & K. Mottus (1995) Dietary modifiers of carcinogenesis. *Environ Health Perspect,* 103 Suppl 8, 177-84.

Kubinyi, H. (1990) Quantitative structure-activity relationships (QSAR) and molecular modelling in cancer research. *J Cancer Res Clin Oncol,* 116, 529-37.

Lin, C. F., T. C. Chang, C. C. Chiang, H. J. Tsai & L. Y. Hsu (2005) Synthesis of selenium-containing polyphenolic acid esters and evaluation of their effects on antioxidation and 5-lipoxygenase inhibition. *Chem Pharm Bull (Tokyo),* 53, 1402-7.

Mabrouk, G. M., S. S. Moselhy, S. F. Zohny, E. M. Ali, T. E. Helal, A. A. Amin & A. A. Khalifa (2002) Inhibition of methylnitrosourea (MNU) induced oxidative stress and carcinogenesis by orally administered bee honey and Nigella grains in Sprague Dawely rats. *J Exp Clin Cancer Res*, 21, 341-6.

Natarajan, K., S. Singh, T. R. Burke, Jr., D. Grunberger & B. B. Aggarwal (1996) Caffeic acid phenethyl ester is a potent and specific inhibitor of activation of nuclear transcription factor NF-kappa B. *Proc Natl Acad Sci U S A*, 93, 9090-5.

Naugler, W. E. & J. M. Schwartz (2008) Hepatocellular carcinoma. *Dis Mon*, 54, 432-44.

Nill, K. R. 2002. *Glossary of biotechnology terms*. Boca Raton, FL: CRC Press.

Ohlson, L. C., L. Koroxenidou & I. Porsch-Hallstrom (2004) Mitoinhibitory effects of the tumor promoter 2-acetylaminofluorene in rat liver: loss of E2F-1 and E2F-3 expression and cdk 2 kinase activity in late G1. *J Hepatol*, 40, 957-62.

Orsolic, N., S. Terzic, Z. Mihaljevic, L. Sver & I. Basic (2005) Effects of local administration of propolis and its polyphenolic compounds on tumor formation and growth. *Biol Pharm Bull*, 28, 1928-33.

Pérez-Carreón, J. I., C. Lopez-García, S. Fattel-Fazenda, E. Arce-Popoca, L. Alemán-Lazarini, S. Hernández-García, V. Le Berre, S. Sokol, J. M. Francois & S. Villa-Treviño (2006) Gene expression profile related to the progression of preneoplastic nodules toward hepatocellular carcinoma in rats. *Neoplasia*, 8, 373-83.

Ramanan, P. N., A. V. Kutty & M. N. Rao (1987) Quantitative structure activity relationship (QSAR) studies on the inhibition of porcine pancreatic amylase by cinnamic acid derivatives. *Indian J Biochem Biophys*, 24, 49-50.

Ramanan, P. N. & M. N. Rao (1987) Antimicrobial activity of cinnamic acid derivatives. *Indian J Exp Biol*, 25, 42-3.

Rosales-Reyes, T., M. de la Garza, C. Arias-Castro, M. Rodríguez-Mendiola, S. Fattel-Fazenda, E. Arce-Popoca, S. Hernández-García & S. Villa-Treviño (2008) Aqueous crude extract of Rhoeo discolor, a Mexican medicinal plant, decreases the formation of liver preneoplastic foci in rats. *J Ethnopharmacol*, 115, 381-6.

Sánchez-Pérez, Y., C. Carrasco-Legleu, C. García-Cuellar, J. Pérez-Carreón, S. Hernández-García, M. Salcido-Neyoy, L. Alemán-Lazarini & S. Villa-Treviño (2005) Oxidative stress in carcinogenesis. Correlation between lipid peroxidation and induction of preneoplastic lesions in rat hepatocarcinogenesis. *Cancer Lett*, 217, 25-32.

Semple-Roberts, E., M. A. Hayes, D. Armstrong, R. A. Becker, W. J. Racz & E. Farber (1987) Alternative methods of selecting rat hepatocellular nodules resistant to 2-acetylaminofluorene. *Int J Cancer*, 40, 643-5.

Solt, D. & E. Farber (1976) New principle for the analysis of chemical carcinogenesis. *Nature*, 701-703.

Son, S. & B. A. Lewis (2002) Free radical scavenging and antioxidative activity of caffeic acid amide and ester analogues: structure-activity relationship. *J Agric Food Chem*, 50, 468-72.

Takabe, W., E. Niki, K. Uchida, S. Yamada, K. Satoh & N. Noguchi (2001) Oxidative stress promotes the development of transformation: involvement of a potent mutagenic lipid peroxidation product, acrolein. *Carcinogenesis*, 22, 935-41.

Uwai, K., Y. Osanai, T. Imaizumi, S. Kanno, M. Takeshita & M. Ishikawa (2008) Inhibitory effect of the alkyl side chain of caffeic acid analogues on lipopolysaccharide-induced nitric oxide production in RAW264.7 macrophages. *Bioorg Med Chem,* 16, 7795-803.

Vásquez-Garzón, V. R., J. Arellanes-Robledo, R. García-Román, D. I. Aparicio-Bautista & S. Villa-Treviño (2009) Inhibition of reactive oxygen species and pre-neoplastic lesions by quercetin through an antioxidant defense mechanism. *Free Radic Res,* 43, 128-37.

Verna, L., J. Whysner & G. M. Williams (1996) N-nitrosodiethylamine mechanistic data and risk assessment: bioactivation, DNA-adduct formation, mutagenicity, and tumor initiation. *Pharmacol Ther,* 71, 57-81.

Vincent, T. L. & R. A. Gatenby (2008) An evolutionary model for initiation, promotion, and progression in carcinogenesis. *Int J Oncol,* 32, 729-37.

Wermuth, C. G. (2006) Similarity in drugs: reflections on analogue design. *Drug Discov Today,* 11, 348-54.

12

Functional Analysis of Natural Polyphenols and Saponins as Alternative Medicines

Hiroshi Sakagami[1], Tatsuya Kushida[2], Toru Makino[3], Tsutomu Hatano[4], Yoshiaki Shirataki[5], Tomohiko Matsuta[1], Yukiko Matsuo[6] and Yoshihiro Mimaki[6]

[1]*Meikai University School of Dentistry, Saitama,*
[2]*Non-Profit Organization Bio-Knowledge Bank, Tokyo,*
[3]*HumaLabo Co., Ltd., Tokyo,*
[4]*Graduate School of Medicine, Dentistry and Pharmaceutical Sciences, Okayama University, Okayama,*
[5]*Faculty of Pharmaceutical Sciences, Josai University, Saitama,*
[6]*Tokyo University of Pharmacy and Life Sciences, School of Pharmacy, Tokyo, Japan*

1. Introduction

Hot water extracts of plants have been utilized to treat various diseases without severe side effects. The presence of numerous kinds of components in the extract made it difficult to identify the causative substances. The hot water extracts contain relatively higher amounts of high-molecular weight polysaccharides and lignin-carbohydrate complexes (LCCs) and relatively lower amounts of low-molecular weight tannins, flavonoids, terpenes and saponins.

Polysaccharides and LCCs are easily extractable by hot-water or alkaline solution and thus be expected to be present in higher amounts in the extract, but the complete determinations of the chemical structures have never been achieved due to the structural complexity. On the other hand, tannins, flavonoids, terpenes and some saponins are mostly difficult to be dissolved in water, but more easily extractable with methanol, and the structures of thousands of compounds have been identified. These low molecular weight compounds are thus expected to be present in lower amounts in the extract. Therefore, the information of how much these lower molecular materials are present in hot-water extract is limited, albeit important.

Based on these circumstances, we analyze the functionality of polysaccharides and LCCs, tannins, flavonoids and saponins as alternative medicines, citing the literatures of other groups and ours, focusing on the following points: (1) yield and putative amounts in methanol and hot-water extracts, (2) biological activity, (3) state in hot-water extract: possible binding to other compounds, (4) site of action, signalling pathway, and receptor identification, and (5) future directions.

2. Lignin-carbohydrate complex (LCC)

Lignins are major class of natural products present in the natural kingdom, and are formed through phenolic oxidative coupling processes in the plant (Davin et al., 1997). Lignins are formed by the dehydrogenative polymerization of three monolignols: *p*-coumaryl, *p*-coniferyl and sinapyl alcohols (Lewis & Yamamoto, 1990). These monolignols were produced from L-phenylalanine by general phenylpropanoid pathway (Emiliani et al., 2009). Some polysaccharides in the cell walls of lignified plants are linked to lignin to form lignin-carbohydrate complexes (LCCs) (Fig.1). Complete structural determination of LCC has not been achieved yet, due to structural complexity. Polysaccharide portions are composed of various types of sugars. For example, LCCs from pine cone of *Pinus parviflora* Sieb et Zucc. contained 11-40% neutral sugars (galactose > glucose > mannose > arabinose or fucose) and 2-58% uronic acid (Sakagami et al., 1987). Similarly, *Lentinus edodes* mycelia extract (LEM) showed similar sugar composition 32% of neutral sugars (glucose > mannose > galactose > arabinose) and 68% uronic acids. Varying the ratio of polysaccharide to phenylpropenoids produces heterogeneity in the acidity, water-solubility, ethanol-insolubility, and molecular weight. LCCs from bald cypress, birch and rice straw show an extremely broad molecular weight distribution from 1.5 to 85 kDa (Azuma & Koshijima, 1988). In their role as integral cell wall components, lignins help provide mechanical support and defend against pathogens. Although the use of dietary fiber (composed of non-α-glucan polysaccharides and lignin) in the treatment of constipation and uncomplicated diverticular diseases is well established (Kay, 1982), very little attention has been paid to the biological activities of lignins or lignin-containing/derived substances.

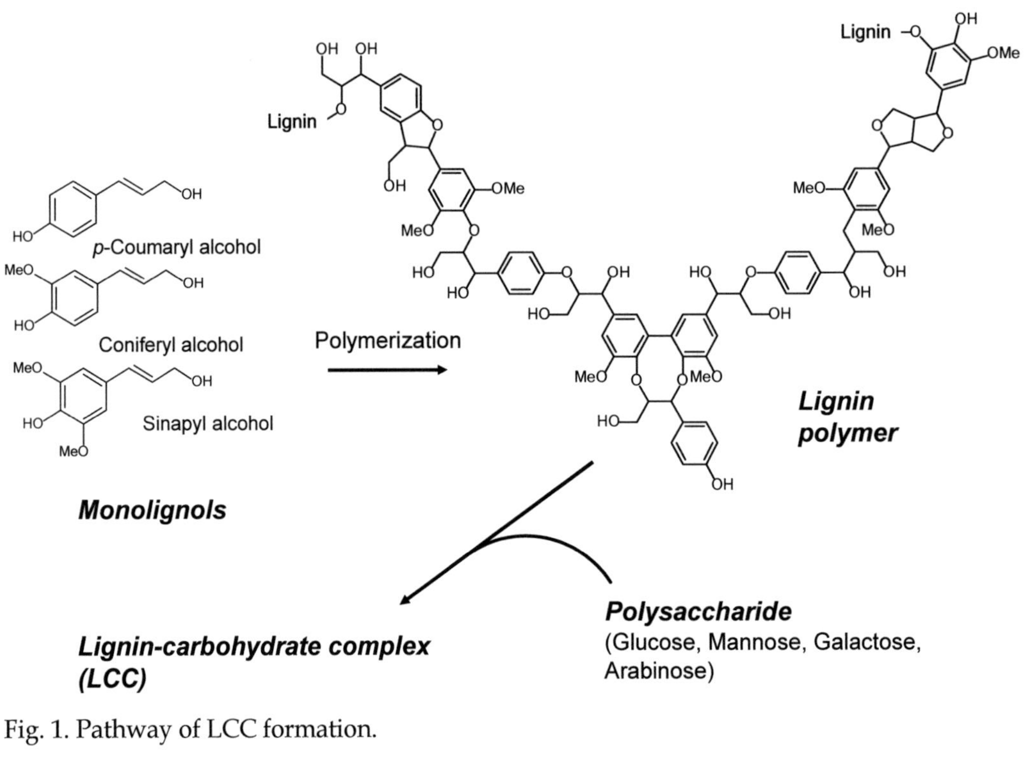

Fig. 1. Pathway of LCC formation.

2.1 Yield and putative amounts in methanol and hot water extracts

Usually, LCCs are extracted by alkaline extract, and concentrated by acid-precipitation. The yield of LCCs are 0.04 to 7.9% of the plant materials (Sakagami et al., 2010a) (Table 2). Gel filtration chromatography of the alkaline extract of *Sasa senanencis* Rehder revealed that LCC represents major parts of the extract (Matsuta et al, 2011). The major part of polyphenols in LCCs from LEM is composed of lignin precursors such as *p*-coumaric acid, vanillic acid, syringic acid and ferulic acid, but not tannin nor flavonoids (Table 1).

	µg/g LEM	µg/g Fr4		µg/g LEM	µg/g Fr4
Lignin precursors			*Tannins and related compounds*		
Vanillic acid	785.5	25.9	Gallic acid	<0.1	<0.1
Syringic acid	638.0	25.7	Catechin	<0.1	<0.1
p-Coumaric acid	277.0	157.7	Epicatechin	<0.1	<0.1
Ferulic acid	74.5	13.4	Epigallocatechin gallate	<0.1	<0.1
Vanillin	59.5	<0.1	Gallocatechin gallate	<0.1	<0.1
Caffeic acid	12.0	<0.1	Epicatechin gallate	<0.1	<0.1
Syringaldehyde	<0.1	<0.1	Catechin gallate	<0.1	<0.1
o-Coumaric acid	<0.1	<0.1	Ellagic acid	<0.1	<0.1
			Theaflavin-3-gallate	<0.1	<0.1
Flavonoids			Theaflavin-3'-gallate	<0.1	<0.1
Fisetin	<0.1	<0.1	Theaflavin-3,3'-gallate	<0.1	<0.1
Daizein	<0.1	<0.1			
Genistein	<0.1	<0.1	*Others*		
Kaempferol	<0.1	<0.1	Eugenol	<0.1	<0.1
Apigenin	<0.1	<0.1	Chlorogenic acid	<0.1	<0.1
Galangin	<0.1	<0.1	Salicylic acid	<0.1	<0.1
Chrysin	<0.1	<0.1	*p*-Hydroxy benzoic acid	737.0	<0.1
Hesperetin	<0.1	<0.1	*o*-Aminobenzoic acid	<0.1	<0.1
Myricetin	<0.1	<0.1	7-Hydroxycoumarin	<0.1	<0.1
LPS		0.0395			

Table 1. Compostion of LCC (Fr4) prepared from *Lentinus edodes* mycelia extract (LEM)

2.2 Biological activity

2.2.1 Immunopotentiating actiivty

Pretreatment of mice with LCC derived from pine cone extract increased the survival time of tumor-bearing mice (Sakagami et al., 1987) and bacterial-inoculated mice, possibly due to the accumulation of polymorphonuclear cells and monocytes/macrophages that produce active oxygens (Harada et al., 1988).

Pretreatment of mice with LCC induced antimicrobial activity against various microorganisms (*Staphylococcus aureus* SH10, *Escherichia coli* GN2411, *Pseudomonas aeruginosa* H7, *Klebsiella pneumoniae* ST101, *Candida albicans* YA2), but not *Salmonella enteritidis* 116-54 (Harada et al., 1988; Oh-hara et al., 1990). When the sugar moiety of LCC was destroyed by treatment with sulfuric acid or trifluoroacetic acid, the antimicrobial activity was significantly reduced. Furthermore, dehydrogenation polymers of phenylpropenoids, which do not contain sugar, showed much lower antimicrobial activity. These data suggest the importance of sugar moiety of LCC for the induction of antimicrobial activity.

Pretreatment with LCCs protected infant mice from *Hymenoleptis nana* (Cestoda) infection. Subcutaneous administration of LCCs (10 mg/kg) to 1 week old mice evoked strong protective immunity against oral infection by *Hymenolepis nana* eggs. Significant antiparasite effects were also induced in 4 week old mice by intraperitoneal or oral administration of LCCs. Injection of LCCs by any root (*s.c, i.p., p.o.*) induced higher antiparasite activity than other natural antitumor polysaccharides [pine cone polysaccharide (Frs. I, II), PSK (protein-bound polysaccharide), Schizophyllan (water-soluble glucan), TAK (water-insoluble glucan), carboxymethyl TAK] (Abe et al., 1989). These data suggest that the conjugation of sugar and polyphenols is essential for the expression of *in vivo* biological activity.

2.2.2 Cytokine production

a. *In vivo* study.

Endogenously produced TNF have been reported to induce resistance against microbial infection (Nakane et al., 1988). When mice were intravenously treated with eliciting agents such as OK-432 (Picibanil)(Sakagami et al., 1990a) or *Lactobacillus casei* (Sakagami et al., 1992a), TNF was induced in the blood, reaching a maximum level after 2-3 hours, and thereafter rapidly declined. Priming the mice with LCC, much higher level of endogenous TNF was induced, accompanied by hepatic accumulation of Kupffer cells. The priming effect of LCC may be involved in the induction of antitumor, antimicrobial and antiparasite activities. The endogenous TNF production primed by LCC decreased during the aging of mice and upon the tumor implantation into the mice (Hanaoka et al., 1989), suggesting the possibility that the resistance of the hosts against microbial infection may decline with aging.

b. *In vitro* study.

In contract, contamination of lipopolysaccharide (LPS) at more than 0.0001% of sample significantly affected cytokine determination *in vitro*. When the biological activity derived from contaminating LPS was subtracted, both cacao mass and husk LCCs lost the stimulation activity of nitric oxide (NO) and cytokine (TNF-α, IL-1β, IFN-γ) production in mouse macrophage-like cell lines (RAW264.7, J774.1). However, cacao mass LCC enhanced LPS-induced iNOS expression in RAW264.7 cells. These data demonstrated several new biological activities of LCC distinct from LPS and further confirmed the promising antiviral and immunomodulating activities of LCCs (Sakagami et al., 2011).

2.2.3 Anti-viral activity

a. Anti-HIV activity:

Anti- human immunodeficiency virus (HIV) activity was assessed quantitatively by a selectivity index (SI=CC_{50}/EC_{50}, where CC_{50} is the 50% cytotoxic concentration against mock-infected MT-4 cells, and EC_{50} is the 50% effective concentration against HIV-infected cells).

LCCs from pine cone from *Pinus parviflora* Sieb et Zucc. and *Pinus elliottii* var. Elliotti (SI=14, 28), bark of *Erythroxylum catuaba* Arr. Cam. (SI=43) (Manabe et al., 1992), husk and mass of *Theobroma cacao* (SI= 311, 46) (Sakagami et al., 2008) and cultured extract of LEM (SI=>94) (Kawano et al. 2010) and mulberry juice (SI=7) (Sakagami et al., 2007; Sakagami and Watanabe, 2011) showed potent anti-HIV activity. The anti-HIV activity of the hot water extract of LEM has been demonstrated also by other groups (Suzuki et al., 1990). The anti-HIV activity of LCCs (Nakashima et al., 1992a) was generally higher than that of lower molecular weight polyphenols, such as tannins (SI=1-11) (Nakashima et al., 1992b), flavonoids (SI=1) (Fukai et al., 2000), gallic acid, (-)-epigallocatechin 3-*O*-gallate (EGCG), curcumin, and natural and chemically modified glucans [*N,N*-dimethylaminoethyl paramylon, *N,N*-diethylaminoethyl paramylon, 2-hydroxy-3-trimethylammoniopropyl paramylon, sodium caroboxymethyl paramylon, carboxymethyl-TAK) (SI=1) except for sulfated polysaccharide (such as paramylon sulfate and dextran sulfate) (Koizumi et al., 1993) (Table 2).

	Yield (%)	Anti-HIV activity (SI)
LCC pine cone of *Pinus parviflora* Sieb. et Zucc.	0.51	14
LCC from pine cone of *Pinus elliottii* var. Elliottii	0.35	28
LCC from seed shell of *Pinus parviflora Sieb. et Zucc.*	0.1	12
LCC from bark of *Erythroxylum catuaba* Arr. Cam.	0.19	43
LCC from husk of *Theobroma cacao*	3.2	311
LCC from mass of *Theobroma cacao*	7.9	46
LCC from cultured *Lentinus edodes* mycelia	0.54	94
LCC from mulberry juice	1.9	7
Dehydrogenation polymers of phenylpropenoids (n=23)		105
Neutral polysaccharide from pine cone	0.1	1
Acidic polysaccharide from pine cone	0.81	1
N,N-dimethylaminoethyl paramylon (SR: 3.7-6.3%)		<1
N,N-diethylaminoethyl paramylon (SR: 10%)		<1
2-hydroxy-3-trimethylammoniopropyl paramylon (SR: 4.3%)		<1
Paramylon sulfate (SR: 0.08%)		<1
Paramylon sulfate (SR: 4.1%)		>274
N,N-dimethylaminoethyl curdlan (SR: 5.0%)		<1
PSK (protein-bound polysaccharide)		1
Hydrolyzable tannins monomer (n=21) (MW: 484-1255)		<1
Hydrolyzable tannins dimer (n=39) (MW: 1571-2282)		<1
Hydrolyzable tannins trimer (n=4) (MW: 2354-2658)		3
Hydrolyzable tannins tetramer (n=3) (MW: 3138-3745)		11
Condensed tannins (n=8) (MW: 290-1764)		<1
Flavonoids (n=160) (MW: 84-648)		<1
Gallic acid (MW170)		<1
(-)-Epigallocatechin 3-*O*-gallate (MW458)		<1
Curcumin		<1

Table 2. Anti-HIV activity of polyphenols.

Limited digestion of lignin structure by $NaClO_2$ resulted in significant loss of anti-HIV activity (from SI=14 to 3), whereas removal of the monosaccharide residues by acid-catalyzed hydrolysis did not significant affect the anti-HIV activity (from SI= 14 to 13) (Lai et al., 1992), suggesting that phenylpropenoid polymer, but not sugar moiety, is important for anti-HIV activity. Dehydrogenation polymers of phenylpropenoids without carbohydrate showed generally higher anti-HIV activity (SI=105) than LCCs (Nakashima et al., 1992a). On the other hand, phenylpropenoid monomers (*p*-coumaric acid, ferulic acid, caffeic acid) were inactive, suggesting the importance of highly polymerized structure. LCCs inhibited HIV adsorption to the cells (Nakashima et al., 1992a) and the HIV-1 reverse transcriptase activity (Lai et al., 1990) and HIV-1 protease activity (Ichimura et al., 1999).

b. Anti-influenza virus activity:

LCCs inhibited the plaque formation and RNA polymerase (enzyme engaged in viral replication) activity of influenza virus (Nagata et al., 1990). Limited digestion demonstrated that phenylpropenoid polymer, but not sugar moiety, is important for anti-influenza virus activity (Harada et al., 1991). This was confirmed by our finding that dehydrogenation polymers of phenylpropenoids without carbohydrate inhibited both the plaque formation and RNA polymerase more effectively than LCCs (Sakagami et al., 1990b).

LCC instantly adsorbed to the influenza virus when mixed *in vitro*, as demonstrated by sucrose gradient centrifugation, and abrogated the infectivity of the influenza virus in mouse infection model (Sakagami et al, 1992b).

c. Anti-HSV activity:

LCCs, isolated from the cones of various pine trees (*Pinus parviflora* Sieb. and Zucc, *Pinus densiflora* Sieb. et Zucc., *Pinus thunbergii* Parl., *Pinus elliottii* var. Elliotti, *Pinus taeda* L., *Pinus caribaea* var. Hondurenses, *Pinus sylvestris* L., and the pine seed shells of *Pinus parviflora* Sieb. et Zucc., and *Pinus armandii* Franch) inhibited the plaque formation of herpes simplex virus types 1 and 2 (HSV-1, HSV-2) strains in African green monkey kidney cells and human adenocarcinoma cells. LCC (pine cone Fr. VI) showed the highest selectivity index (SI=1000) (CC_{50}>300 μg/mL, EC_{50}=0.3 μg/mL) (100% inhibition at 10 μg/mL). On the other hand, neutral polysaccharide (pine cone Fr. I) (0% inhibition at 10 μg/mL) and acidic polysaccharide (rich in uronic acid) (pine cone Fr. II) (0% inhibition), glucans (paramylon, Schizophyllan, TAK), and chemically modified derivatives (*N,N*-dimethylaminoethyl paramylon, sodium carboxymethyl paramylon, sodium paramylon sulfate, carboxymethyl-TAK) and PSK were inactive (Fukuchi et al., 1989a). Tannins such as oenothein B, coriariin A, rugosin D, cornusiin A, tellimagrandin I, casuarictin, penta-*O*-galloyl-β-D-glucose, geraniin, 4,8-tetramer of epicatechin gallate showed potent anti-HSV activity (Fukuchi et al., 1989b), although they showed much weak anti-HIV activity. An experiment using ^{3}H-thymidine labeled virus particles indicated that the anti-HSV effect of both LCCs (Fukuchi et al., 1989a,) and tannins (Fukuchi et al., 1989b) was attributable to interference with virus adsorption to these cells rather than to inhibition of virus penetration into the cells.

Recently, carboxylated lignins, synthesized using 4-hydroxy cinnamic acid scaffold by enzymatic oxidative coupling, have been reported to inhibit the entry of HSV-1 entry into the cells (Thakkar et al., 2010). Sulfated LCC (PPS-2b) (MW8500) also showed anti-HSV activity possibly by inhibiting the viral binding and penetration into host cells. Prunella cream formulated with a semi-purified fraction significantly reduced the skin lesion and mortality induced by HSV-1 infection in Guinea pigs (Zhang et al., 2007) The anti-HSV activity of sulfated lignins depended on their molecular weight, with the maximum at 39.4 kDa (Raghuraman et al., 2007).

d. Clinical application.

A clinical pilot study was carried out to evaluate anti-HSV-1 activity of a pine cone LCC and ascorbic acid treatment, with forty eight healthy patients of both genders between 4 and 61 years old (mean: 31 years), with active lesions of HSV-1. According to the HSV-1 stage at the presentation the patients were classified into the prodromic, erythema, papule edema, vesicle/pustule and ulcer stages. One mg of LCC-ascorbic acid tablet or solution was orally administered three times daily for a month. The patients who began the LCC-ascorbic acid treatment within the first 48 hours did not develop HSV-1 characteristic lesions, whereas those patients who began the treatment later experienced a shorter duration of cold sore lesions and a decrease in the symptoms. The majority of the patients reported the reduction in the severity of symptoms and the reduction in the recurrence episodes after the LCC-ascorbic acid treatment compared with previous episodes, suggesting its possible applicability for the prevention and treatment of HSV-1 infection (López et al., 2009).

2.2.4 Synergistic action with vitamin C

Vitamin C exhibited either antioxidant or prooxidant activity, depending on the concentration (Sakagami et al., 2000b). We have reported that ascorbate derivatives that produced the doublet signal of ascorbate radical (sodium-L-ascorbate, L-ascorbic acid, D-isoascorbic acid, 6-β-D-galactosyl-L-ascorbate, sodium 5,6-benzylidene-L-ascorbate) induced apoptosis (characterized by internucleosomal DNA fragmentation and an increase in the intracellular Ca^{2+} concentration) in HL-60 cells. On the other hand, ascorbate derivatives that did not produce radicals (L-ascorbic acid-2-phosphate magnesium salt, L-ascorbic acid 2-sulfate and dehydroascorbic acid) did not induce apoptosis (Sakagami et al., 1996a, 1996b). This suggests the possible involvement of the ascorbate radical in apoptosis-induction by ascorbic acid-related compounds.

We accidentally found that LCCs from the pine cone of *Pinus parviflola* Sieb et Zucc, pine cone of *Pinus elliottii* var. Elliotti, leaf of *Ceriops decandra* (Griff.) Ding Hou and, thorn apple of *Crataegu Cuneata* Sieb. et Zucc modulated the radical intensity of ascorbate bi-phasically, depending on the concentrations. At higher concentration, LCCs strongly enhanced the radical intensity of sodium ascorbate, which rapidly decayed, possibly due to the breakdown of ascorbic acid or to the consumption of ascorbyl radical. LCCs, not only from pine cones (Fr. VI), but also from Catuaba bark, pine seed shell, *A. nikoense* Maxim. and *C. Cuneata Sieb.* et Zucc. enhanced the radical intensity and cytotoxic activity of sodium ascorbate (Sakagami et al., 2005). On the other hand, tannins such as gallic acid, EGCG, and tannic acid counteracted the radical intensity and cytotoxic activity of sodium ascorbate (Satoh et al, 1999).

Sodium ascorbate rapidly reduced the oxygen concentration in the culture medium, possibly due to oxygen consumption *via* its pro-oxidation action. Simultaneous addition of LCCs further enhanced the ascorbate-stimulated consumption of oxygen (Sakagami et al., 1997). These data suggest that the synergistic enhancement of the cytotoxic activity of LCCs and ascorbate might be due at least in part to the stimulated induction of hypoxia.

Lower concentration of LCC (pine cone Fr. VI) and sodium acorbate showed radical scavenging activity. LCC further stimulated the superoxide anion (O_2^-) and 1,1-diphenyl-2-picrylhydrazyl (DPPH) radical scavenging activity of sodium ascorbate. LCCs from *Ceriops decandra* (Griff.) Ding Hou. and cacao husk scavenged O_2^- and hydroxyl radical, and synergistically enhanced the radical scavenging activity of sodium ascorbate (Sakagami et al., 2005, 2008) .

2.3 State in hot-water extract. Possible binding to other compounds

Solvent fractionation of Alkaline Extract of the Leaves of *Sasa senanensis* Rehder (SE) demonstrated that (i) chlorophyllin in SE was recovered from the water layer, that contains majority of compounds (more than 81%) and inhibited the NO production by macrophages more potently than other *n*-hexane, diethyl ether and ethylacetate layers (Sakagami et al., 2010). Three-dimensional HPLC analysis demonstrated that the majority of SE components are recovered from one major peak. Furthermore, LCC isolated from SE showed the unique greenish color of chlorophyllin (absorption maximum = 452 nm) (Sakagami et al., 2010a). These data strongly suggest the possible association of chlorophyllin with LCC in the native state or during extraction with alkaline solutions.

2.4 Site of action, signaling pathway, and receptor identification

A receptor for LCC, and the related signal transduction pathways had been largely unknown. On the other hand, β-glucans and α-mannans, which constitute the cell wall of fungi and plants, are recognized by dectin-1 and dectin-2, respectively, which are members of C-type lectins, and prominently expressed in the cell membrane of dendritic cells and macrophages as the transmembrane receptors (Brown & Gordon, 2001; McGreal et al., 2006; Vautier et al., 2010). It is also known that dectin-1 and 2 are essential for host defense against fungi, such as, *Pneumocystis carinii*, and *Candia albicans* (Saijo et al., 2007; 2010). Furthermore, genetic and immunological studies have demonstrated the molecular mechanism regarding the immunostimulation and phylaxis recently. It became evident that, in the dendritic cells and macrophages, activated dectin-1 and 2 by β-glucans and α-mannans, respectively, can induce the activation of NFκb thorough signal transduction molecules such as syk and Card9-Bcl10-Malt1 (Gross et al., 2006; Saijo et al., 2010; Vautier et al., 2010).

In order to elucidate their action point, DNA microarray analysis was performed, using mouse macrophage-like J774.1 cells. RNA was isolated with Qiagen RNeasy Plus Mini kit, hydridized with GeneChip MouseGene 1.0 ST arrays, and scanned with Affymetrix GeneChip Command Console software. One of the seven LCC fractions isolated from LEM (Fr4) enhanced the expression of dectin-2 (4.2-fold) and toll-like receptor (TLR)-2 (2.5-fold) prominently, but only slightly modified the expression of dectin-1 (0.8-fold), complement receptor 3 (0.9-fold), TLR1, 3, 4, 9 and 13 (0.8- to 1.7-fold), spleen tyrosine kinase (Syk)b, zeta-chain (TCR) associated protein kinase 70kDa (Zap70), Janus tyrosine kinase (Jak)2 (1.0- to 1.2-fold), nuclear factor (Nf)κb1, NFκb2, reticuloendotheliosis viral oncogene homolog (Rel)a, Relb (1.0- to 1.6-fold), Nfκbia, Nfκbib, Nfκbie, Nfκbi12 Nfκbiz (0.8- to 2.3-fold). On the other hand, LPS did not affect the expression of dectin-2 nor TLR-2 (Fig. 2). These data suggest the significant role of the activation of the dectin-2 signaling pathway in the action of LCC on macrophages (Kushida et al., 2011).

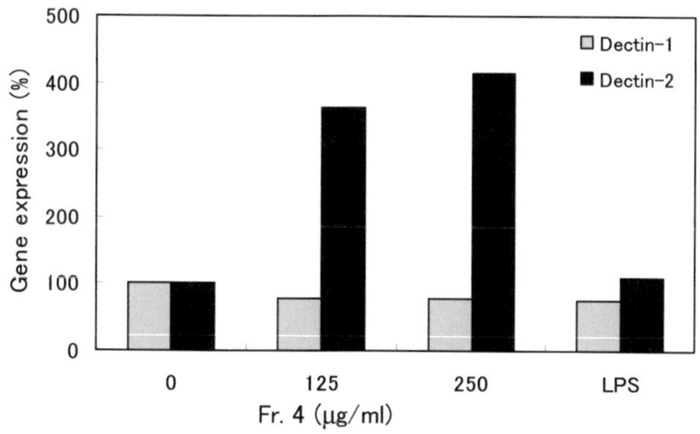

Fig. 2. Enhancement of *dectin-2* gene expression by LCC from LEM. Modified from Kushida et al., 2011, with permission.

2.5 Future directions

We have previously reported that tumor-specificity of oligomeric tannins (both hydrolysable and condensed types) is higher than that of monomeric tannins (Sakagami et al., 2000a), although the tumor-specificity of tannins was much lower than that of chemotherapeutic drugs (Sakagami, 2010a). This suggests the importance of determining the optimal molecular weight of LCC for the expression of the highest biological activity. However, with the increase in the molecular weight, the water-solubility of LCC may decline, and make it difficult to be sterilized by millipore filteration.

There is a possibility that bacterial endotoxin (LPS) in the soil and air may contaminate LCC during the isolation step, since LPS is similarly extracted with alkaline solution and precipitated with acid. Most of previous studies have not paid attention to such LPS contamination in the LCC preparations. Alkaline extraction step that is necessary for the preparation of LCC has both merit and demerit. Merit is the chemical inactivation of LPS. Demerit is the degradation of LCC into its smaller size. Therefore, the conditions for alkaline extraction should be optimized to maximize the LPS inactivation and minimize the loss of biological activity.

It is generally accepted that lignin is linked by various amounts of polysaccharides (polymers of glucose or other sugar), yielding LCCs having broad ranges of molecular weights. Phenylpropenoid polymer portion of LCC have potent anti-vial activity, whereas carbohydrate portion have immunopotentiation activity, possibly *via* activation of TLR pathway and chemokine expression (Fig. 3). After extraction with alkaline solution, the structure of LCC may be either unmodified or modified. When LCC is prepared from the leaves, chlorophyllin may be associated during extraction step with alkaline solution. This association may enhance anti-inflammation activity and inhibition of cytochrome P-450 (CYP). When washing procedure is incomplete, LPS from bacteria in the soil and air may associate with LCC, considering that both LPS and LCC are precipitated by acid. This association may trigger the back-ground level of immune response-related genes expression. The associations with chlorophyllin, LPS and others may produce diverse biological activities, depending on the plant species and preparative procedures.

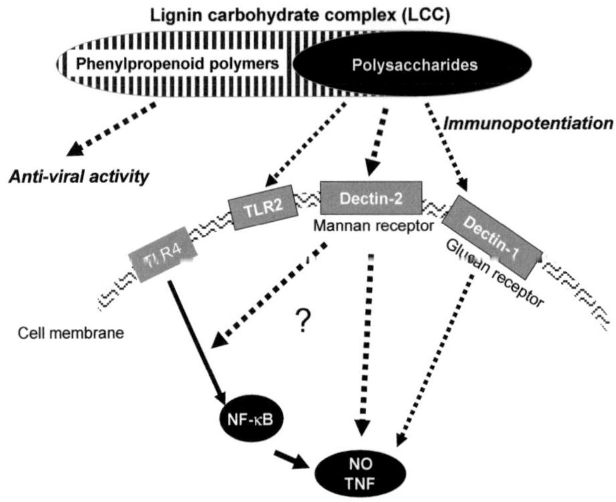

Fig. 3. Possible site of action of LCC

3. Tannins

3.1 Yield and putative amounts in methanol and hot water extracts

Tannins are defined to be naturally occurring polyphenols with potent binding activity with proteins and other biomolecules such as polysaccharides and lipids. The binding of tannins with those molecules is attributed to the hydrogen bonding and/or hydrophobic interaction, in addition to electrostatic interaction. In some cases covalent bonding also attributes to the interaction with proteins. Tannins are structurally classified into two major groups. Those belonging to one group are called hydrolysable tannins: i.e., esters of gallic acid and its oxidative derivatives with glucose or related sugars. The other ones are belonging to condensed tannins: i.e., flavan oligomers or polymers where their constituent monomeric flavans are connected mainly by C-4 - C-8 or C-4 - C-6 linkages. Some other types of polyphenolic compounds such as those containing several caffeic acid units (caffeetannins), and phloroglucinol oligomers or polymers (phlorotannins) are also regarded to be tannins. The binding properties of tannins, and therefore their biological and/or pharmacological properties attributed to the binding, vary depending on their structures. Since tannins bind strongly with cellulose and lignin of plant cells with hydrogen bonding and hydrophobic interaction, combinations of acetone and water are used as the solvents for extraction of tannins to release them from the plant cells. Some examples for the extractability of tannins from plant materials are shown below.

Geranium thunbergii is a plant species belonging to the family Geraniaceae, and its aerial part has been used as a folkmedicine for treatments of intestinal disorders including diarrhoea in Japan. Geraniin, the major constituent of this medicinal herb, is the representative hydrolysable tannin composed of galloyl, hexahydroxydiphenoyl (HHDP), and dehydrohexahydroxydiphenoyl (DHHDP) groups, in addition to a glucopyranose core. Several other tannins with related structures, including didehydrogeraniin, furosin, furosinin, elaeocarpusin (=ascorgeraniin), and geraniinic acids B and C, were also isolated from the same source plant species. Quantitative analysis of this medicinal herb using methylene blue for the estimation of total tannin indicated that the tannin contents vary 0.9

% - 2.4 % of the aerial part, depending on the collected month. The quantitative experiments applied to several *Geranium* species indicated that the extractability for tannins with methanol is lower than that with the mixture of acetone and water (ca. 30-50% lower). The quantitative analysis of geraniin, the major tannin of *G. thunbergii*, by high-performance liquid chromatography (HPLC) of the aqueous acetone extracts indicated that the contents were 0.6 % - 1.8 % of the aerial parts of the plant species (Okuda et al., 1980).

Most of the medicinal herbs have been extracted with hot water used in the traditional medicine, although some types of constituents are decomposed in hot water to give various products. Geraniin is also easily hydrolyzed in water to give several lower molecular weight polyphenols, such as corilagin, gallic acid, ellagic acid, and brevifolin (Fig. 4). Thus, the behaviour of geraniin during the extraction of the constituents from this medicinal herb with hot water was investigated. The first increment of the geraniin concentration was then followed by its decrease accompanied by the increase of corilagin, a hydrolysis product from geraniin. The highest concentration of geraniin during the decoction was observed at the time just after the boiling.

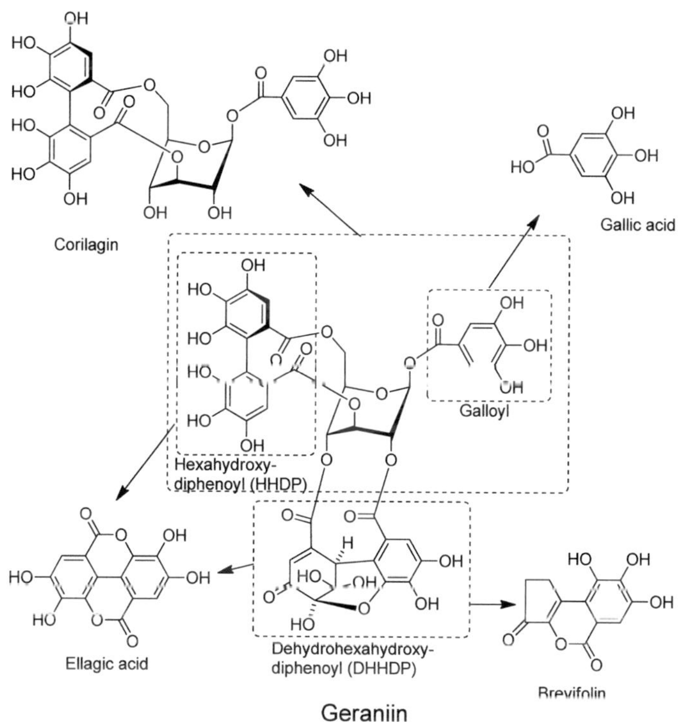

Fig. 4. Structural changes of geraniin in hot water

Analogous quantitative analysis was also performed for the extraction of rosmarinic acid (Fig. 5), called Labiatae-tannin, from dried leaves of *Perilla frutescens*. As a result, the concentration of this polyphenolic compound increased until the time of the boiling. The concentration did not decrease during the continuous heating of the aqueous solution, while rosmarinic acid was quite unstable when preparing the dried herb by heated air (Okuda et al., 1986).

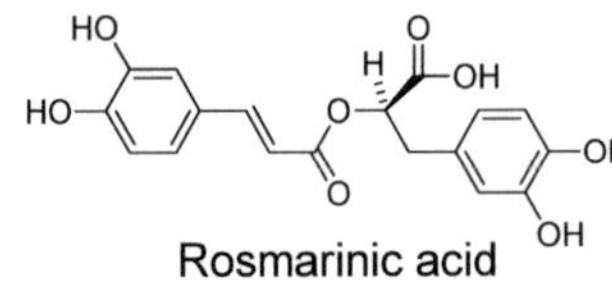

Fig. 5. Structure of rosmarinic acid

3.2 Biological activity

3.2.1 Anti-tumor activity

Some hydrolysable tannins with high molecular weights, including oenothein B, have been shown to have potent host-mediated anti-tumor activity. Recently, we found that several hydrolysable tannins isolated from plants belonging to the family Tamaricaceae, such as nilotinin D8 (Fig. 6), showed remarkable cytotoxic effects on cultured cell lines from oral tumors (Orabi et al. 2010).

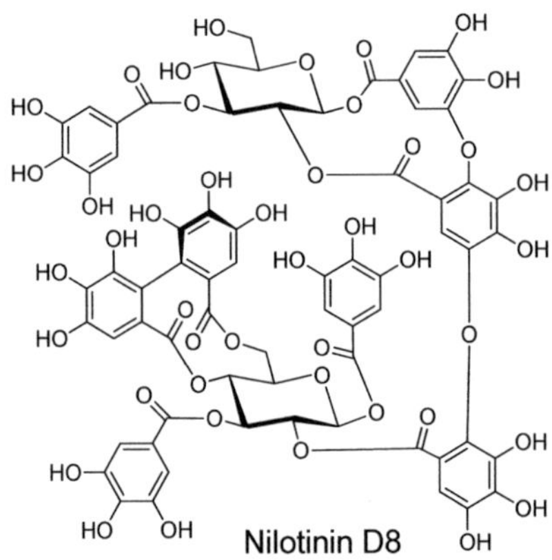

Fig. 6. Structure of a *Tamarix* tannin effective on the tumor cells

3.2.2 Anti-bacterial activity

Antibacterial effects of polyphenolic compounds including tannins have been revealed for various bacterial species. One of the important problems concerning the infectious disease is the menace of antibiotic resistance. Clinical usages of antibiotics against infectious diseases have caused developments of antibiotic resistance of the bacteria. Among various antibiotic-resistant bacteria species, methicillin-resistant *Staphylococcus aureus* (MRSA) causes about 20 000 or more patients in a year in Japan. Tannins showed potent effects on the antibiotic resistance of bacteria as shown below.

Clinical isolates of MRSA found in Okayama University Hospital, which acquired antibiotic resistance against β-lactams, aminoglycosides, macrolides, and some other antibiotics, were used as target bacteria. The addition of (-)-epicatechin gallate (25 mg/L), isolated from green tea leaves, decreased the minimum inhibitory concentration (MIC) of oxacillin, 128-512 mg/L for four MRSA strains, to 0.5-1 mg/L (Shiota et al., 1999). An analogous decrease of MIC of oxacillin was found for the addition of tellimagrandin I, a hydrolysable tannin isolated from rose petals. The addition of tellimagrandin I also brought the decrease of the

MIC of tetracycline for two MRSA strains, from 2 to 0.25, and 8 to 1 mg/L, respectively (Shiota et al., 2000). Corilagin, isolated from leaves of *Arctostaphyllos uva-ursi*, also caused noticeable decreases of the MIC values of several β-lactam antibiotics. The mechanisms of the effects of the hydrolysable tannins were also examined, and the suppression of the function of penicillin-binding protein 2a (PBP-2a), and also the inhibitory effects on β-lactamase have been suggested (Shimizu et al., 2001).

Further investigation revealed that a product obtained by incubation of (-)-epigallocatechin gallate (EGCG) in solution showed lowering effects on MIC of β-lactam antibiotics. Since EGCG is unstable even in neutral solution, we investigated the changes in the structure of EGCG, and found formation of dimeric products. Among the products, theasinensin A (Fig. 7) caused marked decrease of MIC of oxacillin, and related β-lactam antibiotics. MIC of streptomycin for the MRSA strains and for a methicillin-sensitive *Staphylococcus* strain decreased upon the addition of theasinensin A (Hatano et al., 2003a). Condensed proanthocyanidin obtained from pericarpus of Japanese pepper (*Zanthoxylum piperitum*) also decreased MIC of β-lactam antibiotics (Kusuda et al., 2006).

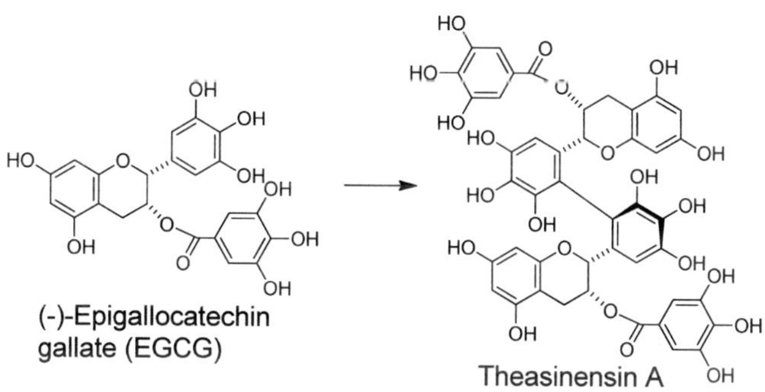

Fig. 7. Structural changes of EGCG into theasinensin A

3.3 State in hot-water extract: Possible binding to other compounds

Although some hydrolysable tannins such as geraniin were unstable in water as mentioned above, the stability of hydrolysable tannins in water is dependent on their structures. Structural changes of different oligomeric hydrolysable tannins during the hot water treatment were investigated, and differences in the instability of those tannins have also been shown. For example, isorugosin D, which is a regio-isomer of rugosin D concerning the orientation of valoneoyl group, was more stable, relative to rugosin D, against the hot water treatment. Oenothein B, which has a macrocyclic structure with two valoneoyl groups in the molecule, was much more stable relative to those dimers (Fig. 8) (Yoshida et al., 1992).

Investigation on the metabolic profiles after oral administration of galloylglucoses revealed formation of 4-O-methylgallic acid. The HHDP group in ellagitannins is metabolised into urolithins A and B, and some compounds structurally related to them (Ito et al., 2008). On the other hand, metabolism of catechins and related oligomeric flavanoids gives protocatechuic acid, and its methyl derivatives (Fig. 9). Our investigation of the binding of EGCG and those low-molecular-weight metabolites revealed that they affects the bindings of site-I- and site-II-binding drugs to human serum albumin, depending on their structures (Nozaki et al., 2009).

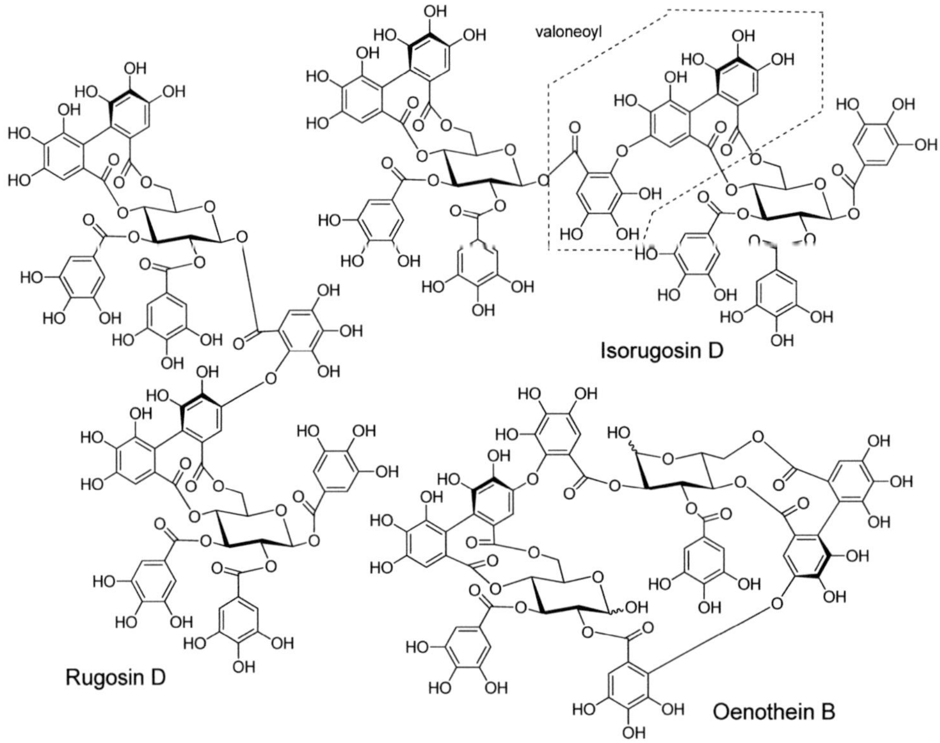

Fig. 8. Structures of rugosin D, isorugosin D, and oenothein B

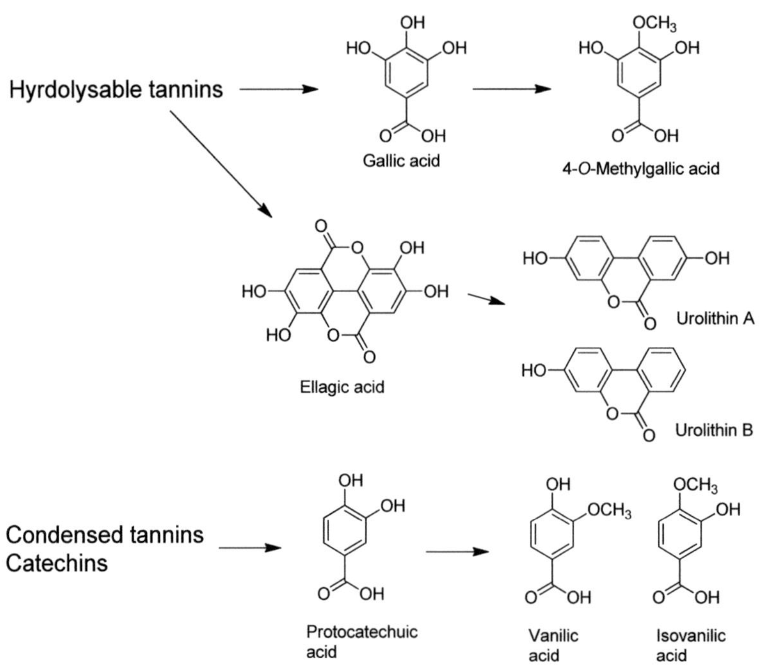

Fig. 9. Metabolism of tannins

3.4 Site of action, signaling pathway, and receptor identification

Pentagalloyglucose has been reported to induce autophagic cell death in prostate cancer cells (Hu et al., 2009) and inhibit its bone metastasis by transcriptionally repressing EGF-induced metalloproteinase secrtion (Kuo et al., 2009). On the other hand, proanthocyanidines induce apoptotic cell death in human non-small cell lung cancer cells, at least in part due to inhibition of COX-2, PGE_2 and PGE_2 receptor expression (Shama et al., 2010).

3.5 Future directions

Many researchers have reported various pharmacological and biological activity of polyphenolic compounds including tannins. However, some of those compounds, especially several tannins and condensed proanthocyanidins or catechins are unstable in water and/or on heating. Therefore, the actual pharmacologically active compounds may be different from the administered compounds. The changing procedures should be clarified. Our study on the structural changes of catechins will give a solution of the problem (Taniguchi et al., 2008).

Binding of polyphenolic compounds, especially the binding of tannins, to biomolecules should be further investigated, too, since their pharmacological activity starts with the association or complex formation of the polyphenols and biomolecules. Our study on the formation of complex from tannins and related polyphenols with serum albumin revealed that the formed supermolecule has the "molecular weight" of 9.5×10^5 for a combination (Hatano et al., 2003b). The structural details of those supermolecules are still in an enigma.

4. Flavonoids

Flavonoids are important secondary metabolites in higher plants, and classified into flavones, isoflavones, flavonols, flavanones, catechins and anthocyanidins, based on the skeletons of aglycone moieties (Fig. 10). Backbone structures of all flavonoids are derived from two metabolites, malonyl-CoA and *p*-coumaroyl-CoA, and the biosynthetic pathway of flavonoids are the condensation of three molecules of malonyl-CoA with one molecule of *p*-coumaroyl-CoA (Martens & Mithöfer, 2005).

Flavone glycosides are classified into *O*- and *C*-glycoside, and flavone *C*-glycosides are found in several plants such as *sasa* genus (Nakajima et al., 2003, Park et al., 2007), *cucurbitaceae* (Abou-Zaid et al., 2001) and buckwheat seedling (Watanabe and Ito, 2002). Flavonols such as kaempferol and quercetin glycosides, flavones such as apigenin and luteolin glycosides and anthocyanidins (Fig. 10) display several biological activities.

4.1 Yield and putative amounts in methanol and hot water extracts

Flavonoids of yellow pigment are usually extracted by methanol, ethanol or alcohol-water mixtures, and fractionated by diethyl ether and ethyl acetate. Anthocyanines of red pigment are usually extracted by methanol and hydrochloric acid or trifluoroacetic acid mixtures (with yield of about 1-5%). The use of mineral acid can lead to the loss of attached acyl group.

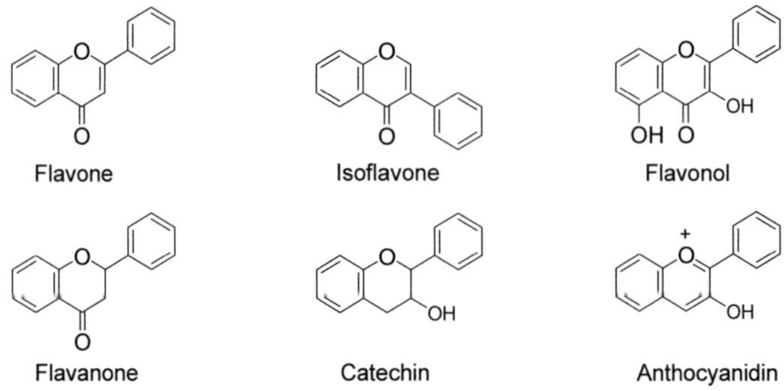

Fig. 10. Basic structures of flavonoids.

4.2 Biological activity

4.2.1 Anti-osteoporosis activity

Osteoporosis is considered to be one of the hormonal deficiency diseases observed in the menopausal women and elderly persons. When estrogen is reduced in the body, the production of pro-inflammatory cytokines such as IL-1β and IL-6 are elevated, and the osteoclastogenesis enhanced, leading to the bone resorption. Glucosidic isoflavones of PIII (Isocal, glucosidic isoflavones extracted from *Sophorae fructus*) stimulated the osteoblastic proliferation by suppressing the IL-1β and IL-6 production and elevating the NO level. In bone marrow primary culture, PIII effectively suppressed the osteoclastogenesis. These effects of PIII was slightly lower than 17β-estradiol, but higher than two soybean isoflavones [daidzin (**1**), genistin (**2**)]. PIII may preferentially induce anti-osteoporosis response by attenuating their osteoclastic differentiation and by upregulating the NO (Fig.11) (Joo et al., 2003).

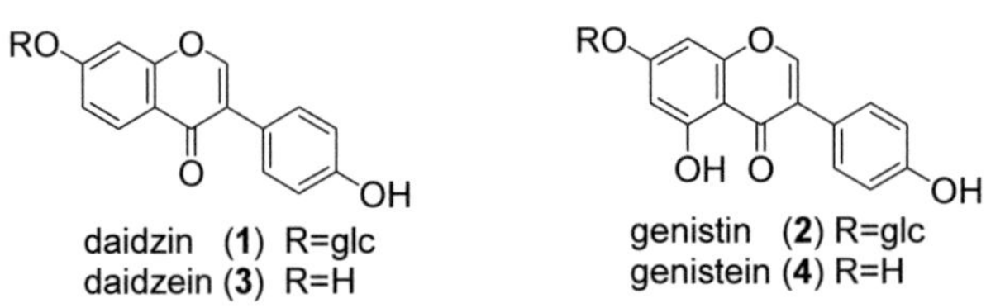

Fig. 11. Two glucosidic isoflavones of daidzin (1) and genistin (2)

4.2.2 Tumor-specificity evaluated in vitro

Prenylflavanones [sophoraflavanone G (**5**), sophoraflavanone B, sophoraflavanone A, euchrestaflavanone A, sophoraflavanone H (**6**), sophoraflavanone I (**7**)](Fig. 12) showed higher cytotoxicity agaist two human oral tumor cell lines (HSC-2, HSG), as compared with normal gingival fibroblast (HGF) . Prenylflavanones having either prenyl-, lavandulyl- or geranyl groups on A-ring, and two flavonostilbenes having stilbene (resveratrol) on B-ring showed tumor-specific cytotoxicity, radical generation and O_2^- scavenging activity.

Isoflavones with two isoprenyl groups (one in A-ring and the other in B-ring) such as tetrapterol G and isosophoranone, and isoflavanones with α,α-dimethylallyl group at C-5' of B-ring such as secundifloran, secundiflorol A, secundiflorol D and secundiflorol E had their relatively higher cytotoxic activity. Secundiflorol A had the highest tumor-specific cytotoxicity (tumor specicicity index (TS)=2.8), followed by genistein (TS=2.4) (**4**), secundiflorol D (TS=1.9), secundiflorol E (TS=1.9), secundiflorol F (TS=1.9) > sophoraisoflavanone A (TS=1.8), sophoronol (TS=1.7), secundifloran (TS=1.7) > tetrapterol G (TS=1.6) > isosophoranone (TS=1.5) > daidzein (TS=1.1) (**3**). 6,8-Diprenylation of genistein further enhanced the cytotoxicity *via* radical-mediated oxidation mechanism, but reduced the tumor-specificity.Their cytotoxicity became maximum at a log P value of around 4 (Shirataki et al., 2001a, 2001b).

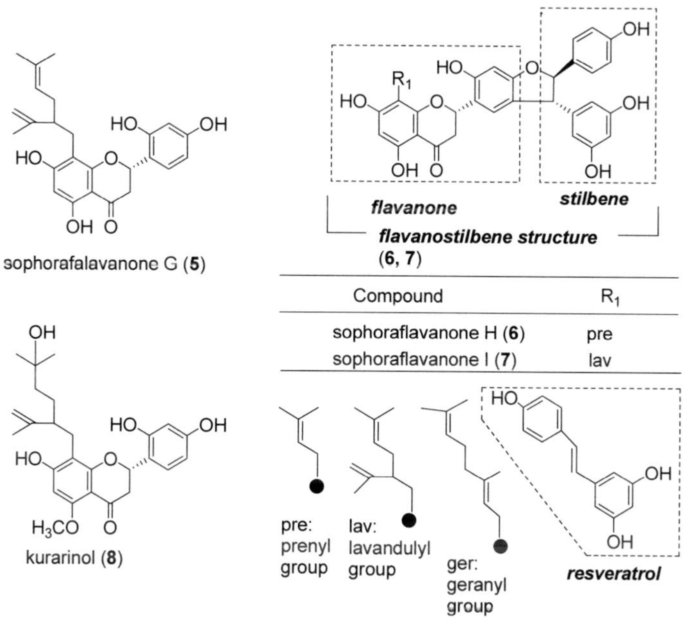

Fig. 12. Prenylflavanones (**5-8**) from *Sophora* plants and its relates

4.2.3 Antimicrobial activity

Among ten prenylflavanones of *Sophora tomentosa* and *Sophora moorcroftiana*, sophoraflavanone G (**5**) showed the highest antimicrobial activity against three Gram-positive bacteria such as *Staphylococcus aureus* 6571, 8530 and 8531, followed by euchrestaflavanone A, sophoraflavanone H (**6**) and sophoraflavanone I (**7**). Sophoraflavanone G (5) also was effective against *Shigella dysenteria* 1, *Escherichia coli* R832 and *Vibrio cholerae* 865. Moreover, sophoraflavanone I (**7**) had the highest anti-*Helicobacter pylori*, followed by sophoraflavanone H (**6**) and sophoraflavanone G (**5**) (Shirataki et al., 2001a). Combined treatment of sophoraflavanone G (**5**) and ampicillin gave synergistic effects against *Streptococcus mutans*, *S. sanguinis*, *S. sobrinus*, *S. gordonii*, *Actinobacillus actinomycetemcomitans*, *Fusobacterium nucleatum*, *Prevotella intermedia*, and *Porphylomonas gingivalis*, whereas the combination treatment of sophoraflavanone G (**5**) and gentamicin was synergistic against *Streptococcus* sanguinis, *S. criceti*, *S. anginosus*, *Actinobacillus actinomycetemcomitans*, *Fusobacterium nucleatum*, *Prevotella intermedia*, and *P. gingivalis*. In particular, the minimum inhibitory concentrations/minimum bactericidal concentrations (MICs/MBCs) for all the bacteria could be reduced to 1/2-1/16 by their drug combinations.

Sophoraflavanone G (**5**) combined with other antibiotics might be microbiologically beneficial (Cha et al., 2007).

Eleven isoflavonoids were examined for their possible antimicrobial property against twelve known Gram-positive and Gram-negative sensitive bacteria. Daidzein (**3**) and calycosin failed to show antimicrobial activity and formononetin, genistein (**4**), biochanin A, irisolidone, 7,4'-dihydroxy-3'-methoxyisoflavone, licoisoflavone A and licoisoflavone B had moderate antimicrobial action. Sophoraisoflavone A and 6,8-diprenylgenistein showed higher antimicrobial activity *in vitro* against 214 strains of bacteria. Their MIC ranged from 25 to 200 mg/L in most strains. At the concentrations of 30 and 60 μg/mouse, sophoraisoflavone A and 6,8-diprenylgenistein significantly protected the mice from 50 median lethal dose (MLD) of a virulent strain of *Salmonella Typhimurium* (Dastidar SG et al., 2004).

4.2.4 Anti-HIV activity

Among ten prenylflavanones, sophoraflavanone G **(5)** (selectivity index (SI) showed weak anti-HIV activity, followed by euchrestaflavanone A (SI=3) and sophoraflavanone H **(6)** (SI=3). Prenylflavanones having either prenyl-, lavandulyl- or geranyl groups on A-ring and/or B-ring, and flavonostilbenes having stilbene (resveratrol) on B-ring showed anti-HIV activity. A good relationship between their anti-HIV activity and radical generation or O_2^- scavenging activity was observed. Eleven isoflavones failed to induce their anti- HIV activity (Shirataki et al., 2001a, 2001b).

4.2.5 Radical generation and radical O_2^- scavenging activity

Among ten prenylflavanones, 6-prenylnaringenin and sophoraflavanone G (**5**), sophoraflavanone H (**6**), sophoraflavanone I (**7**) and euchrestaflavanone A showed radical generation and O_2^- scavenging activity (Shirataki et al., 2001a). Sophoraflavanone G (**5**) and Kurarinone **(9)** protected renal epithelial LLC-PK(1) cells from 2,2'-azobis(2-amidinopropane)dihydrochloride (AAPH)-induced injury, possibly by their antioxidative activity (Piao et al., 2006). Prenylated chalcones such as kuraridin and kuraridinol scavenged DPPH radical. Five flavanones such as kushenol E, leachianone G, kurarinol (**8**), sophoraflavanone G (**5**), and kurarinone (**9**) inhibited *t*-BHP-induced NF-κB activation and exhibited significant antioxidant potentials against 2,2'-azino-*bis*-3-ethylbenzothiazoline-6-sulfonic acid (ABTS), peroxynitrite ($ONOO^-$), and reactive oxygen species (ROS). Prenylated chalcones or flavonol showed higher scavenging and inhibitory activities than prenylated flavanones. Additionally, the results showed that *Sophora flavescens* and its prenylated flavonoids could have their good anti-inflammatory activity, possibly due to their significant antioxidant activity (Jung et al., 2008).

Five compounds such as *trans*-hexadecyl ferulic acid, *cis*-octadecyl ferulic acid, *trans*-hexadecyl sinapic acid, (-)-4-hydroxy-3-methoxy-(6a*R*,11a*R*)-8,9-methylenedioxypterocarpan and desmethylanhydroicaritin exhibited their DPPH and $ONOO^-$ scavenging activities (Jung et al., 2005). All isoflavones [daidzein (**3**), genistein (**4**)] and isoflavanones did not stimulate their NO production by mouse macrophage-like Raw264.7 cells, but almost completely inhibited their NO production by the LPS-activated Raw264.7 cells. Secundifloran and secundiflorol D most potently inhibted the NO production, but also efficiently scavenged the O_2^- and NO radicals.

The inhibition of macrophage NO production by these isoflavanones might, at least in part, be explained by their radical scavenging or reduction activity (Shirataki et al., 2004).

4.2.6 Enzyme inhibitory activity

Sophoflavescenol with a C-8 prenylated flavonol inhibited cyclic guanosine monophosphate (cGMP)-specific phosphodiesterase type 5 (PDE5), more efficiently than PDE3 and PDE4. Among twelve prenylated flavonoids with the resorcinol moiety, kuraridin (**10**), sophoraflavanone G (**5**), kurarinone (**9**) and norkurarinol inhibited the tyrosinase activity more effectively than kojic acid, a tyrosinase inhibitor. The substitution of a lavandulyl or hydroxylavandulyl group at the C-8 position and a methoxy or hydroxy group at the C-5 position (Fig. 13) may be required for their inhibitory effect (Son et al., 2003, Kim et al., 2003)

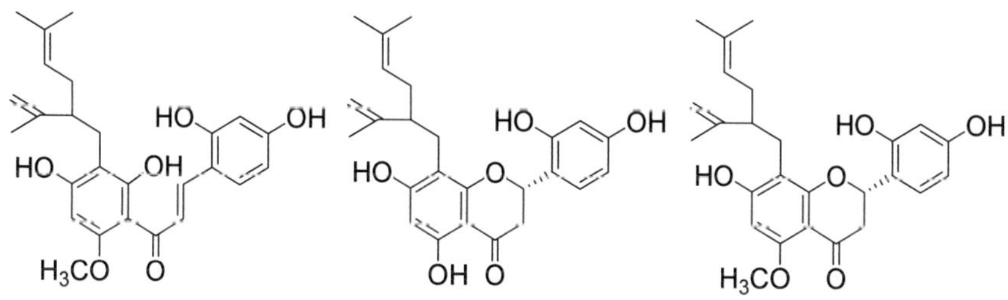

kuraridin (**10**) sophorafalavanone G (**5**) kurarinone (**9**)

Fig. 13. *Sophora flavescens* that inhibit tyrosinase activity

4.3 State in hot-water extract: Possible binding to other compounds

Neutral aqueous solutions in anthocyanins are unstable and quickly decolorized. The copigmentation reaction, first reported by Robinson, is a colour-stabilizing mechanism (Oszmianski et al., 2004) and regarded as significant factors for stabilizing the structure of anthocyanins (Marcovic et al., 2000). The copigmentation reaction occurs, when planar molecule interaction between anthocyanin and other pigments occurs to form the complex. The common copigment compounds are flavonoids such as rutin and quercetin (Bakowska et al., 2003), other polyphenols, amino acids and organic acids.

4.4 Site of action, signaling pathway, and receptor identification

It has been recently reported that baicalin, a flavone, induced the osteoblastic differentiation *via* the activation of Wnt/β-catenin signalling pathway (Guo et al, 2011). Apigenin induced cell growth retardation *via* leptin/leptin receptor pathway in human A549 adenocarcinoma cell line (Bruno et al., 2011).

4.5 Future direction

Flavonoids are distributed into virtually all parts of the plant, the root, heartwood, sapwood, bark, leaf, fruit and flower. Although various pharmacological and biological activities of flavonoids are reported, the reason why biosynthesis of prenylflavonoids is restricted in Leguminosae, Moraceae and a few species of plants is unclear. Further chemical and physiological investigations are needed to answer this question.

5. Saponins

Saponins are naturally occurring glycosides with the ability of forming a soapy lather when shaken with water, and classified as triterpene saponins or steroidal saponins on the basis of the structural features of the aglycone moieties. Triterpene saponins are found in a wide variety of dicotyledonous plants, but are rare in monocotyledons (Dinda et al., 2010). On the other hand, steroidal saponins are mainly distributed among a limited species of monocotyledonous plants (Mahato et al., 1982). Some marine organisms are known to produce saponins with unique chemical structures and biological properties (Minale et al., 1996).

Several important Chinese herbal medicines such as Astragalus Root, Licorice Root, Polygala Root, Ginseng, Bupleurum Root, Anemarrhena Rhizome and Ophiopogon Tuber contain saponins as the main secondary metabolites, which may be responsible for their specific pharmacological activities. Depending on the fundamental skeletons of the aglycone moieties, triterpene saponins have been classified into more than 10 types, oleanane-type, ursane-type, lupan-type, dammarane-type, and so on. As for steroidal saponins, they have been classified as being spirostan-type, furostan-type, or cholestane-type. Cardiac glycosides and pregnane glycosides are parts of steroidal glycosides, but are not usually included in the saponin category.

In this section, the current aspects of a potent cytotoxic saponin of a cholestane-type, 17α-hydroxy-16β-[(*O*-(2-*O*-*p*-methoxybenzoyl-β-D-xylopyranosyl)-(1→3)-2-*O*-acetyl-α-L-arabinopyranosyl)oxy)]cholest-5-en-22-one (OSW-1) (Fig. 14), are mainly described according to the concept of this Chapter.

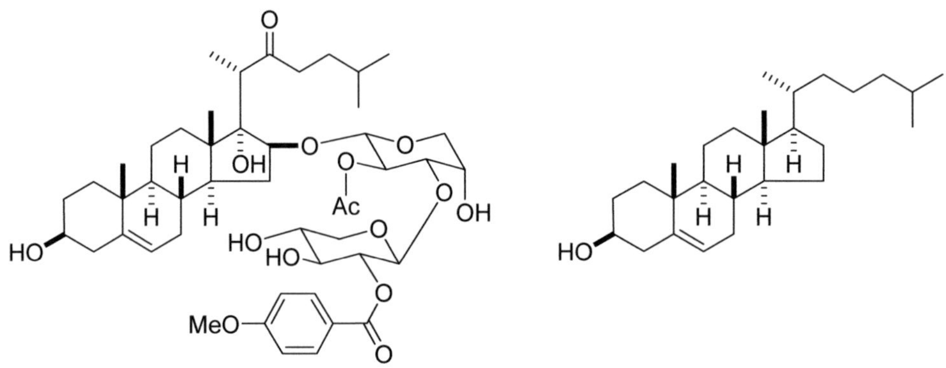

Fig. 14. Structures of OSW-1 (left) and cholesterol (right)

5.1 Yield and putative amounts in methanol and hot water extracts

Saponins can to be extracted with hot water. However, since saponins are structurally composed of a hydrophobic aglycone unit and a hydrophilic sugar moiety, methanol and a mixture of ethanol and water (4:1, v/v) allow saponins, including cardiac and pregnane glycosides with deoxysugar residues, to be exhaustively extracted from crude materials. OSW-1 was quantitatively extracted from a plant material using methanol. Pure ethanol fails to extract saponins with high polar properties such as glycyrrhizinic acid whose sugar moiety is composed of two glucuronic acid units (Kuroda et al., 2010).

5.2 Biological activity

5.2.1 Cytotoxic and antitumor activities of OSW-1

Isolation and identification of OSW-1: OSW-1 was isolated from the methanol extract of the bulbs of *Ornithogalum saundersiae*, a Liliaceae plant native to South Africa. The structure of OSW-1 was determined by conventional spectroscopic analysis and hydrolysis, and was revealed to be a cholestane-type saponin with an acylated sugar unit at the C-16β hydroxy group of the cholestane skeleton (Kubo et al., 1992).

Cytotoxic activities: OSW-1 exhibited significantly potent cytotoxic activities against various cultured malignant tumor cells such as mouse mastocarcinoma, human pulmonary adenocarcinoma, human pulmonary large cell carcinoma and human pulmonary squamous cell carcinoma, including adriamycin (ADM)-resistant P388 leukemia and camptothecin (CPT)-resistant P388; the activities are around 10-100 times more potent than those of the clinically used anticancer drugs, mitomycin C (MMC), ADM, cisplatin (CDDP), CPT and taxol (TAX). To the contrary, normal human pulmonary fibroblasts are little sensitive to OSW-1 (Mimaki et al., 1997).

Panel screening: Evaluation of OSW-1 in the Japanese Foundation for Cancer Research 38 cell-line assay (Yamori et al., 1999) showed that the mean concentration required to achieve GI_{50} against the panel cells tested was 5.6 nM. OSW-1 displayed differential cytotoxicities, with breast cancer, CNS cancer and lung cancer subpanel cell lines showing particular sensitivity, but with colon cancer, ovarian cancer, stomach cancer and prostate cancer subpanel cell lines being relatively resistant to it. The pattern of the differential cytotoxicities of OSW-1 was evaluated using the Compare Program and was revealed not to correlate with those shown by any of the other compounds, including currently used anticancer drugs; correlation coefficient values were less than 0.5. This indicates that OSW-1 must have a unique mode of action and the potentiality as the lead of a new anticancer agent.

In vivo evaluation: OSW-1 was not haemolytic in human erythrocytes at 100 μg/mL. In *in vivo* evaluations, OSW-1 was effective versus mouse P388 with an increased life span of 59% by one-time administration (i.p.) of 0.01 mg/kg. As for the response of Hep134 rat xenograft to OSW-1, administration of OSW-1 on the second day and the fourth day (each 0.04 mg/kg, i.p.) significantly reduced tumor growth compared to the non-treated group (unpublished data).

OSW-1 analogues: O. saundersiae yielded several OSW-1-related compounds, which were slightly different from OSW-1 in the structures of the aromatic acid moieties. A few more polar analogues having a glucosyl unit at C-4 of the terminal xylosyl moiety were also isolated and identified. Phytochemical studies of *Ornithogalum thyrsoides* and *Galtonia candicans*, which are taxonomically related to *O. saundersiae*, resulted in the isolation of a series of OSW-1 derivatives, possessing a glucosyl, diglucosyl, or triglucosyl unit at the C-3 hydroxy group of the aglycone moiety without exceptions (Mimaki, 2006). These OSW-1 analogues, together with those partially modified by hydrolysis and reduction, were useful for elucidating the structure-activity relationship (SAR) of OSW-1.

Total synthesis of OSW-1: Since the potentiality of OSW-1 as a new lead compound for a new anticancer agent was evident, OSW-1 has been an attractive synthetic target for organic chemists. Furthermore, a number of OSW-1 analogues with modified acylated diglycosides, side-chains and/or steroidal nuclei have been obtained by means of chemical synthesis for SAR studies. Guo and Fuchs reported the first synthesis of the protected aglycone of OSW-1 (Guo & Fuchs, 1999). By employing the same approach, Deng and his co-workers established the first total synthesis of OSW-1 in 1999 (Deng et al., 1999). Yu and Jin reported a total synthesis of OSW-1 based on their own new strategy (Yu & Jin, 2001). Most recently, Xue and his co-workers have succeeded in the gram scale total synthesis of OSW-1 in 10 linear steps with an overall yield of 6.1%, starting from (+) dehydroisoandrosterone (Xue et al., 2008).

Panel/cell line		log GI_{50}	Panel/cell line		log GI_{50}
Breast Cancer	HBC-4	-8.03	Melanoma	LOX-IMVI	-9.44
	BSY-1	-9.20			
	HBC-5	-8.73	Ovarian Cancer	OVCAR-3	-6.86
	MCF-7	-9.42		OVCAR-4	-8.27
	MDA-MB-231	-8.70		OVCAR-5	-8.27
				OVCAR-8	-6.00
CNS Cancer	U251	-9.51		SK-OV-3	-7.70
	SF-268	-7.48			
	SF-295	-10.00	Renal Cancer	RXF-631L	-8.79
	SF-539	-10.00		ACHN	-6.39
	SNB-75	-10.00			
	SNB-78	-9.31	Stomach Cancer	St-4	-8.06
				MKN1	-6.07
Colon Cancer	HCC2998	-7.42		MKN7	-7.26
	KM-12	-8.98		MKN28	-6.24
	HT-29	-8.24		MKN45	-6.00
	HCT-15	-8.17		MKN74	-9.30
	HCT-116	-8.48			
			Prostate Cancer	DU-145	-6.44
Lung Cancer	NCI-H23	-7.69		PC-3	-7.28
	NCI-H226	-7.15			
	NCI-H522	-9.01	Mean value		-8.25
	NCI-H460	-10.00			(GI_{50} 5.6 nM)
	A549	-8.76			
	DMS273	-10.00			
	DMS114	-9.20			

Table 3. The log GI_{50} values of OSW-1 against the 38 cell lines. The GI_{50} value is the concentration that yields 50% growth.

SAR of OSW-1: The aglycone of OSW-1 is a cholesterol (cholest-5-en-3β-ol) derivative with a β-hydroxy group at C-16, an α-hydroxy group at C-17 and a carbonyl group at C-22. The sugar moiety attached to C-16 of the aglycone was assigned as *O*-(2-*O*-*p*-methoxybenzoyl-β-D-xylopyranosyl)-(1→3)-2-*O*-acetyl-α-L-arabinopyranosyl. The acylated sugar moiety is essential for the exhibition of the potent cytotoxic activities of OSW-1 (Morzycki et al., 2004; Tang et al., 2007). Slight differences in the aromatic acid structure gave no effects on the activities (Mimaki et al., 1997), but the following modifications, 1) deacylation (Mimaki et al, 1997), 2) glucosylation at C-4 of the xylosyl unit (Kuroda et al., 2001), 3) removal of the C-4 hydroxy group of the arabinosyl unit (Tschamber et al., 2007), 4) change in the linkage position of the xylosyl unit from C-3 of the arabinosyl moiety to its C-4 (Zheng et al., 2010, 2011), significantly reduced its cytotoxicities.

Although replacement of the aglycone by disparate steroids led to inactive compounds (Ma et al., 2000, 2001a, 2001b), the steroidal aglycone moiety tolerate certain modifications without a significant loss in cytotoxic potency. The C-17α hydroxy group was shown to be of little importance for the cytotoxicities (Zheng et al., 2010, 2011). The C-22 carbonyl group was reported to be a pharmacophore requirement (Wojtkielewicz et al., 2007); however, a current SAR study concluded that it is not necessary for the cytotoxic activities (Zheng et al., 2011). A number of the side chain modified analogues of OSW-1 have been synthesized, and some C-23-oxa analogues have been found to be significantly cytotoxic (Deng et al., 2004; Shi et al., 2005). The steroidal A- and B-rings can be generally modified without a loss of cytotoxic potency, as was evident when the 3-*O*-glucopyranosyl- (Mimaki, 2006), 3-*O*-biotinyl- (Kang et al., 2009) and 5,6-dihydro- (Guan et al., 2011) OSW-1 derivatives were as active as the parent. However, the activity of a derivative with an aromatic A-ring was exceptionally much less than that of OSW-1 (Tschamber et al., 2007). The linkage of the acylated diglycoside to the C-16β hydroxy group of the aglycone is essential for the potent cytotoxicity (Ma et al., 2001b), except in the case of a few synthetic analogues (Guan et al., 2011; Zheng et al., 2011).

5.2.2 Other biological activities of OSW-1

At first, OSW-1 was isolated from a cyclic AMP phosphodiesterase inhibitor from *O. saundersiae* bulbs (Kubo et al., 1992). Tamura and his co-workers found that OSW-1 inhibited ovarian E_2 secretion. The decrease in the levels of ovarian steroid induced by OSW-1 was shown to be due to its direct inhibitory action on the gene expression of the steroidal enzyme and the proliferation of granulose cells in the ovary (Tamura et al., 1997).

5.2.3 Other cholestane-type saponins with cytotoxic activities

O. saundersiae bulbs produced a novel 24(23→22)*abeo*-cholestane glycoside named saundersioside B, which has a six-membered hemiacetal ring between C-16 and C-23, and a five-membered acetal ring between C-18 and C-20. Saundersioside B possesses an aromatic acid ester group at the sugar moiety attached to C-3 of the aglycone and inhibited HL-60 cell growth through induction of apoptosis (Kuroda et al., 1997).

Candicanoside A, isolated from *G. candicans*, has two epoxy functional groups between C-16 and C-23, and between C-18 and C-23 in its rearranged cholestane skeleton (Mimaki et al., 2000). A novel polyoxygenated 5β-cholestane glycoside, designated as galtonioside A, has also been isolated from *G. candicans* (Kuroda et al., 2000). These cholestane-type saponins also display potent cytotoxic activities against cultured tumor cells with differential cytotoxicities in panel screenings. The obtained cytotoxic profiles are related to that of OSW-1.

5.3 State in hot-water extract: Possible binding to other compounds

Although some spirostan-type saponins such as digitonin are characterized by the formation of complex with cholesterol, it has not been reported that cholestane-type saponins interact with other compounds. When OSW-1 is dissolved in water, methanol, or other alcohols and the solution is allowed to stand for a few days, OSW-1 gradually decomposes to afford deacyl derivatives.

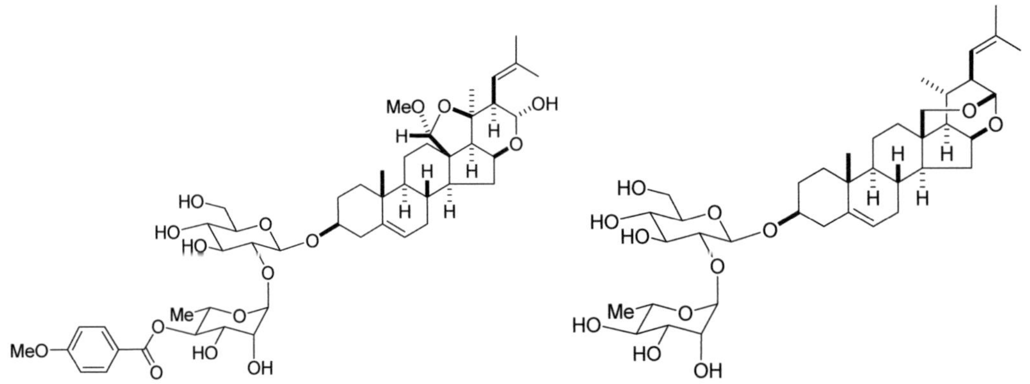

Fig. 15. Structures of saundersioside B (left) and candicanoside A (right)

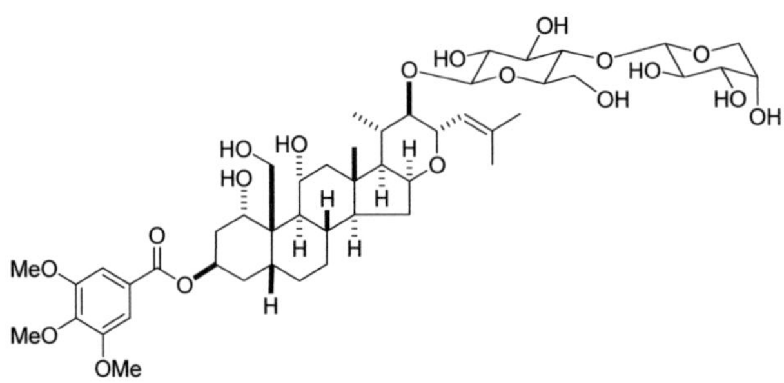

Fig. 16. Structure of galtonioside A

5.4 Site of action, signaling pathway, and receptor identification

The action mechanism of OSW-1 has been recently disclosed to damage the mitochondrial membrane and cristae in human leukemia and pancreatic cancer cells, leading to losses of transmembrane potential, increases in cytosolic calcium contents, and activation of calcium-dependent pathways. No anticancer compounds reported to date have this mechanism (Zhou et al., 2005). Furthermore, OSW-1 has been shown to induce apoptosis in mammalian cells through the mitochondrial pathway, involving the caspase-8-depending cleavage of Bcl-2 (Zhu et al., 2005).

5.5 Future directions

A number of crude drugs, including those used in Kampo prescriptions, are known to contain saponins. However, the pharmacological roles of saponins in Kampo prescriptions remain to be elucidated, except for glycyrrhizinic acid in Licorice Root. Manifestation of the specific pharmacological effects of each saponin will lead to providing evidence on the efficacy of Kampo medicines.

It is notable that *O. saundersiae*, an ornamental plant without a folkloric medicinal background, produces OSW-1, a cholestane-type steroidal saponin with high apparent potential for effectively treating some cancers that are resistant to available medicines. Thus, OSW-1 clearly warrants further chemical and biological investigations for its clinical applications.

6. Conclusion

This review summarizes unique biological properties of LCCs, tannins, flavonoids and saponins, suggesting their functionality as alternative medicines. LCCs showed broad and potent anti-viral activity and synergism with vitamin C. Since virus is one of major risk factor of oral cavity cancer (Sakagami; 2010a), anti-viral action of LCC may reduce the incidence of virus-triggered diseases such as cancer. The use of a genetic algorithm-kernel partial least squares algorithm combined with an artificial neural network (Jalai-Heravi, 2008) may be useful to predict the optimal structure of LCCs for the expression of biological activities. Identification of dectin-2 as LCC receptor awaits further confirmation with siRNA and gene overexpression experiments. Tannins are found to be relatively unstable in hot water, and easily decomposed and associated with serum albumin. Biological significance of such degradation products and associates remains to be investigated. Saponins with high polarity can to be extracted with hot water, and therefore should be present in many herbal extracts and Kampo medicines. The antitumor potentital of OSW-1 should be further pursued. .

7. Acknowledgment

This study was supported in part by a Grant-in-Aid from the Ministry of Education, Science, Sports and Culture of Japan (Sakagami No.14370607, 2002-2004, Sakagami No. 19592156, 2007-2009, Hatano No 22580128, 2010~, Mimaki No. 14572013, 2002-2005, Mimaki No. 21590023, 2009-).

8. References

Abe, M., Okamoto, K., Konno, K. & Sakagami, H. (1989). Induction of antiparasite activity by pine cone lignin-related substances. *In vivo* Vol.3, pp. 359-362.

Abou-Zaid, M.M., Lombardo, D.A., Kite, G.C., Grayer, R.J., & Veitch, N.C. (2001). Acylated flavone C-glycosides from *Cucumis sativus*. *Phyotochemistry* Vol.58. pp. 167-172.

Azuma, J-I. & Koshijima, T. (1988). Lignin-carbohydrate complexes from various sources. *Methods Enzymol* Vol.161. pp. 12-18.

Bakowska, A., Kucharska, A.Z. & Ozmianski, J. (2003). The effects of heating, UV and storage on stability of the anthocyanin-polyphenol copigment complex. *Food Chem* Vol.81. pp. 349-355.

Brown, G.D. & Gordon, S. (2001). Immune recognition. A new receptor for beta-glucans. *Nature* Vol.413(6851), pp. 36-37

Bruno, A., Siena, L., Gerbino, S., Ferraro, M., Chanez, P., Giammanco, M., Gjomarkaj, M. & Pace, E. (2011). Apigenin affects leptin/leptin receptor pathway and induces cell apoptosis in lung adenocarcinoma cell line. *Eur J Cancer*, in press.

Cha, J.D., Jeong, M.R., Jeong, S.I. & Lee, K.Y. (2007). Antibacterial activity of sophoraflavanone G isolated from the roots of Sophora flavescens. *J Microbiol Biotechnol* Vol.17, pp.858-864.

Dastidar, S.G., Manna, A., Kumar, K.A., Mazumdar, K., Dutta, N.K., Chakrabarty, A.N., Motohashi, N. & Shirataki, Y. (2004). Studies on the antibacterial potentiality of isoflavones. *Int J Antimicrob Agents* Vo.23, pp. 99-102.

Davin, L.; Wang, H.B., Crowell A.L.,Bedgar, D.L., Martin, D.M., Sarkanen, S. & Lewis, N.G. (1997). Stereoselective biomolecular phenoxy radical coupling by an auxiliary (dirigent) protein without an active center. *Science* Vol.275, pp. 362-366.

Deng, S., Yu, B., Lou, Y. & Hui, Y. (1999). First total synthesis of an exceptionally potent antitumor saponin, OSW-1. *J Org Chem* Vo.64, pp. 202-208.

Deng, L., Wu, H., Yu, B., Jiang, M. & Wu, J. (2004). Synthesis of OSW-1 analogs with modified side chains and their antitumor activities. *Bioorg Med Chem Lett* Vo.14, pp. 2781-2785.

Dinda, B., Debnath, S., Mohanta, B.C. & Harigaya, Y. (2010). Naturally occurring triterpenoid saponins. *Chem Biodivers* Vo.7, pp. 2327-2580.

Emiliani, G., Fondi, M., Fani, R. & Gribaldo, S. (2009). A horizontal gene transfer at the origin of phenylpropanoid metabolism: a key adaptation of plants to land. *Biology Direct* Vol.4, 4 (https://www.biology-direct.com/content/4/1/7)

Fukai, T., Sakagami, H., Toguchi, M., Takayama, F., Iwakura, I., Atsumi, T., Ueha, T., Nakashima, H. & Nomura, T. (2000). Cytotoxic activity of low molecular weight polyphenols against human oral tumor cell lines. *Anticancer Res* Vol.20, pp. 2525-2536.

Fukuchi, K., Sakagami, H., Ikeda, M., Kawazoe, Y., Oh-hara, T., Konno, K., Ichikawa, S., Hata, N., Kondo, H. & Nonoyama, M. (1989a). Inhibition of herpes simplex virus infection by pine cone antitumor substances. *Anticancer Res* Vol.9, pp. 313-318.

Fukuchi, K., Sakagami, H., Okuda, T., Hatano, T., Tanuma, S., Kitajima, K., Inoue, Y., Inoue, S., Ichikawa, S., Nonoyama, M. & Konno, K. (1989b). Inhibition of herpes simplex virus infection by tannins and related compouneds. *Antiviral Res* Vol.11, pp. 285-298.

Gross, O., Gewies, A., Finger, K., Schäfer, M., Sparwasser, T., Peschel, C., Förster, I. & Ruland, J. (2006). Card9 controls a non-TLR signalling pathway for innate anti-fungal immunity. *Nature Vo.*442(7103), pp. 651-656.

Guan, Y., Zheng, D., Zhou, L., Wang, H., Yan, Z., Wang, N., Chang, H., She, P. & Lei, P. (2011). Synthesis of 5(6)-dihydro-OSW-1 analogs bearing three kinds of disaccharides linking at 15-hydroxy and their antitumor activities. *Bioorg Med Chem Lett* Vol.21: pp. 2921-2924.

Guo, A.J.Y., Choi, R.C.Y., Cheung, A.W.H., Chen, V.P., Xu, S.L., Dong, T.T.X., Chen, J.J., & Tsim, K.W.K. (2011). Baicalin, a flavone, induces the differentiation of cultured osteoblasts: an action via the WNT/β-catenin signaling. *J Biol Chem* in press.

Guo, C. & Fuchs, P.L. (1998). The first synthesis of the aglycone on the potent anti-tumor steroidal saponin OSW-1. *Tetrahedron Lett* Vol.39, pp. 1099-1102.

Hanaoka, A., Sakgami, H. & Konno, K. (1989). Pine cone antitumor substances stimulate cytotoxic factor production in young mice, but not in aged or tumor-bearing mice. *Showa Univ J Med Sci,* Vol.1, pp. 57-63.

Harada, H., Sakagami, H., Konno, K., Sato, T., Osawa, N., Fujimaki, M. & Komatsu, N. (1988). Induction of antimicrobial activity by antitumor substances from pine cone extract of *Pinus parviflora* Sieb. et Zucc. *Anticancer Res,* Vol. 8, pp. 581-588

Harada, H., Sakagami, H., Nagata, K., Oh-hara, T., Kawazoe, Y., Ishihama, A., Hata, N., Misawa, Y., Terada, H. & Konno, K. (1991). Possible involvement of lignin structure in anti-influenza virus activity. *Antiviral Res* Vol.15, pp. 41-50.

Hatano, T., Hori, M., Hemingway, R., & Yoshida, T. (2003a). Size exclusion chromatographic analysis of polyphenols-serum albumin complexes. *Phytochemistry*, Vol.63, pp. 817-823.

Hatano, T., Kusuda, M., Hori, M., Shiota, S., Tsuchiya, T. & Yoshida, T. (2003b). Theasinensin A, a tea polyphenols formed from (-)-epigallocatechin gallate, suppresses antibiotic resistance of methicillin-resistant *Staphylococcus aureus*. *Plant Med*, Vol.69, pp. 984-989.

Hu, H., Chai, Y., Wang, L., Zhang, J., Lee, H.J., Kim, S.H. & Lü, J. (2009). Pentagalloylglucose induces autophagy and caspase-independent programmed cell deaths in human PC-3 and mouse TRAMP-C2 prostate cancer cells. *Mol Cancer Ther*, Vol.8, pp. 2833-2843.

Ichimura, T., Otake, T., Mori, H. & Maruyama, S. (1999). HIV-1 protease inhibition and anti-HIV effect of natural and synthetic water-soluble lignin-like substances. *Biosci Biotechnol Biochem*, Vol.63, pp. 2202-2024.

Ito, H., Iguchi, A. & Hatano, T. (2008). Identification of urinary and intestinal bacterial metabolites of ellagitannin geraniin in rats. *J Agric Food Chem*, Vol.56, pp. 393-400.

Jalali-Heravi, M. (2008). Neural networks in analytical chemistry. *Methods Mol Biol*, Vol.458, pp. 81-121.

Joo, S.S., Kang, H.C., Lee, M.W., Choi, Y.W. & Lee, D.I. (2003). Inhibition of IL-1β and IL-6 in osteoblast-like cell by isoflavones extracted from Sophorae fructus. *Arch Pharm Res*, Vol.26, pp. 1029-1035.

Jung, H.J., Kang, S.S., Woo, J.J. & Choi, J.S. (2005). A new lavandulylated flavonoid with free radical and ONOO- scavenging activities from Sophora flavescens . *Arch Pharm Res*, Vol.28, pp. 1333-1336.

Jung, H.A., Jeong, D.M., Chung, H.Y., Lim, H.A., Kim, J.Y., Yoon, N.Y. & Choi, J.S. (2008). Re-evaluation of the antioxidant prenylated flavonoids from the roots of Sophora flavescens. *Biol Pharm Bull*, Vol.31, pp. 908-915.

Kang, Y., Lou, C., Ahmed, K.B., Huang, P. & Jin, Z. (2009). Synthesis of biotinylated OSW-1. *Bioorg Med Chem Lett*, Vol.19, pp. 5166-5168.

Kubo, S., Mimaki, Y., Terao, M., Sashida Y, Nikaido T & Ohmoto, T (1992): Acylated cholestane glycosides from the bulbs of *Ornithogalum saundersiae*. *Phytochemistry*, Vol.31, pp. 3969-3973.

Kawano, M., Sakagami, H., Satoh, K., Shioda, S., Kanamoto, T., Terakubo, S., Nakashima, H. & Makino, T. (2010a). Lignin-like activity of *Lentinus edodes* mycelia Extract (LEM). *In Vivo*, Vol.24, pp. 543-552.

Kay, R.M. (1982). Dietary fiber. *J Lipid Res*, Vol.23, pp. 221-242.

Kim, S.J., Son, K.H., Chang, H.W., Kang, S.S. & Kim, H.P. (2003). Tyrosinase inhibiting prenylated flavonoids from Sophora flavescens. *Biol Pharm Bull*, Vol.26, pp. 1348-1350.

Koizumi, N., Sakagami, H., Utsumi, A., Fujinaga, S., Takeda, M., Asano, K., Sugawara, I., Ichikawa, S., Kondo, H., Mori, S., Miyatake, K., Nakano, Y., Nakashima, H., Murakami, T., Miyano, N. & Yamamoto, N. (1993). Anti-HIV (human immunodeficiency virus) activity of sulfated paramylon. *Antiviral Res*, Vol.21, pp.1-14.

Kuo, P.T., Lin, T.P., Liu, L.C., Huang, C.H., Lin, J.K., Kao, J.Y. & Way, T.T. (2009). Penta-*O*-galloyl-beta-D-glucose suppresss prostate cancer bone metastasis by transcriptionally repressing EGF-induced MMP-9 expression. *J Agric Food Chem*, Vol.57, pp3331-3339.

Kuroda, M., Mimaki, Y., Sashida, Y., Hirano, T., Oka, K., Dobashi, A., Li, H.Y. & Harada, N. (1997). Novel cholestane glycosides from the bulbs *Ornithogalum saundersiae* and their cytostatic activity on leukemia HL-60 and MOLT-4 cells. *Tetrahedron*, Vol.53, pp. 11549-11562.

Kuroda, M., Mimaki, Y., Sashida, Y., Yamori, T. & Tsuruo ,T. (2000). Galtonioside A, a novel cytotoxic cholestane glycoside from *Galtonia candicans*. *Tetrahedron Lett*, Vol.41, pp. 251-255.

Kuroda, M., Mimaki, Y., Yokosuka, A., Sashida, Y. & Beutler, J.A. (2001). Cytotoxic cholestane glycosides from the bulbs of *Ornithogalum saundersiae*. *J Nat Prod*. Vol.64, pp. 88-91.

Kuroda, M., Mimaki, Y., Honda, S., Tanaka, H., Yokota, S. & Mae, T. (2010). Phenolics from *Glycyrrhiza glabra* roots and their PPAR-γ ligand-binding activity. *Bioorg Med Chem*, Vol.18, pp. 962-970.

Kushida, T., Makino, T., Tomomura, M., Tomomura, A. & Sakagami, H. (2011). Enhancement of dectin-2 gene expression by lignin-carbohydrate complex from Lendinus edodes extract (LEM) in mouse macrophage-like cell line. *Anticancer Res*, Vol.31, pp. 1241-1248

Kusuda, M., Inada, K., Ogawa, T., Yoshida, T., Shiota, S., Tsuchiya, T. & Hatano, T. (2006). Polyphenolic constituents of *Zanthoxylum piperitum* fruit and the antibacterial effects of its polymeric proanthocyanidins on methicillin-resistant *Staphylococcus aureus*. *Biosc Biotechnol Bochem*, Vol.70, pp. 1423-1431.

Lai, P.K., Donovan, J., Takayama, H., Sakagami, H., Tanaka, A., Konno, K. & Nonoyama, M. (1990). Modification of human immunodeficiency viral replication by pine cone extacts. *AIDS Res Human Retroviruses*, Vol.6, pp. 205-217

Lai, P.K., Oh-hara, T., Tamura, Y., Kawazoe, Y., Konno, K., Sakagami, H., Tanaka, A. & Nonoyama, M. (1992). Polymeric phenylpropenoids are the active components in the pine cone extract that inhibit the replication of type-1 human immunodeficiency virus *in vitro*. *J Gen Appl Microbiol*, Vol.38, pp. 303-323.

Lewis, N.G. & Yamamoto, E. (1990). Lignin. Occurrence, biogenesis and biodegradation. *Ann Rev Plant Physiol Plant Nol Biol*, Vol.41, pp. 455-496.

López, B.S.G., Yamamoto, M., Utsumi, K., Aratsu, C. & Sakagami, H. (2009). Clinical pilot study of lignin-ascorbic acid combination treatment of herpes simplex virus. *In Vivo*, Vol.23, pp. 1011-1016, 2009

Ma, X., Yu, B., Hui, Y., Xiao, D. & Ding, J. (2000). Synthesis of glycosides bearing the disaccharide of OSW-1 or its 1→4-linked analogue and their antitumor activities. *Carbohydr Res*. Vol.329, pp. 495-505.

Ma, X., Yu, B., Hui, Y., Miao, Z. & Ding, J. (2001a). Synthesis of steroidal glycosides bearing the disaccharide moiety of OSW-1 and their antitumor activities. *Carbohydr Res*, Vol.334, pp. 159-164.

Ma, X., Yu, B., Hui, Y., Miao, Z. & Ding, J. (2001b). Synthesis of OSW-1 analogues and a dimer and their antitumor activities. *Bioorg Med Chem Lett*. Vol.11, pp. 2153-2156.

Mahato, S.B., Ganguly, A.N. & Sahu, N.P. (1985). Steroid saponins. *Phytochemistry*, Vol.21, pp. 959-978.

Manabe, H., Sakagami, H., Ishizone, H., Kusano, H., Fujimaki, M., Wada, C., Komatsu, N., Nakashima, H., Murakami, T. & Yamamoto, N. (1992). Effects of Catuaba extracts on microbial and HIV infection. *In Vivo*, Vol.6, pp. 161-166.

Marcovic, J.M., Petranovic, N.A. & Baranac, J.M. (2000): A spectrophotometric study of the copigmentation of malvin with caffeic and ferulic acid. *J Agric Food Chem*, Vol.48, pp. 5530-5536.

Martens, S. & Mithöfer, A. (2005). Flavones and flavone systhases. *Phytochemistry*, Vol.66, pp. 2399-2407.

Matsuta, T., Sakagami, H., Satoh, K., Kanamoto, T., Terakubo, S., Nakashima, H., Kitajima, M., Oizumi, H. & Oizumi T. (2011): Biological activity of luteolin glycosides and tricin from *Sasa senanensis* Rehder. *In Vivo*, Vol. 25, pp. 757-762.

McGreal, E.P., Rosas, M., Brown, G.D., Zamze, S., Wong, S.Y., Gordon, S., Martinez-Pomares, L. & Taylor, P.R. (2006). The carbohydrate-recognition domain of Dectin-2 is a C-type lectin with specificity for high mannose. *Glycobiology*, Vol.16(5), pp. 422-430.

Mimaki, Y., Kuroda, M., Kameyama, A., Sashida, Y., Hirano, T., Oka, K., Maekawa, R., Wada, T., Sugita, K. & Beutler, J.A. (1997). Cholestane glycosides with potent cytostatic activities on various tumor cells from *Ornithogalum saundersiae* bulbs. *Bioorg Med Chem Lett*, Vol.7, pp. 633-636.

Mimak,i Y., Kuroda, M., Sashida, Y., Yamori, T. & Tsuruo, T. (2000). Candicanoside A, a novel cytotoxic rearranged cholestane glycoside from *Galtonia candicans*. *Helv Chim Acta*, Vol. 83, pp. 2698-2704.

Mimaki, Y. (2006). Structures and biological activities of plant glycosides: cholestane glycosides from *Ornithogalum saundersiae, O. thyrsoides* and *Galtonia candicans*, and their cytotoxic and antitumor activities. *Nat Prod Commun*, Vol.1, pp. 247-253.

Minale, L., Iorizzi, M., Palagiano, E. & Riccio, R. (1996). Steroid and triterpenoid oligoglycosides of marine origin. *Adv Exp Med Biol*, Vol.404, pp. 335-356.

Mohamed, A. A. O., Taniguchi, S., Yoshimura, M., Yoshida, T., Kishino, K., Sakagami, H. & Hatano, T. (2010). Hydrolyzable tannins of tamaricaceous plants. III. Hellinoyl- and macrocyclic-type ellagitannins from *Tamarix nilotica*. *J Nat Prod*, Vol.73, pp. 870-879.

Morzycki, J.W., Wojtkielewicz, A. & Wołczyński, S. (2004). Synthesis of analogues of a potent antitumor saponin OSW-1. *Bioorg Med Chem Lett*, Vol.14, pp. 3323-3326.

Nagata, K., Sakagami, H., Harada, H., Nonoyama, M., Ishihara, A. & Konno, K. (1990). Inhibition of influenza virus infection by pine cone antitumor substances. *Antiviral Res*, Vol.13, pp. 11-22.

Nakajima, Y., Yun, Y. S. & Kunugi, A. (2003). Six new flavonolignans from *Sasa veitchii* (Carr.) Rehder. *Tetrahedron*, Vol.59, pp. 8011-8015.

Nakane, A., Minagawa, T. & Kato, K. (1988). Endogenous tumor necrosis factor (cachectin) is essential to host resistance against *Listeria monocytogenes* infection. *Infect Immun*, Vol.56, pp. 2503-2506.

Nakashima, H., Murakami, T., Yamamoto, N., Naoe, T., Kawazoe, Y., Konno, K. & Sakagami, H. (1992a). Lignified materials as medicinal resources. V. Anti-HIV (human immunodeficiency virus) activity of some synthetic lignins. *Chem Pharm Bull*, Vol.40, pp. 2102-2105

Nakashima, H., Murakami, T., Yamamoto, N., Sakagami, H., Tanuma, S., Hatano, T., Yoshida, T. & Okuda, T. (1992b). Inhibition of human immunodeficiency viral replication by tannins and related compounds. *Antiviral Res,* Vol.18, pp. 91-103

Nozaki, A., Kimura, T., Ito, H. & Hatano, T. (2009). Interaction of polyphenolic metabolites with human serum albumin: a circular dichroism study. *Chem Pharm Bull,* Vol.57, pp. 1019-1023.

Oh-hara, T., Sakagami, H., Kawazoe, Y., Kaiya, T., Komatsu, N., Ohsawa, N., Fujimaki, M., Tanuma, S. & Konno, K. (1990). Antimicrobial spectrum of lignin-related pine cone extracts of *Pinus parvilofra* Sieb. et Zucc. *In Vivo,* Vol.4, pp. 7-12.

Okuda, T., Mori, K. & Hatano, T. (1980). The distribution of geraniin and mallotusinic acid in the order Geraniales. *Phytochemistry,* Vol.19, pp. 547-551.

Okuda, T,, Hatano, T., Agata, I. & Nishibe, S. (1986). The constituents of tannic activities in labiatae plants. I. Rosmarinic acid from labiatae plants in Japan. *Yakugaku Zasshi,* Vol.106, pp. 1108-1111.

Oszmianski, J., Bakowska, A. & Piacente, S. (2004). Thermodynamic characteristics of copigmentation reaction of acylated anthocyanin isolated from blue flowers of *Scutellaria baicalensis* Georgi with copigments. *J Sci Food and Agric,* Vol.84, pp. 1500-1506.

Park, H., Lim, J.H., Kim, H.J., Choi, H.J. & Lee, I. (2007). Antioxidant flavone glycoside from the leaves of *Sasa borealis. Arch Pham Res,* Vol. 30, pp. 161-166.

Piao, X,L,, Piao, X.S., Kim, S.W., Park, J.H., Kim, H.Y. & Cai, SQ. (2006) .Identification and characterization of antioxidants from Sophora flavescens. *Biol Pharm Bull,* Vol.29, pp. 1911-1915.

Raghuraman, A,, Tiwari, V., Zhao, Q., Shukla, D., Debnath, A.K. & Desai, U.R. (2007). Viral inhibition studies on sulfated lignin, a chemically modified biopolymer and a potential mimic of heparin sulfate. *Biomacromolecules,* Vol.8, pp. 1759-1763.

Saijo, S,, Ikeda, S., Yamabe, K., Kakuta, S., Ishigame, H., Akitsu, A., Fujikado, N., Kusaka, T., Kubo, S., Chung, S.H., Komatsu, R., Miura, N., Adachi, Y., Ohno, N., Shibuya, K., Yamamoto, N., Kawakami, K., Yamasaki, S., Saito, T., Akira, S. & Iwakura, Y. (2010). Dectin-2 recognition of alpha-mannans and induction of Th17 cell differentiation is essential for host defense against Candida albicans. *Immunity,* Vol.32(5), Vol. 681-691.

Sakagami, H., Ikeda, M., Unten, S., Takeda, K., Murayama, J., Hamada, A., Kimura, K., Komatsu, N. & Konno, K. (1987). Antitumor activity of polysaccharide fractions from pine cone extract of *Pinus parviflora* Sieb. et Zucc. *Anticancer Res,* Vol7, pp. 1153-1160.

Sakagami, H., Kohno, S., Tanuma, S. & Kawazoe, Y. (1990a). Induction of cytotoxic factor in mice by lignified materials combined with OK-432 (Picibanil). *In Vivo,* Vol.4, pp. 371-376.

Sakagami, H., Nagata, K., Ishihama, A., Oh-hara, T. & Kawazoe, Y. (1990b). Anti-influenza virus activity of synthetically polymerized phenylpropenoids. *Biochem Biophys Res Commun,* Vol.172, pp. 1267-1272.

Sakagami, H., Kuroiwa, Y., Takeda, M., Ota, H., Kazama, K., Naoe, T., Kawazoe, Y., Ichikawa, S., Kondo, H., Yokokura, T. & Shikita, M. (1992a). Distribution of TNF endogenously induced by various immunopotentiators and *Lactobacillus casei* in mice. *In Vivo,* Vol.6, pp. 247-254

Sakagami, H., Takeda, M., Kawazoe, Y., Nagata, K., Ishihama, A., Ueda, M. & Yamazaki, S. (1992b). Anti-influenza virus activity of a lignin fraction from cone of *Pinus parviflora* Sieb. et Zucc. *In Vivo*, Vol.6, pp. 491-496.

Sakagami, H., Kuribayashi, N., Iida, M., Hagiwara, T., Takahashi, H., Yoshida, H., Shiota, F., Ohata, H., Momose, K. & Takeda, M. (1996a). The requirement for and mobilization of calcium during induction by sodium ascorbate and by hydrogen peroxide of cell death. *Life Sciences*, Vol.58, pp. 1131-1138.

Sakagami, H., Satoh, K., Ohata, H., Takahashi, H., Yoshida, H., Iida, M., Kuribayashi, N., Sakagami, T., Momose, K. & Takeda, M. (1996b). Relationship between ascorbyl radical intensity and apoptosis-inducing activity. *Anticancer Res*, Vol.16, pp. 2635-2644.

Sakagami, H., Satoh, K., Aiuchi, T., Nakaya, K. & Takeda, M. (1997). Stimulation of ascorbate-induced hypoxia by lignin. *Anticancer Res*, Vol.17, pp. 1213-1216.

Sakagami, H., Jiang, Y., Kusama, K., Atsumi, T., Ueha, T., Toguchi, M., Iwakura, I., Satoh, K., Ito, H., Hatano, T. & Yoshida, T. (2000a) Cytotoxic activity of hydrolysable tannins against human oral tumor cell lines - A possible mechanism. *Phytomedicine*, Vol.7, pp. 39-47.

Sakagami, H., Satoh, K., Hakeda, Y. & Kumegawa, M. (2000b). Apoptosis-inducing activity of vitamin C and vitamin K. *Cell Mol Biol*, Vol.46, pp. 129-143.

Sakagami, H., Hashimoto, K., Suzuki, S., Ogiwara, T., Satoh, K., Ito, H., Hatano, T., Yoshida, T. & Fujisawa, S. (2005). Molecular requirement of lignin for expression of unique biological activity. *Phytochemistry*, Vol.66 (17), pp. 2107-2119.

Sakagami, H., Asano, K., Satoh, K., Takahashi, K., Kobayashi, M., Koga, N., Takahashi, H., Tachikawa, R., Tashiro, T., Hasegawa, A., Kurihara, K., Ikarashi, T., Kanamoto, T., Terakubo, S., Nakashima, H., Watanabe, S. & Nakamura, W. (2007). Anti-stress, anti-HIV and vitamin C-synergized radical scavenging activity of mulberry juice fractions. *In Vivo*, Vol.21, pp. 499-506

Sakagami, H.. Satoh, K., Fukamachi, H., Ikarashi, T., Simizu, A., Yano, K., Kanamoto, T., Terakubo, S., Nakashima, H., Hasegawa, H., Nomura, A., Utsumi, K., Yamamoto, M., Maeda, Y. & Osawa, K. (2008). Anti-HIV and vitamin C-synergized radical scavenging activity of cacao husk lignin fractions. *In Vivo*, Vol.22, pp. 327-33

Sakagami, H., Kushida, T., Oizumi, T., Nakashima, H. & Makino, T. (2010a). Distribution of lignin carbohydrate complex in plant kingdom and its functionality as alternative medicine. *Pharmacology & Therapeutics*, Vol.128, pp. 91-105.

Sakagami, H., Zhou, L., Kawano, M., Thet, M.M., Takana, S., Machino, M., Amano, S., Kuroshita, R., Watanabe, S., Chu, Q., Wang, Q.T., Kanamoto, T., Terakubo, S., Nakashima, H., Sekine, K., Shirataki, Y., Hao, Z.C., Uesawa, Y., Mohri, K., Kitajima, M., Oizumi, H. & Oizumi, T. (2010b). Multiple biological complex of alkaline extract of the leaves of *Sasa senanensis* Rehder. *In Vivo*, Vol.24, pp. 735-744.

Sakagami, H., Kawano, M., Thet, M.M., Hashimoto, K., Satoh, K., Kanamoto, T., Terakubo, S., Nakashima, H., Haishima, Y., Maeda, Y. & Sakurai, K. (2011). Anti-HIV and immunomodulation activities of cacao mass lignin carbohydrate complex. *In Vivo*, Vol.25, pp. 229-236.

Sakagami, H. & Watanabe, S. (2011). Beneficial effects of mulberry on human health. In: Phytotherapeutics and Human Health: Pharmacological and Molecular Aspects, ed. Farooqui AA, in press, Nova Science Publishers, Inc, Hauppauge, NY.

Satoh, K., Ida, Y., Ishihara, M. & Sakagami, H. (1999). Interaction between sodium ascorbate and polyphenols. *Anticancer Res*, Vol.19, pp. 4177-4186.

Sharma, S.D., Meeran, S.M. & Katiyar, S.K. (2010). Proanthocyanidins inhibit in vitro and in vivo growth of human non-small cell lung cancer cells by inhibiting the prostaglandin E2 and prostaglandin E2 receptors. *Mol Cancer Ther*, Vol.9 (3), pp.569-580.

Shi, B., Tang, P., Hu, X., Liu, J.O. & Yu, B. (2005). OSW saponins: Facile synthesis toward a new type of structures with potent antitumor activities. *J Org Chem*, Vol.70, pp. 10354-10367.

Shimizu, M., Shiota, S., Mizushima, T., Ito, H., Hatano, T., Yoshida, T. & Tsuchiya, T. (2001). Marked potentiation of activity of β-lactams against methicillin-resistant *Staphylococcus aureus* by corilagin. *Antimicrob Agents Chemother*, Vol.45, pp. 3198-3201.

Shiota, S., Shimizu, M., Mizushima, T., Ito, H., Hatano, T., Yoshida, T. & Tsuchiya, T. (1999). Marked reduction in the minimum inhibitory concentration (MIC) of β-lactams in methicillin-resistant *Staphylococcus aureus* produced by epicatechin gallate, and ingredient of green tea (*Camellia sinensis*). *Biol Pharm Bull*, Vol.22, pp. 1388-1390.

Shiota, S., Shimizu, M., Mizusima, T., Ito, H., Hatano, T., Yoshida, T. & Tsuchiya, T. (2000). Restoration of effectiveness of β-lactams on methicillin-resistant *Staphylococcus aureus* by tellimagrandin I from rose red. *FEMS Microbiol Lett*, Vol.185, pp. 135-138.

Shirataki, Y., Motohashi, N., Tani, S., Sakagami, H., Satoh, K., Nakashima, H., Mahapatra, S.K., Ganguly, K., Dastidar, S.G. & Chakrabarty, A.N. (2001a). In Vitro Biological Activity of Prenylflavanones. *Anticancer Res*, Vol.21, pp.275-280.

Shirataki, Y., Tani, S., Sakagami, H., Satoh, K., Nakashima, H., Gotoh, K. & Motohashi, N. (2001b). :Relationship between cytotoxic activity and tadical intensity of isoflavones from Sophora Species. *Anticancer Res*, Vol.21, pp.2643-2648.

Shirataki, Y., Wakae, M., Yamamoto, Y., Hashimoto, K., Satoh, K., Ishihara, M., Kikuchi, H., Nishikawa, H., Minagawa, K., Motohashi, N. & Sakagami, H. (2004). Cytotoxicty and radical modulating activity of isoflavones and isoflavanones from Sophora Species. *Anticancer Res*, Vol.24, pp. 14811488.

Son, J.K., Park, J.S., Kim, J.A., Kim, Y., Chung, S.R. & Lee, S.H. (2003). Prenylated flavonoids from the roots of Sophora flavescens with tyrosinase inhibitory activity. *Planta Med*, Vol.69, pp. 559-561.

Suzuki, H., Iiyama, K., Yoshida, O., Yamazaki, S., Yamamoto, N. & Toda, S. (1990). Structural characterization of the immunoreactive and antiviral water-solubilized lignin in an extract of the culture medium of *Lentinum edodes* Mycelia (LEM). *Agric Biol Chem*, Vol.54, pp.. 479-487

Tamura, K., Honda, H., Mimaki, Y., Sashida, Y. & Kogo, H. (1997). Inhibitory effect of a new steroidal saponin, OSW-1, on ovarian functions in rats. *Br J Pharmacol*, Vol.121, pp. 1796-1802.

Taniguchi, S., Kuroda, K., Doi, K., Tanabe, M., Shibata, T., Yoshida, T. & Hatano, T. (2008). Dimeric flavans from gambir and their structural correlations with (+)-catechin. *Heterocycles*, Vol.76, pp. 1171-1180.

Tang, P., Mamdani, F., Hu, X., Liu, J.O. & Yu, B. (2007). Synthesis of OSW saponin analogs with modified sugar residues and their antiproliferative activities. *Bioorg Med Chem Lett*, Vol.17, pp. 1003-1007.

Thakkar, J.N., Tiwari, V. & Dessai, U.R. (2010). Nonsulfated, cinnamic acid-based lignins are potent antagonists of HSV-1 entry into cells. *Biomacromolecules*, Vol.11, pp. 1412-1416.

Tschamber, T., Adam, S., Matsuya, Y., Masuda, S., Ohsawa, N., Maruyama, S., Kamoshita, K., Nemoto, H. & Eustache, J. (2007). New analogues of the potent cytotoxic saponin OSW-1. *Bioorg Med Chem Lett*, Vol.17, pp. 5101-5106.

Vautier, S., Sousa Mda, G. & Brown, G.D. (2010). C-type lectins, fungi and Th17 responses. *Cytokine Growth Factor Rev*, Vol.21(6), pp. 405-412.

Watanabe, M. (1999). Antioxidative phenolic compounds from Japanese barnyard millet (Echinochloa utilis) grauns. *J Agric Food Chem*, Vol.47, pp. 4500-4505.

Watanabe, M. & Ito, M. (2002). Changes in antioxidative activity and flavone comosition of extracts from aerial parts of buckwheat during growth period. *Nippon Shokuhin Kagaku Kogaku Kaishi* Vol.49, pp. 119-125 (in Japanese).

Wojtkielewicz, A., Długosz, M., Maj, J., Morzycki, J.W., Nowakowski, M., Renkiewicz, J., Strnad, M., Swaczynová, J., Wilczewska, A.Z. & Wójcik, J. (2007). New analogues of the potent cytotoxic saponin OSW-1. *J Med Chem*, Vol.50, pp. 3667-3673.

Xue, J., Liu, P., Pan, Y. & Guo, Z. (2008). A total synthesis of OSW-1. *J Org Chem*, 73: pp. 157-161.

Yamori, T., Matsunaga, A., Sato, S., Yamazaki, K., Komi, A., Ishizu, K., Mita, I,. Edatsugi, H., Matsuba, Y., Takezawa, K., Nakanishi, O., Kohno, H., Nakajima, Y., Komatsu, H., Andoh, T. & Tsuruo, T. (1999). Potent antitumor activity of MS-247, a novel DNA minor groove binder, evaluated by an *in vitro* and *in vivo* human cancer cell line panel. *Cancer Res*, Vol.59, pp. 4042-4049.

Yoshida, T., Hatano, T., Kuwajima, T. & Okuda, T. (1992). Oligomeric hydrolyzable tannins – their ^{1}H NMR spectra and partial degradation. *Heterocycles*, Vol.33, pp.463-482.

Yu, W. & Jin, Z. (2001). A new strategy for the stereoselective introduction of steroid side chain via α-alkoxy vinyl cuprates: Total synthesis of a highly potent antitumor natural product OSW-1. *J Am Chem Soc*, Vol.123, pp. 3369-3370.

Zhang, Y., But, P.P., Ooi, V.E., Xu, H.X., Delaney, G.D., Lee, S.H. & Lee, S.F. (2007). Chemical properties, mode of action, and in vivo anti-herpes activities of a lignin-carbohydrate complex from Prunella vulgaris. *Antiviral Res*, Vol.75, pp. 242-249.

Zheng, D., Zhou, L., Guan, Y., Chen, X., Zhou, W., Chen, X. & Lei, P. (2010). Synthesis of cholestane glycosides bearing OSW-1 disaccharide or its 1→4-linked analogue and their antitumor activities. *Bioorg Med Chem Lett*, Vol.20, pp. 5439-5442.

Zheng, D., Guan, Y., Chen, X., Xu, Y., Chen, X. & Lei, P. (2011). Synthesis of cholestane saponins as mimics of OSW-1 and their cytotoxic activities. *Bioorg Med Chem Lett*, Vol.21, pp. 3257-3260.

Zhou, Y., Garcia-Prieto, C., Carney, D.A., Xu, R.H., Pelicano, H., Kang, Y., Yu, W., Lou, C., Kondo, S., Liu, J., Harris, D.M., Estrov, Z., Keating, M.J., Jin, Z. & Huang, P. (2005). OSW-1: a Natural compound with potent anticancer activity and a novel mechanism of action. *J Natl Cancer Inst*, Vol.97, pp. 1781-1785.

Zhu, J., Xiong, L., Yu, B. & Wu, J. (2005). Apoptosis induced by a new member of saponin family is mediated through caspase-8-dependent cleavage of Bcl-2. *Mol Pharmacol,* Vol.68, pp. 1831-1838.